LIVING WITH
HEARING LOSS

The Sourcebook for
Deafness and Hearing Disorders

LIVING WITH HEARING LOSS

The Sourcebook for Deafness and Hearing Disorders

Carol Turkington and
Allan Sussman, Ph.D.

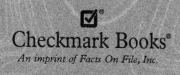

Checkmark Books®
An imprint of Facts On File, Inc.

Living with Hearing Loss: The Sourcebook for Deafness and Hearing Disorders

Checkmark Books
An imprint of Facts On File, Inc.
11 Penn Plaza
New York, NY 10001

Library of Congress Cataloging-in-Publication Data

Turkington, Carol.
  Living with hearing loss: The sourcebook for deafness and hearing disorders /
  Carol Turkington and Allen Sussman.
    p. cm.
  Includes bibliographical references.
  ISBN 0-8160-4140-7 (pbk.: acid-free paper)
    1. Deafness. 2. Hearing disorders. I. Sussman, Allen E. II. Title.

  RF290 T934 2000
  617.8—dc21

                                                            00-022731

Text design by Evelyn Horovicz
Cover design by Cathy Rincon

Printed in the United States of America

MP Hermitage 10 9 8 7 6 5 4 3 2

This book is printed on acid-free paper.

CONTENTS

PREFACE

One out of 10 Americans has some degree of hearing loss, and one out of every 400 is profoundly deaf. Yet many hard-of-hearing and deaf people in this country do not consider themselves handicapped, at a disadvantage or lacking in any way. They do not believe their hearing loss makes them less—just different—and they look upon the deaf community as a separate culture, as rich and diverse as that of the hearing world.

The Encyclopedia of Deafness and Hearing Disorders reflects the continuing struggle within the deaf community to maintain its integrity following years of segregation and misunderstanding. Although educators, linguists, experts in the field of deafness and deaf and hard-of-hearing people have come a long way toward replacing antagonism with cooperation, there still remain areas of controversy.

Where there are conflicting philosophies on a particular point, we have tried to identify and explain all sides. An extensive bibliography at the end of the book will assist anyone who wishes to explore any specific topic in further depth.

In addition, we made a great effort to include comprehensive appendixes that reflect the diverse range of organizations and support services available to deaf and hard-of-hearing people. We have tried to list as many of these special groups and services as we could find, together with current addresses and phone/TDD numbers.

Entries include all facets of deafness and hearing disorders: physiology of the ear; experts in education, science, linguistics and communication; famous deaf individuals; organizations and groups for deaf people; brief outlines of deaf culture in foreign countries; and more. All entries are cross-referenced to related subjects.

Although information presented in this book comes from the most recent sources available, readers should keep in mind that changes can occur very rapidly in medicine and technology. The very latest technical information on hearing aids and on assistive and telecommunications devices should be obtained from specialists. The authors would also like to stress that information in any medical entry should not be substituted for prompt medical attention.

—Carol Turkington
Morgantown, PA

—Allen E. Sussman, Ph.D.
Washington, DC

ACKNOWLEDGMENTS

The authors would like to thank the staff members at Gallaudet University who so generously offered their time during this project. In particular, we wish to thank the staffs at the university's library, public relations office, university press, information center and law center.

In addition, we appreciate the efforts of countless people from national organizations, services and government agencies concerned with deaf and hard-of-hearing people who offered a great deal of helpful information, statistics and support.

Thanks also to Elca Swigart, Ph.D., director of the Speech and Hearing Center at Reading Hospital and Medical Center, and audiologist Robert Gance for their valuable technical assistance and review; and to staffers at the National Library of Medicine and the medical libraries of Hershey Medical Center, the University of Pennsylvania Medical Center and Reading Medical Center. Hats off as well to public relations personnel at the National Institute of Mental Health and the National Institutes of Health.

We would also like to thank our editor at Facts On File, Jim Chambers, for his thoughtful suggestions and editorial guidance. We are also grateful to Bert Holtje of James Peter Associates for his valuable support.

Finally, thanks to friends and family for their patience and understanding. And a very special thank you to Michael and Kara.

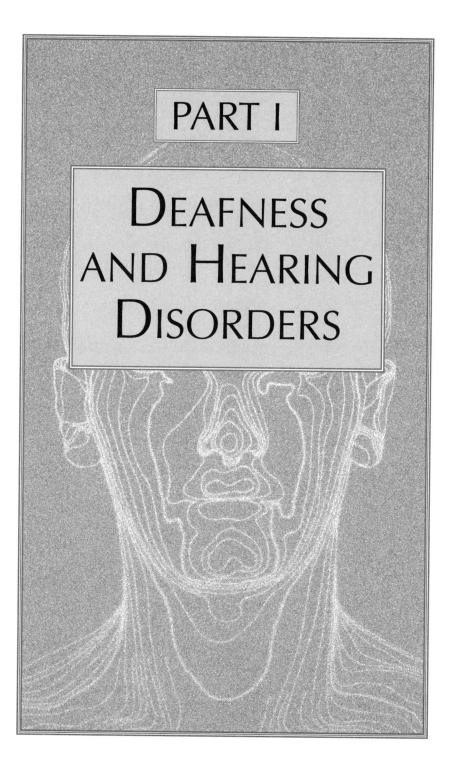

PART I

DEAFNESS AND HEARING DISORDERS

CHAPTER 1
DO YOU HAVE A HEARING LOSS?

If you live long enough, almost everyone will develop a hearing problem. For most of us, loss of hearing begins around age 55 to 65, although it can begin in the early 30s in men and in the late 30s for women. Of course, hearing loss also can occur at any age—from birth due to toxic conditions or heredity, in childhood as a result of diseases, or at any time from disease, accident or noise damage. Age-related hearing loss is known as presbycusis, and it's not a symptom of any particular medical problem—it's simply a function of age.

Estimate of the Prevalence of Hearing Impairments by Age Group (1990–91)

AGE	NUMBER OF HEARING IMPAIRED	% OF POPULATION
3–17 years	968,000	1.8%
18–34 years	2,309,000	3.4%
35–44 years	2,380,000	6.3%
45–54 years	2,634,000	10.3%
55–64 years	3,275,000	15.4%
65 years and older	8,729,000	29.1%
TOTAL	20,295,000	8.6%

Estimate of the Prevalence of Hearing Impairments by Age, Group and Gender (1990–91)*

AGE GROUP	MEN	WOMEN
3–17	541,000	427,000
18–44	3,018,000	1,672,000
45–64	3,946,000	1,963,000
65 and older	4,497,000	4,232,000

*National Center for Health Statistics, Data from the National Health Interview Survey, Series 10, Number 188, Table 1, 1994)

TYPES OF HEARING LOSS

Three people in one room may all have some problems in hearing, but they may have very different types of loss:

Conductive Hearing Loss

A problem with the transfer of sound to the inner ear, usually because of damage to the eardrum or the three bones of the middle ear. In an adult, conductive hearing loss may be caused by earwax blocking the ear or by a disease such as otosclerosis. In a child, it's most commonly caused by ear infections with fluid. Sometimes, a conductive loss may be due to damage to the eardrum or because of sudden pressure changes or a punctured eardrum.

Sensorineural Hearing Loss

Hearing loss caused by sounds that reach the inner ear but don't go on to the brain because of damage to the structure of the inner ear or the auditory ("hearing") nerve. Its effects are almost always irreversible, and tend to progress slowly with age, affecting one or both ears. Commonly called "nerve deafness," hearing aids often don't help understanding even loud speech.

Central Hearing Loss

Hearing loss caused by damage to the nerves or nuclei of the central nervous system, either in the pathways to the brain or in the brain itself. Central hearing loss may be caused by a congenital brain abnormality, tumor or lesion of the central nervous system, stroke or from some medications that specifically harm the ear.

Mixed Hearing Loss

A combination of conductive and sensorineural loss that is often treatable, depending on the cause.

PRESBYCUSIS

More than 12 million Americans experience some form of hearing loss as they age—and about half of everyone over age 74 has some hearing loss. These late-deafened adults make up the vast majority of the elderly with hearing problems. They are usually not profoundly deaf and aren't likely to know sign language or consider themselves part of the deaf community.

Hearing loss among older people is much more common among men than women, among whites than blacks, among those earning less than

$7,000 a year and among those who didn't graduate from high school. One explanation for these characteristics could be that those in lower economic brackets are likely to become sick more often, and chronic health conditions can lead to or worsen hearing problems.

Most people think of age-related hearing loss as a problem for senior citizens in their 70s and 80s, but it often begins much sooner than that. Surprisingly, by age 30 most men and women can't hear frequencies over 15,000 cycles per second. By about age 50, that drops to 12,000—when most people report some loss of the ability to hear. By age 60, the maximum range drops to 10,000 and at 70, to 6,000 cycles (well below the upper limit of everyday speech).

Hearing loss among this group can be caused by a number of things, including ear infections, blood clots, loud noises, inherited conditions, bony growths in the middle ear and adverse reactions to medications. But the most common cause of deafness is presbycusis, a type of sensorineural hearing loss that comes with age. ("Presby" meaning *old* and "cusis" meaning *hearing*.) Presbycusis is a progressive deterioration of the hearing organ leading to an intolerance for loud noises, but not total deafness. "Presbycusis" is not an ear disease, however—it's simply a process that often occurs with age. If we all lived long enough, we'd all eventually develop this problem.

Cause of Presbycusis

Presbycusis is caused by changes in the hair cells within the cochlea or the nerves attached to it, where high-frequency sound is perceived; this damage means that sound signals can't be transmitted as efficiently, leading to hearing loss.

Studies have shown that as you age, you lose nerve cells in the base of the cochlea. But researchers don't know whether this degeneration is primarily due to aging, or whether it is caused by a decrease in the specific frequencies supplying those cells. Some researchers suspect that prolonged exposure to loud noise, reduced blood flow to the inner ear and hardening of the arteries may contribute to presbycusis.

Some older people with hearing problems have nothing more seriously wrong than a simple buildup of wax in the ear canal—or it could be related to damage to the inner ear from infection, disease or trauma. Some experts think that too much noise accounts for more hearing loss in old age than all the other factors combined.

Symptoms

Each person experiences the development of presbycusis differently. It usually involves a slow decline in hearing ability, beginning with the high-pitched sounds followed by a loss of hearing in the middle frequencies, followed by the lowest.

Because normal speech covers all these frequencies, the ability to understand conversation may vary according to the extent of the presbycusis. Perhaps you have noticed that you have a harder time understanding conversations with women or children (whose voices are of higher frequency). You may find you have a hard time understanding conversation in a group.

Warning Signs of Age-Related Hearing Loss

As you get older, you're likely to begin noticing signs of hearing loss. Here's what to look for:

- Tinnitus (ringing of the ears)
- Talking louder than you used to do
- Turning up the TV or radio
- Others starting to sound as if they're mumbling
- Confusing words with similar sounds
- Trouble hearing high-pitched sounds
- Trouble hearing soft sounds

Treatment

This type of hearing loss as a result of aging can't be surgically reversed, but hearing aids may help. If you have started to notice hearing loss, you should immediately see an otologist (specialist in diseases of the ear), an otolaryngologist (specialist in diseases of the ear, nose and throat) or an audiologist (professional who often works with a physician to assess hearing loss and provide auditory training). Unfortunately, most people with presbycusis wait an average of five years before doing anything about it.

Although hearing aids can help most people, not everyone will benefit from them (such as people who can't discriminate different speech sounds, for instance). For those who can, an aid should not be prescribed or fitted before an examination and hearing test are given.

SYMPTOMS

As a person begins to lose the ability to hear, others may notice changes in personality, or attitude, as the ability to communicate begins to deteriorate. A child may begin to stop paying attention in class or grades may start to slip. Adults may begin to feel isolated, and start missing parts of conversations. They may begin to think people are talking about them. It's not uncommon for people with failing hearing not to realize that gradual decline is taking place, and to react with disbelief or hostility when the possibility is pointed out to them.

While the symptoms of a hearing loss vary quite a lot from one person to the next, there are some basic signs of significant ear disease that require referral to an otolaryngologist. These signs have been compiled by the National Hearing Aid Society:

- Visible deformity of the ear
- Drainage from the ear
- Sudden or rapidly progressive hearing loss in one or both ears
- Dizziness or tinnitus (ringing of the ear)
- Hearing test results that reveal a significant hearing loss
- Visible earwax buildup or a foreign object in the ear canal
- Pain or discomfort in the ear

There are other signs of potential hearing loss:

Speech Deterioration

Since the ears help you modulate loudness and pronunciation, it's not surprising that a hearing loss can seriously affect the quality of human speech. If you begin to slur words or drop word endings (or if the speech sounds oddly "flat") this could be a sign of hearing loss.

Fatigue

If you start to feel exhausted or irritable while listening to a conversation or a speech, it might be caused by straining to hear what's being said.

Indifference

If you can't hear what's being said around you, it's easy to feel depressed and disinterested. What many people with hearing loss discover is that while folks in a group will make an initial effort, people sometimes find that it becomes too much trouble to speak loudly and clearly. Unintentionally, people with a hearing problem might find themselves being excluded from group conversations.

Social Withdrawal

Not being able to hear conversation and sensing that others don't have the patience to try to communicate can worsen social isolation. It can also make you want to avoid situations to avoid potential embarrassment.

Insecurity

Knowing that it's easy to make communication mistakes when your hearing isn't normal can lead some people to develop a real fear of making mistakes. No matter how well or how poorly we hear, no one likes to say or do things that might be held up to ridicule or that make us feel foolish.

TAKE THIS TEST

It's not really possible for you to accurately test your own hearing, but there are some guidelines you can follow to see if you have a hearing problem. Many times, hearing loss is so gradual we don't realize it's happening. Take this simple test and see if you answer yes to any of these questions. Do you:

- Let your spouse or friend do most of your talking?
- Get tired after a long conversation?
- Notice friends seem to be avoiding conversations with you?
- Have to ask people to repeat what they say again and again?
- Often misunderstand others?
- Tune out when more than one person is talking?
- Nod your head as if you are following the conversation when you actually don't understand what has been said?
- Notice people seem embarrassed by your answers, as if they don't fit the questions?
- Have a ringing or roaring in your ears (tinnitus)?

The symptoms listed above suggest you may need to visit an ear specialist—but some people with a hearing loss resist seeking this type of help. Many still fear that poor hearing is a sign of old age, or that wearing a hearing aid carries a social stigma. However, since there's no way for you to tell for sure if your problem is related to presbycusis or any of the other causes, it's important to visit a doctor for a correct diagnosis.

Diagnosis

Your doctor can diagnose your problem with a painless exam. It is especially important to see your doctor right away if you also experience dizziness, ringing or roaring noises in your ears, pain, a feeling of pressure or drainage from your ear. These symptoms could be a sign of a serious medical problem.

Basically, hearing tests measure sensitivity (the level at which you can first detect sound) and discrimination. Your hearing loss is measured in decibels (dB); however, two people with the same decibel loss may actually perceive speech quite differently, depending on the amount of structural damage to the ear and the age at onset of the hearing loss.

Many methods have been used in the past to measure hearing, but today there are several basic types of hearing tests: routine diagnostic audiometry, acoustic-immitance audiometry, special audiometric tests and electrophysiologic tests.

WHO TREATS HEARING LOSS?

You can either visit your family doctor first for a referral to a specialist for routine diagnostic audiometry—or you can make an appointment yourself with an otolaryngologist (also called an ear, nose and throat [ENT] specialist, otorhinolaryngologist or head-and-neck surgeon). Specialists who limit their practice to the ears (excluding neck, nose or throat) are known as otologists. In fact, before getting a hearing aid, the law requires you must first consult a doctor to certify that there is no medical reason why you should not be able to wear an aid.

To qualify for the American Board of Otolaryngology certification exam, an otolaryngologist must complete five or more years of post-M.D. specialty training in otolaryngology. These specialists treat problems ranging from common conditions such as ear infections and minor hearing loss to more complex problems like Ménière's disease or otosclerosis. In addition, they are expert in the diagnosis and treating of different types of hearing loss. The specialist can advise you whether a hearing aid will help you hear better, and if so, what kind will be suitable.

An otologist/neurologist is a physician who specializes in the treatment of the ear and brain. After completing medical school, general surgery training and otolaryngology training, an otologist/neurologist completes fellowship training in diagnosing and treating diseases of the ear and skull base. People who consult an otologist/neurologist usually are referred by an otolaryngologist because the case is complicated and because the patient has not responded to conventional treatment.

Your First Visit

During your first visit, the doctor will take a detailed medical history of your hearing problems and look inside your ears with an otoscope, the lighted scope with which you are probably familiar. Your doctor will be looking for any evidence of infection, blockage or other problem in the ear canal and eardrum.

This "nasopharynx" exam can reveal infections that can obstruct the eustachian tubes, causing abnormalities in the middle ear. It can also uncover problems such as middle ear effusion (production of a sticky fluid in the middle ear), a retracted eardrum, ear infections, sinusitis, allergy and inflamed or enlarged adenoids. The doctor can look at the nasopharynx by looking through your mouth with a mirror placed behind the free edge of the soft palate, or a right-angle telescope can be used through the mouth to look around the soft palate. Other ways to examine this area include using a nasopharyngoscope (a thin right-angle telescope passed through the nose) or a flexible fiber-optic endoscope to look through the nose or mouth. Feeling with the finger can also be helpful, but it's usually performed under general anesthesia.

Next, you may be tested for balance and coordination problems in order to rule out any neurological problems underlying your hearing loss. The doctor may use a tuning fork to see if it's possible to make a rough estimate about your ability to hear.

Depending on what this initial examination reveals, your doctor may want you to be evaluated by an audiologist—a professional trained in evaluating hearing. While an ENT specialist is highly trained in the pathology of the ear and fully understands medical and surgical techniques, most aren't usually trained in the special skills of hearing rehabilitation.

Your ENT specialist may have an audiologist or audiometrist on staff, or you may be given a referral and asked to return once the testing is done. An audiologist is not a medical doctor, but may have a doctorate in audiology and thus be referred to as "Dr." An audiometrist is a person without a degree in audiology who has been given informal training in the administration of hearing tests. An audiometrist must work under the supervision of an audiologist or a physician, and can neither diagnose hearing disorders nor interpret audiograms.

Audiograms

An audiogram is a graph produced as part of some hearing tests that can be used to represent at what level of loudness you can hear different frequencies. The audiogram form is arranged so that octave and half-octave frequencies range across the top, with the frequency increasing from left to right. The hearing-level scale on the left side of an audiogram shows the strength of the test sound in decibels (dB).

Audiologist

The audiologist will want to give you a complete examination and conduct a series of hearing tests; depending on the results, the audiologist can recommend hearing aids and provide counseling and therapy to help you deal with hearing loss.

An audiologist is a licensed and/or certified professional trained to identify and measure hearing loss, and to rehabilitate those with hearing or speech problems. Audiologists are trained to determine where hearing loss occurs, and they can assess the effect of the loss on your ability to communicate. They can offer hearing aid evaluation and orientation, auditory training, training in speechreading techniques and speech conservation and counseling. Audiologists are not doctors, however, and can't treat infections or other ear diseases.

"Dispensing audiologists" usually have more training than "hearing aid dispensers," who are licensed by their state but who have no college degree.

You'll find audiologists working in a wide variety of settings, including universities, hospitals, schools, medical offices and private practices. When employed by a university, audiologists may teach, supervise clinical practice, and direct clinical services. At medical centers, hospitals, and rehabilitation agencies, they test hearing, including the pre- and postoperative evaluation of surgical patients. Referrals come from a wide variety of professionals, including otolaryngologists, neurologists, neurosurgeons, pediatricians, geriatricians, family doctors and internists. In hospitals with acute care pediatric nurseries, audiologists direct hearing screening programs for infants at risk for hearing problems.

Since most school districts require some type of hearing screening for students, audiologists may serve as directors of these programs and work with teachers to help with special educational needs of students with hearing problems. In schools with special classes for those with hearing problems, audiologists equip and maintain classroom amplification systems.

You may also find an audiologist working in a private practice with your physician (especially an otolaryngologist), where they will test hearing, evaluate vestibular function and dispense hearing aids.

Recently, audiologists have begun branching out into private practice themselves, primarily to dispense hearing aids directly to clients with hearing problems. What separates them from commercial hearing aid dealers is the in-depth professional rehabilitation programs they can offer their customers.

Community hearing and speech centers employ audiologists to work with adults and children as rehabilitation specialists to test hearing, select hearing aids and help improve speech and reading skills.

TESTS

When you go for your visit with an audiologist, you'll find that these specialists may use both formal and informal tests to determine your ability to hear and understand. Although these tests usually measure hearing abilities, the audiologist may also test your skill at interpreting gestures and facial expressions.

Your audiologist routinely tests three aspects of your hearing: the *degree* of hearing ability, the *kind* of hearing loss and the *ability* to understand speech under different conditions. He or she will usually provide these services:

- *Hearing evaluation:* a set of tests to gauge the amount and degree of hearing loss
- *Hearing aid evaluation:* to decide what type of hearing aid will be the best choice for you
- *Counseling:* to help you learn to communicate more effectively, and to cope with the emotional side of your problem

When you arrive for your appointment with an audiologist, he or she will first take a detailed case history. After your ears are checked with an otoscope to rule out infection or obstruction, you'll be given a pair of headphones. The hearing tests take place in a soundproof booth designed to screen out background noise.

Pure Tone Air Conduction

First, the audiologist will administer a basic screening test called a *pure tone air conduction test.* This is a subjective method of estimating hearing sensitivity by evoking your responses to air-conducted "pure tones" (a single frequency). "Air conduction" refers to the process by which sound travels through the air to your conductive mechanism, which stimulates nerve endings in the eighth cranial nerve. The test evaluates how softly you can hear across the spectrum of frequencies, and measures the lowest hearing level at which you can respond correctly to pure tones 50% of the time.

During the test, a series of tones like music notes will be played through your headphones in one ear at a time. The decibel loudness when these sounds can first be heard is called the "pure tone hearing threshold" (or hearing level) for that frequency. People with normal hearing will usually hear each pure tone frequency at the zero point, or close to it; if you have a hearing loss, you will only hear pure tones much louder than zero.

You'll be asked to respond by raising your hand or pushing a button each time you first hear the tone. You should raise your hand whenever you detect this tone, even if it is very faint, since the purpose of the test is to find the softest sound you can hear in all frequency ranges. Since hearing loss may occur at some frequencies but not others, it's important to determine how well you hear across all frequencies.

Pure tones are usually in octave or half-octave steps, and cover the frequencies between 250 and 8,000 hertz (Hz). Because speech falls within this range, it is possible (in a limited way) to measure your ability to hear a conversation by testing with pure tones. The disadvantage of testing hearing with pure tones is that the sounds heard every day are not pure tones, but complex ones.

When you hear much better in one ear than in the other, the audiologist will mask the better ear to prevent it from responding and giving a false reading while the poorer ear is tested. The better ear is masked by presenting a band of noise through the earphone at about the same frequency as the one being tested.

Pure Bone Conduction

Next, the audiologist might remove the headphones for a *pure bone conduction test*. Bone conduction is the process by which sound vibrates the skull, and thus the cochlea (bypassing the conductive structures of your ears). This test assesses the sensitivity of the inner ear. For this test, the audiologist will place a small vibrator behind your ear or on your forehead, and again you will be asked to indicate which sounds you can hear. The "air bone gap" is the difference between how well you hear by air conduction and bone conduction.

If you have normal bone conduction results but significant hearing loss as measured by air conduction tests, this indicates that your hearing loss is a conductive loss, not sensorineural ("nerve related"). Therefore, you may be a candidate for surgical or medical treatment of your hearing loss.

With the electronic audiometer, it's possible to measure a person's threshold of hearing for a series of pure tones at 11 different frequency points, starting at 125 cycles per second and ending at 8,000. This includes the three octaves between 500 and 4,000 Hz that are most important for speech.

The Weber test can determine which ear (if either) hears a tuning fork better by bone conduction. The base of the vibrating fork is held on the center of the forehead or upper front teeth, and the patient is asked in which ear the fork sounds louder. If hearing isn't the same in both ears, the fork's tone will be heard in only one ear, or appear to be displaced to one side of the head. A person complaining of hearing loss in one ear who can hear the fork in the good ear may have a sensorineural hearing loss. If the sound is heard in the poor ear, a conductive loss may be suspected. A mixture of both types of hearing loss will not be accurately revealed by the Weber test.

The average level of thresholds elicited for each ear for frequencies believed to be essential for understanding speech (500, 1,000 and 2,000 hertz) is called the "pure tone average" (PTA). The PTA is used to determine the level at which to start presenting words to find a person's speech reception threshold.

Speech Audiometry Tests

Speech reception (or speech recognition) threshold tests and speech discrimination (word recognition) tests are considered to be types of speech audiometry tests. While pure tones may reveal the nature and extent of your hearing loss, they don't reveal the extent of communication problems. In addition to pure tone tests, a hearing evaluation often includes "speech audiometry"—a measure of how sensitive you are to speech (or the lowest level at which speech can be heard).

These tests are important because patients with hearing loss in one ear with poor discrimination at high loudness levels may need more audiometric or X-ray studies to rule out the possibility of a tumor on the hear-

Discrimination Score	
DISCRIMINATION SCORE	INTERPRETATION
90–100%	Excellent understanding of speech
80–89%	Good understanding of speech
70–79%	Fair understanding of speech
60–69%	Poor understanding of speech
0–59%	Markedly reduced understanding of speech

ing nerve. In addition, speech discrimination results may help predict the extent to which a person with a sensorineural hearing loss will benefit from a hearing aid.

The *speech discrimination (word recognition) test* measures your ability to understand important sounds (primarily consonants). In this test, the audiologist is trying to find out how clearly you can discriminate one-syllable words while listening at a comfortable level and measures how well you can discriminate speech at intensities 30 to 40 dB above your speech reception threshold. You'll be read a list of about 50 one-syllable words and asked to repeat them. As you repeat what you hear, the words gradually become fainter. This is your speech reception threshold.

Acoustic-Immitance Tests

There are a few other tests you might be given. Immitance tests evaluate the middle ear, measuring the response of the eardrum, ossicles and small muscles attached to the ossicles. Specifically, "immitance" is a measure of how easy it is to transfer sound from the external ear through the middle ear to the cochlea.

The measure of acoustic immitance (called "tympanometry") is a function of air pressure in the ear canal; it can be defined as either "acoustic admittance" or "acoustic impedance." Admittance refers to how easily energy flows through a system, while impedance represents the opposition to the flow of energy. A system with high acoustic impedance to the flow of sound will have low acoustic admittance, and vice versa.

The most common acoustic immitance test is tympanometry, a measure of eardrum stiffness as a function of air pressure change. It can determine with fairly good accuracy whether there is fluid behind the eardrum or whether air pressure in the middle ear is abnormal. The tympanogram is the graphic representation of acoustic admittance or acoustic impedance as a function of this air pressure. In a person with normal hearing, the acoustic impedance (opposition to air flow) is least when the air pressure is close to zero (atmospheric level). As the air pressure changes from this level, acoustic impedance increases and acoustic immitance decreases. The air pressure changes stiffen the eardrum and ossicles, reducing energy transfer through the middle ear. In a patient with a middle ear disorder, acoustic immitance measures are different, and the specific disease can be diagnosed depending on the tympanogram configuration. For example, a middle ear infection with fluid creates a "flat" tympanogram; a disrupted ossicular chain will produce a tympanogram with an abnormally sharp peak.

Another acoustic immitance test is the *acoustic reflex test,* which helps to test young children. This test measures the reflex contraction of muscle in the middle ear.

These tests are used in addition to hearing tests, since it's possible to have significant ear disease with little hearing loss. Most hearing tests can uncover the type and degree of hearing loss, but they may not be good at diagnosing specific ear diseases. Unlike most hearing tests, acoustic-immitance tests can reveal middle ear disorders without requiring active participation on the part of the client.

Acoustic Impedance Tests

This type of test measures hearing at the level of the cochlea and brain stem, to determine how well the cochlea and auditory pathways of the medulla are functioning. In this test, two tubes are placed into the external ear canal, and sound is sent from a small loudspeaker through one tube. The sound reflected from the eardrum is picked up by the other tube, which leads to a microphone, amplifier and recorder. When a sudden intense sound is applied to the other ear, the stapedium muscle contracts, the impedance is increased, and the recorder indicates when more sound is picked up.

This does not measure the actual acoustic impedance of the ear. This is tested by using an acoustic bridge, which allows an otologist to listen to a sound as it is reflected from a patient's eardrum. At the same time, a similar sound of the same intensity is reflected in an artificial cavity that is adjusted to equal that of the external canal of the ear.

When the two sounds are matched by changing the acoustic impedance of the cavity, the otologist can then read the impedance of the ear from the scale of the instrument. This test can uncover conductive defects of the middle ear.

Tone Decay Test

This test measures tone decay (auditory fatigue) that can be caused by pressure or damage to the auditory nerve. In the test, constant tones are presented at the client's threshold. When the sound fades, the tone is increased five decibels. The amount of decay is determined by subtracting the intensity of the initial signal from the intensity at the end of the test. Clients with a disorder of the auditory nerve will show a difference greater than 10 dB to 15 dB.

Alternate Binaural Loudness Balance (ABLB)

This test measures "recruitment" (the abnormal rapid increase in loudness above the threshold level). It's measured with a device that allows the client to set controls, so that the loudness of a tone heard by the defective ear matches the tone heard in the normal ear.

By repeating this comparison at several intensity levels, the presence or absence of recruitment can be identified. This test is used to diagnose a sensorineural hearing loss (nerve deafness) that affects mostly one ear.

Electrophysical Tests

Other tests that don't require the client to give a conscious response include electroencephalic (EEG) audiometry and evoked response audiometry. For the very young, hearing thresholds for pure tones can be deciphered from these methods. (See Chapter 3.)

What Happens Next

After your hearing tests have been completed, the audiologist will discuss whether or not a hearing aid might be of help. If these tests show you have a hearing problem in the middle or outer ear, you might be able to correct the problem with medical treatment or surgery. However, if the hearing loss is a result of problems in the inner ear, such as the loss that occurs with age, your only option may be a hearing aid. While an aid cannot restore normal function to your ears, it can improve your hearing.

If the audiologist believes a hearing aid may be of help, you'll be asked to come back for a hearing aid evaluation (see Chapter 4). At this time, further tests will help pinpont which type of hearing aid will be best for your particular type of hearing loss. In the meantime, if you haven't already done so, you should make an appointment with an ENT specialist to make sure there is no other medical problem causing your hearing loss. Your audiologist will write a report of the results of your test and forward them to your ENT specialist. You may have a copy of this report if you wish.

Percent of Hearing Loss

The percent of hearing loss used for medical and legal purposes can be estimated by approximating the number of damaged hair cells within the cochlea. Because it is impossible to count the damaged cells among the 15,000 in the ear, a percent of loss is made by using the tympanogram.

The amount of hearing loss is based on threshold levels at 500, 1,000 and 2,000 Hz. Hearing sensitivity better than 26 dB is not considered a loss; hearing worse than 93 dB is a total loss. Therefore, the percentage (0 to 100) of hearing loss covers a range of 67 dB. Each decibel above 26 dB is rated as a 1.5% loss. To calculate the percentage of hearing loss, an audiologist averages the thresholds at 500, 1,000, and 2,000 Hz and subtracts 26 dB from this average. The remainder is multiplied by 1.5.

Although percentage is used to describe hearing loss, it doesn't give a clear picture of actual hearing deficits. For example, a 40% hearing loss doesn't specify whether the loss is within the high, low or middle frequencies for speech recognition. But this is important to know, since *where* the damage occurs in a frequency range determines the ability to hear speech.

A group of people all with a 40% hearing loss won't each have the same ability to understand speech; one person's loss may be in the low frequencies, one in the high, and another in the middle, with uncounted degrees in between.

Degree of Hearing Loss

There are specific terms used to define how much hearing loss has been sustained:

- *mild loss:* Loss of some sounds
- *moderate loss:* A loss of enough sounds so that a person's ability to understand his surrounding environment is affected, including some speech
- *significant bilateral loss:* Loss of hearing in both ears with the better ear having some difficulty hearing and understanding speech
- *severe loss:* Many sounds aren't heard, including most speech sounds.
- *profound loss:* An inability to hear almost all sound, generally over 90 dB
- *Deafness:* In this sense, the ability to hear is disabled to an extent that precludes the understanding of speech through the ear alone, with or without use of a hearing aid. This definition was adopted in 1974 by the Conference of Educational Administrators Serving the Deaf.

ADAPTING TO A HEARING LOSS

If you're in a relationship with someone with a hearing loss—close friend, parent, spouse or child—you may think you understand their emotional responses. Odds are you still struggle yourself with the ways the person is responding to hearing loss. Actually, it's hard to understand what it's like to lose your hearing, and why there is so often an emotional component to the experience.

If you're the one who has begun to lose the ability to hear, you may feel a range of emotions, including frustration, tension, fatigue and fear of embarrassment. First of all, it's frustrating not to be able to understand normal conversation, and it's frustrating to have to ask people to repeat themselves. Constantly feeling you must be alert to catch the drift of the conversation also creates quite a bit of tension. You don't want to miss important points or lose the thread of the discussion altogether. All that alertness is enormously draining, requiring constant effort to "fill in" the missed words and to try to predict what's coming next. Finally, the fear of making an inappropriate comment fills some people with such anxiety that they stop interacting at all.

If you're the family member of someone losing their hearing and you've ever been tempted to dismiss these feelings as overreactions, imagine how you would feel in similar circumstances. Anyone who has ever traveled to a foreign country and tried to communicate without being able to speak the language has encountered some of these same feelings. If you want to imagine what it's like for people with hearing loss to handle their fear of embarrassment at making an inappropriate comment, think how it would feel for you to walk into a party filled with people of a group of which you're not a member. Everyone else is chatting knowledgeably, and you're filled with nervousness at the thought of making an inappropriate comment.

This is why communication with hearing friends can simply be seen as too much effort by the person with hearing loss, and why sometimes the person withdraws from social situations completely. This is also one reason why many people in the deaf community feel, quite rightly, that they have been treated with prejudice and misconceptions.

How to Communicate Effectively

There are several things to keep in mind when communicating with a person who is hard of hearing:

Get the person's attention. Before you start speaking, make sure the person who is hard of hearing is paying attention; call her name or touch him. By watching your face, he or she can deduce valuable cues to help in understanding your words.

Decrease background noise. It's very difficult for a person with a hearing problem to understand conversation if there are competing noises in the background—other people talking, dogs barking, stereos playing. Turn off the TV set or radio and close the windows if there is outside traffic noise. If you can't avoid background noise, try moving to a quieter area.

Move in closer. Especially in the presence of background noise, move within two to three feet of the person with whom you are talking so your speech will be louder than other distracting noises. Don't talk from another room.

Don't shout. Remember to keep your speech at a normal level if the person is wearing a hearing aid. If the persons isn't wearing an aid and you know he or she has a hearing problem, you can speak a little louder than normal, but don't shout.

Articulate. Speak clearly and articulate well, but don't exaggerate your mouth movements.

Hold still. Don't make lots of gestures or move your head around, which can be distracting

Be alert. While communicating, be aware of slight facial nuances that might mean the person is not understanding what you are saying. Many people who are hard of hearing will sometimes nod as if they understand to avoid having to keep asking you to repeat yourself.

Watch pitch. Keep the pitch of your conversation fairly low, since a lower-pitched voice is easier to understand. Don't mumble.

Concentrate. Don't do other things at the same time, and don't talk when you're too busy.

Gesture. Use appropriate body language and facial expressions.

If the person to whom you're speaking doesn't understand you, don't say "Turn up your hearing aid!" or accuse the person of only paying attention when it pleases him or her. In the first place, many people with hearing loss (especially age-related hearing loss) often hear speech as distorted. Turning up the volume on the hearing aid can't make distorted sound any more clear; it can actually make it worse. It can also be painful.

Instead, if you haven't been understood, try these suggestions:

- Repeat the sentence, using the same words ("Where are my glasses?")
- Try to rephrase the sentence ("Have you seen my specs?")
- Break up your sentence into two phrases. ("I need my eyeglasses. Do you know where they are?")
- Write down the key words.
- Make sure you're looking at the person and speaking clearly.

Remember that even if the hard-of-hearing person is fairly good at speechreading (reading lips), almost no one can follow a complete conversation just by using this method. At best, speechreading can give a person *clues* about what is being said. There are too many speech sounds that can't be detected by reading the lip movements, and too many words that look identical when spoken.

CHAPTER 2

CAUSES OF DEAFNESS IN ADULTS

The complexity of the ear means that it's vulnerable to damage from a wide variety of sources—disease, genetic disorders, infection, noise or trauma. A number of ear diseases can result in hearing loss as well, including auditory neuritis, cholesteatoma, labyrinthitis and otosclerosis.

Leading Causes of Hearing Loss in Adults, 1990–91	
CAUSE	PERCENT DUE TO CAUSE
Aging	28%
Noise	23.4%
Other	16.8%
Ear infection	12.2%
Loud brief noise	10.3%
Ear injury	4.9%
Birth	4.4%

National Center for Health Statistics, data from the National Health Interview Survey, 1994

INFECTIONS AND HEARING LOSS

A healthy immune system is crucial to the defense against infection of both the middle and the inner ear, protecting against hearing loss and the progression of chronic ear infections. Certain diseases that affect the immune system (such as AIDS) can also result in hearing loss, and a faulty immune system may be related to other disorders for which no cause has been found (such as Ménière's disease).

Auditory Neuritis

Neuritis (the inflammation of the auditory nerve) can follow infections such as scarlet fever or typhoid fever, or any other infection with a high fever. Deafness usually progresses over several days or weeks, although an immediate hearing loss after such an infection is possible. The gradual development of inflammation can cause a sensorineural deafness very much like the hearing loss that appears in old age, but it occurs much earlier in life and is usually attributed to loss of oxygen, anemia, viruses or labyrinthitis (inflammation of the fluid-filled chambers of the inner ear).

Cholesteatoma

This chronic middle ear inflammatory disease is a rare condition in which skin cells and debris collect inside the middle ear, usually after the eardrum bursts following a middle-ear infection. A cholesteatoma that appears later in life may be caused by a persistent narrowing of the eustachian tube that eventually pulls the upper part of the eardrum back, forming a sac in the middle ear. It also may result from a tiny hole in the eardrum that allows skin cells of the external ear canal to move into the middle ear.

Untreated, a cholesteatoma may grow and damage the small bones in the middle ear and the surrounding bone structures, causing a conductive or a mixed hearing loss. While a cholesteatoma is benign and won't spread to other sites in your body, it could lead to serious complications such as a secondary infection, meningitis or a brain abscess.

Therefore, it must be removed either through the eardrum or by a mastoidectomy (removal of the mastoid bone behind the ear, together with the cholesteatoma). Repeat operations may be required, because the cyst can grow back. The operation may also require the rebuilding the bones of the middle ear to restore hearing. Ear bone transplants or artificial devices may be used to reconstruct the bones.

Encephalitis

This inflammation of the brain itself can cause many different symptoms of brain injury, including a central hearing loss. The impairment is usually related to the brain itself, not the hearing mechanism, although there may be some cochlear dysfunction as well. (For a more complete discussion of encephalitis, see Chapter 3.)

Labyrinthitis

Infection of the labyrinth, the fluid-filled maze of inner ear chambers that sense balance, can cause nausea, vomiting, tinnitus (ringing of the ears), vertigo and deafness. Also called "otitis interna," labyrinthitis is almost always caused by either a bacterial or viral infection that enters the inner ear from the middle ear. Bacterial labyrinthitis may be caused by an untreated acute or chronic ear infection, especially if a cholesteatoma (infected skin debris) has developed. The bacteria enters the inner ear through the eroded labyrinthine capsule. Infection may also reach the inner ear from a head injury or through the bloodstream from elsewhere in the body.

Infection also may occur as a result of contamination during certain ear operations. This type of labyrinthitis requires immediate treatment with antibiotics in order to prevent the spread of infection that might lead to meningitis or profound sensorineural hearing loss, violent vertigo, and total deafness.

Viral labyrinthitis attacks the inner ear during illnesses such as measles, mumps, chickenpox, shingles or flu. With this type of sensorineural hearing loss, onset is sudden and may cause a severe or profound hearing problem. Eventually the inflammation will fade away, although symptoms can be relieved with antihistamines.

Syphilitic labyrinthitis is usually caused by congenital syphilis and results in a sudden, flat sensorineural hearing loss or a sudden increasing fluctuation of sensorineural hearing loss. Acquired syphilitic labyrinthitis is rare.

Mastoiditis

This inflammation of the mastoid bone (the bone behind the ear) is caused by a spreading infection from the middle ear, resulting in severe pain, swelling and tenderness behind and inside the ear, together with a fever, creamy discharge and progressive hearing loss. The real danger is that infection may spread to *inside* the skull, causing meningitis, a brain abscess, or a stroke. The infection could also spread outward, damaging the facial nerve and paralyzing the facial muscles.

Mastoiditis has become uncommon since the use of antibiotic drugs for the treatment of ear infections. Because it can be difficult to drain the infected material from the mastoid cells, it can be hard to cure this infection. High-dose antibiotic treatment for several weeks will usually clear up the problem, but a mastoidectomy (removal of the infected air cells within the mastoid bone) may be needed if it doesn't.

Tympanosclerosis

This middle ear problem is caused by a chronic ear infection. Often seen as a white area in the eardrum, it is caused when new bone is formed by calcification of the tissue in the lining of the middle ear.

Typhoid Fever

This infectious disease transmitted by food or water contaminated with the bacteria salmonella typhosa may cause a hearing loss. The infection is found in the feces of an infected person and can be spread by drinking water contaminated by sewage, by flies carrying the bacteria from infected feces, or by eating food handled by typhoid carriers. Epidemics still occur in developing countries, and immunization against the disease is recommended for anyone traveling to these areas. Because the vaccine doesn't provide complete protection, tourists should drink only boiled water when traveling to these areas.

Middle Ear Infections

Because middle ear infections are such a common occurrence in childhood, a full discussion of the problem is found in Chapter 3.

External Ear Infections

Also known as otitis externa (or "swimmer's ear"), this ear problem is an infection of the ear canal that is usually caused by swimming in polluted water. Other causes may include:

- excessive washing
- perspiration
- irritation of the ear canal after removing a foreign object
- allergies
- generalized skin disease (such as seborrheic dermatitis)

In general, the risk of getting swimmer's ear rises with the frequency of swimming, the longer the person stays in the water, and the more often the head is submerged. It usually causes swelling and inflammation of the ear canal, a discharge and sometimes eczema around the ear opening. Itching may become painful, and deafness can occur if pus blocks the ear. It can be treated by drying the ear, followed by applying antibiotic drops or antifungal or anti-inflammatory drugs.

Malignant Otitis Externa

This disorder inflames and damages the bones and cartilage at the base of the skull, caused by spread of infection from an external ear infection (otitis externa). Malignant otitis externa is a relatively uncommon complication of both acute and chronic otitis externa (also known as swimmer's ear). It occurs in approximately 5 out of 10,000 people, and is more common among diabetics and those whose immune system are compromised from diseases or medications.

The infection, often caused by difficult-to-treat germs such as Pseudomonas, spreads from the floor of the ear canal to nearby tissue and into the bones of the base of the skull. The bones may be damaged or destroyed from the resulting infection and inflammation. The infection may further spread and affect the cranial nerves, the brain, or other parts of the body.

Symptoms include draining from the ear, yellow or foul-smelling pus, itching ear or ear canal, deep ear pain that may worsen on head movement and persistent hearing loss. The head around and behind the ear may be tender to touch. Neurological examination may show involvement of cranial nerves. A culture of drainage may show bacteria or fungus (usually Pseudomonas). A head CT scan, skull X rays, MRI scan of the head, or radionuclide scan may show bone infection adjacent to the ear canal.

Treatment is often prolonged, lasting several months, because of the difficulty of treating the involved bacteria and the problems in reaching an infection within bone tissue. Antibiotics that are effective against the involved microorganism are given for prolonged periods until tests show a marked reduction in the inflammation.

Occasionally, surgery is needed to allow drainage and to reduce deterioration of the skull bone. Malignant otitis externa usually responds to prolonged treatment, but it may recur. Complications include damage to the cranial nerves, skull or brain; spread of infection to the brain or other parts of the body.

To prevent malignant ear infection, it's important to treat an acute external ear infection completely and not to stop treatment sooner than recommended. You should dry ears thoroughly after exposure to moisture, avoid swimming in polluted water, and if susceptible to external ear infection, you should protect the ear canal with cotton or lamb's wool while applying hair spray or hair dye. After swimming, one or two drops of a mixture of 50% alcohol and 50% vinegar in each ear will help to dry the ear and prevent infection.

EAR CONDITIONS

Acoustic Neuroma

A rare benign tumor called an *acoustic neuroma* (also called auditory nerve tumor or Schwannoma) can cause a hearing loss on the affected side. This usually slow-growing tumor occurs most often in women between ages 40 and 50, and makes up between 5 and 7% of all brain tumors.

The tumors arise from the Schwann cell sheath of the cranial or spinal nerve roots, most often involving the hearing (eighth cranial) nerve. Symptoms begin with tinnitus in one ear and a progressive high-frequency hearing loss. There is often a loss of speech discrimination out of proportion with the hearing loss, probably due to the lessened ability of the cochlear nerve to conduct sound because of the tumor's pressure. Compression of the blood vessels within the internal auditory canal may also cause hearing loss, because of the reduced blood flow to and from the cochlea. As the tumor enlarges, it may press on the brain stem and cerebellum, causing lack of coordination. Unsteadiness or vertigo may appear as the nerve cells within the internal auditory canal degenerate.

The diagnosis is confirmed by hearing and balance tests, an auditory brain stem response test and by brain scans. Most acoustic neuromas affect the size and shape of the internal auditory canal by eroding the bone, which can be detected by scanning. While these tumors rarely become malignant, early detection is imperative to prevent more serious hearing loss.

Today it's possible to identify even small acoustic neuromas. If routine auditory tests reveal loss of hearing and speech discrimination (hearing sound in that ear, but not understanding what is being said), an auditory brain stem response test may be done. This test provides information on how sound passes along the path from the ear to the brain. A detailed "imaging scan" is usually ordered if there is an abnormality in the ABR test, which suggests the presence of an acoustic neuroma. The CT scan is a powerful tool in locating acoustic neuromas. Although small tumors still confined to the internal auditory canal may not show up on a simple CT scan, a scan using contrast dye will enhance the image of the tumor.

Magnetic Resonance Imaging (MRI) is a newer diagnostic test that is very effective in identifying acoustic neuromas. MRI combines modern computer technology with harmless magnetic pulses and radio frequency waves passed through the portion of the body being studied. The image that is formed clearly defines any acoustic neuroma. A contrast material is required to enhance the tumor, making it easier to see. Currently, an MRI with gadolinium contrast is the preferred study for diagnosing an acoustic neuroma.

At this time, the only treatment that can totally eradicate the tumor is microsurgical removal, which is the treatment of choice for acoustic neuromas.

Within the last three decades, microsurgical techniques have been refined so that the risk in total tumor removal has been greatly reduced. Microsurgical instruments and an operating microscope are routinely used, and damage to the surrounding nerve tissue has been markedly decreased. The death rate is extremely low. In addition, facial nerve function is routinely monitored during surgery, which has reduced the frequency and severity of facial nerve injury. The surgeon will also monitor the cochlear nerve where it appears feasible to preserve hearing. According to the National Institutes of Health, patients do best if they are treated at medical centers with surgeons who have a specific interest in these tumors and sufficient continuing experience to develop, refine and maintain proficiency.

After the surgery, the patient is observed in the intensive care unit for one or two days with careful monitoring. Possible postsurgical problems include headache, nausea, vomiting, decreased mental alertness, cerebrospinal fluid leak and meningitis. Patients usually stay in the hospital between four to seven days, and recover at home for between four to six weeks. In the hands of an experienced microsurgeon, regrowth rates after microsurgery are less than 5%.

Alternatively, some patients have radiation instead of microsurgery. Conventional radiation of most tumors involves multiple doses of radiation delivered over three to six weeks. The treatment team usually consists of a neurosurgeon, radiophysicist and a radiation oncologist working together to develop a treatment plan based on the size and shape of the tumor.

Follow-up studies are important because 5% to 10% of tumors will continue to grow after this treatment or at some time in the future. It appears that the tumor will be controlled throughout life following radiation treatment in at least 90 percent of patients. A tumor that has been irradiated and grows may be more difficult to remove than an unradiated tumor, just as a tumor that recurs after microsurgery may be more difficult to remove.

Symptoms such as dizziness and disturbances of balance get better quicker after microsurgical treatment than after radiation because the effects of radiation may require up to 18 months. Many patients have some residual dizziness and disturbed balance after either radiation or microsurgical treatment, but this is commonly less after microsurgical treatment.

In patients with useful hearing before radiation, about 50% will still have useful hearing two years later. Among patients with normal facial movement and sensation before treatment, 10% will develop some degree of facial weakness or numbness, which usually recovers in several months. These early statistics compare very favorably with microsurgical tumor removal.

In the short term, radiation is less expensive than microsurgery. Most patients are treated on an outpatient basis; many patients return home several hours after treatment is complete, and they can return to work within a few days. A few patients experience headaches, nausea and tiredness, but these side effects are considerably less than after microsurgical tumor removal. Patients treated with radiation are usually able to return to their job within a matter of days. Radiation requires follow-up MRIs over the years, and there is the potential for additional treatment in cases of continued growth or later regrowth. Microsurgery is initially more expensive, with follow-up MRIs suggested at one and five years if the tumor has been completely removed. The National Institutes of Health recommends that radiation therapy is a treatment option limited to patients unable or unwilling to undergo otherwise indicated surgery.

In small tumors (usually up to an inch), it may be possible to save some hearing. In larger tumors (those that protrude from the internal auditory canal into the brain stem), the hearing usually has been partially or totally lost and cannot be restored. This loss means that problems locating the direction of sound, hearing a person speaking softly on the deaf side, and understanding speech over a high level of background noise will continue. For some, a CROS hearing aid will be helpful.

Since the facial nerve, which controls muscles of facial expression, is in close contact with acoustic neuromas, it is usually necessary for the surgeon to manipulate and sometimes to remove portions of this nerve. In some instances nerve damage or swelling may cause facial paralysis. This paralysis resolves with time, but some permanent weakness may persist.

Nerve regeneration is a slow process, and it may take up to a year for recovery. If facial paralysis doesn't improve, a second operation may be performed to connect the healthy portion of the facial nerve to a nerve in the neck.

Studies show that long-term eye discomfort and other eye problems affect at least half of those who have had an acoustic neuroma removed, particularly if the tumor was medium or large. It is important to be under the care of an eye specialist if problems occur. Loss of eyelid function or altered tear production cause much of the scratchiness and irritation because the eye becomes dry and is unprotected.

Ménière's Disease

This inner ear disorder of unknown origin causes hearing loss, dizziness or vertigo, and ringing in the ears. Ménière's disease affects more than 1 million Americans and can be extremely incapacitating.

First described by the French physician Prosper Ménière in 1861, the disease is characterized by dizziness in which people feel either they or their surroundings are spinning. This occurs together with hearing loss, nausea and vomiting, tinnitus and fullness or pressure within the ear. Symptoms may last from a few minutes to eight hours or more, and can be profoundly disturbing. The attacks of vertigo may occur every so often every few weeks.

There are several less common variants of the condition. While most patients with Ménière's disease experience vertigo, hearing loss and tinnitus, those with cochlear Ménière's disease have symptoms that include tinnitus *without* vertigo. Another variant—vestibular Ménière's disease—causes vertigo without hearing loss.

Ménière's disease tends to come and go, but the vertigo usually gets progressively worse until it peaks after several years; symptoms will then become less severe until the vertigo finally disappears. By this time, however, the patient is usually severely deaf. Normally, only one ear is affected, and the sensorineural hearing loss may get worse and worse over the years, although a few people have experienced hearing loss in both ears. The loss may start with low frequencies and then involve higher frequencies, eventually becoming permanent. Hearing tests can usually reveal loudness recruitment and poor speech discrimination.

While the exact cause of Ménière's disease is unknown, researchers believe the problem is related to a change in pressure of the fluid in the inner ear, but the cause isn't understood. As excess fluid accumulates in the inner ear, delicate nerve endings become damaged. One of the strangest things about the disorder is its unpredictability; remissions come and go, lasting anywhere from six months to six years.

Researchers at the House Ear Institute in California have found a wide range of potential links to the disorder, including allergies, endocrine problems and trauma. Treating these separate conditions may improve the Ménière's symptoms, but not everyone will get relief this way. Recent research at the University of Southern California at Los Angeles suggests that allergy-related immune problems may help trigger symptoms of the disease. These researchers found that for many Ménière's patients, allergy shots for airborne allergies or special diets (for food-related allergies) can be very effective in controlling vertigo and tinnitus. This could be because the anatomy of the inner ear makes it a target of histamine and other chemicals released during an allergic reaction. Airborne allergies to dust, mold and pollen, and food allergies (especially wheat) are often associated with Ménière's.

House Ear Institute researchers found that by severely restricting diet, some patients may find their symptoms subside and hearing increases by as much as 20 dB. Unfortunately, diet restrictions are severe, including no wheat, flour, eggs, chocolate, corn or mayonnaise. Some patients at the institute who temporarily disregard the diet restrictions notice an immediate return of symptoms. Ménière's patients who have abnormal insulin levels and/or impaired glucose tolerance should eat six small meals of low-carbohydrate, low-cholesterol food.

Other treatments vary. Some doctors recommend lifestyle changes, including less stress, no cigarettes or alcohol, regular exercise and a different diet (in addition to the above restrictions, less salt and more low-fat foods).

Strategies to deal with vertigo generally involve ways to minimize stimulation of the balance system by limiting head movements. This allows the eyes, looking at a stationary object, to convince the brain that the body is not rotating. In general, head movements or closing the eyes will make the vertigo worse. Patients should lie or sit as still as possible, while trying to keep eyes fixed on a stationary object some distance away. Movements should be slow and even.

For the relief of nausea and the stress associated with vertigo, one of the following drugs may be prescribed:

- *prochlorperizine (Compazine):* controls nausea, vomiting and anxiety.
- *promethazine (Phenergan):* controls nausea, vomiting, motion sickness.
- *diazepam (Valium):* suppresses anxiety.
- *meclizine (Antivert):* controls nausea, vomiting and motion sickness. Another H1-blocking antihistamine.
- *scopolamine:* controls nausea and vomiting.

While most of these drugs are generally aimed at treating the effects of vertigo in Ménière's disease, they may also play a role in controlling the disease by reducing anxiety, since stress is an important factor in triggering Ménière's attacks.

Many physicians prescribe steroids such as prednisone or dexamethasone, which may work by suppressing the immune response (some believe that Ménière's is a form of autoimmune disease). However, glucocorticoids also affect carbohydrate and protein metabolism, lipid metabolism, electrolyte balance, inflammatory responses and immune responses.

Surgical options include placing a tympanostomy tube, a relatively minor albeit controversial procedure that is widely used in children and adults for the relief of middle-ear infections (otitis media). The purpose of the tube is to maintain a tiny hole through the eardrum. Although the medical community has been skeptical that this treatment would have any bearing on Ménière's disease, many doctors are finding that they are very effective with success rates as good as endolymphatic shunt surgery. Studies indicate a high proportion of Ménière's patients get relief from vertigo by this procedure. However, some physicians remain unconvinced.

In addition, there are many surgical procedures involving the endolymphatic sac:

- *Endolymphatic sac decompression:* Drilling away the bone overlying the endolymphatic sac to make a larger "cavity" for the sac to occupy.
- *Endolymph-subarachnoid shunt:* Placing a tube between the endolymphatic sac and the cranium
- *Endolymph-mastoid shunt:* placing a tube between the endolymphatic sac and the mastoid cavity of the middle ear to avoid potential problems of opening the cranium in the endolymph-subarachnoid shunt.

However, endolymphatic sac surgery is extremely controversial. Based on a published study, many doctors regard endolymphatic sac surgery as a "placebo" surgery (i.e. the patient gets the same outcome whether or not the sac is actually shunted) and will no longer perform it. Others regard surgery of the sac as a step between nonsurgical therapies and more invasive procedures.

An alternative, less invasive method to destroy the vestibular system is by using certain antibiotics that are known to destroy the vestibular hair cells. By destroying these cells, the brain is no longer sent "incorrect" information that the head is rotating. The techniques rely on the fact that for antibiotics such as gentamycin, the sensory cells of the vestibular system are more sensitive to damage than are the cells of the cochlea. This means that at the right dose, vestibular function can be reduced without damaging hearing. The antibiotic is usually injected into the middle ear space through the eardrum, and enters the inner ear through the round and oval windows. This method can be effective, but it is difficult to avoid some damage to hearing. For this reason, many doctors use just enough treatments to ease vertigo without necessarily destroying all vestibular function.

Surgical removal of either a portion or the entire labyrinth can be performed when there is no useful hearing in the affected ear, since collateral damage to the cochlea may produce significant hearing loss.

Vestibular nerve section surgery is a more invasive type of surgery, but it can dramatically cure vertigo. The goal of the surgery is to cut the nerve from the vestibular apparatus while leaving the auditory nerve intact, thereby preserving hearing. During the recovery period, the brain adapts to manage without vestibular input from the operated side, so that normal activity can be resumed.

Mondini's Dysplasia

This developmental problem of the inner ear is characterized by malformations of the cochlear and semicircular canals that may cause a severe sensorineural hearing loss, perilymph fistulas, or recurrent meningitis. In a Mondini malformation, only one and a half turns of the normal two and one half turns of the cochlea is completed. The defect occurs during the seventh week of pregnancy after development of the ear begins. The vestibule and semicircular canals may or may not be normal. A problem with development between the fourth and fifth week of pregnancy will lead to a common cavity between the cochlea and vestibule. The semicircular canals may or may not be normal, and hearing loss is usually profound. The diagnosis is confirmed by a high-resolution CT scan of the temporal bone.

For patients without symptoms, most otologists recommend a "wait and see" approach before treating the condition. Patients with symptoms may require surgical exploration and packing of the ear. Research suggests that a multichannel cochlear implant may be of some benefit to those who have lost hearing due to Mondini dysplasia; at worst, the condition is not a contraindication for cochlear implantation.

Osteogenesis Imperfecta

In about half the people with this "brittle bone" disease (related to otosclerosis), there is a conductive hearing loss and a blue tinge to the whites of the eyes. The conductive hearing loss occurs because of fractures in the stapes.

Otosclerosis

This disorder occurs when an overgrowth of spongy bone immobilizes the stapes (the innermost bone of the middle ear), preventing sound vibrations from passing to the inner ear and resulting in conductive hearing loss. In most cases, both ears are usually affected. Eventually, this soft, spongy bone will harden and become as dense as surrounding bone.

While the problem can occur anywhere on the temporal bone, it usually begins in front of the oval window, gradually spreading to the oval window and then the footplate of the stapes. Eventually, this will imbed the stapes to the surrounding tissue, restricting movement. In addition, otosclerosis can affect the cochlea, causing a sensorineural hearing loss.

The disease, which begins in early adulthood (between age 15 and 35), is the most frequent cause of middle ear hearing loss in young adults, and affects about one in every 200 people. Often occurring during pregnancy, it tends to run in families and is more common in women than in men, in whites than in blacks, Native Americans or Asians.

People with otosclerosis tend to speak softly and hear muffled sound more clearly when there is background noise. Hearing loss progresses slowly over a period of 10 to 15 years, often accompanied by tinnitus and sometimes by vertigo. The rate of hearing loss may increase during pregnancy. Eventually, there may be some sensorineural hearing loss caused by damage spreading to the inner ear, which makes high tones hard to hear.

Hearing tests can uncover otosclerosis, showing a conductive hearing loss greater in lower frequencies. There is no medication or treatment that will improve the hearing in people with otosclerosis, although in some cases a medication known as Florical (sodium fluoride and calcium carbonate) is prescribed to prevent further nerve hearing loss. Ideally, Florical should be taken twice a day for two years, followed by an assessment of the degree of tinnitus and the severity of imbalance. If these conditions have stabilized, Florical may be reduced or stopped. Florical should be avoided during pregnancy.

Hearing aids can help, although the conductive deafness can only be cured by a stapedectomy (an operation in which the stapes, or stirrup, is replaced with an artificial substitute). The stapedectomy is performed under local or general anesthesia with the use of laser and microscopic techniques either as an outpatient or inpatient procedure. During the operation, the surgeon uses a laser to open a small hole in the bottom of the stapes bone to make way for the artificial stapes.

There may be some dizziness after surgery, which usually disappears. Hearing usually returns fairly quickly, although occasionally a blood clot will appear in the middle ear, which can block sound conduction. These usually break up within a few weeks. Convalescence at home for about a week or so is recommended. Nearly 90% of these operations are successful in improving the conductive hearing loss, but there is also some small risk. While it can help most people, between 1 and 2% of patients lose all hearing in the ear. This is why people with otosclerosis in both ears often choose to undergo surgery for only one ear at a time, waiting at least a year between surgeries. Once the inner ear is damaged, a stapedectomy may not help the problem.

Tumors (Middle Ear)

Tumors of the middle ear are rare growths that can remain undetected until they have become quite invasive. Both cancerous and noncancerous tumors in the middle ear can cause a conductive hearing loss by blocking the middle ear and external auditory canal, destroying the ossicles and interfering with the eardrum's movement. Malignant tumors also can cause a sensorineural loss as the growth protrudes into the inner ear.

Symptoms include dizziness, bleeding, deep ear pain, drainage and paralysis of the facial nerve. Middle ear tumors include choristoma, congenital cholesteatoma, dermoid cysts, meningioma, facial nerve neuroma, acoustic neuroma, glomus tympanicum and glomus jugulare.

Generally, it's rare to find a malignant tumor in the middle ear; if it does occur, it is usually a squamous cell carcinoma or glomus tumor. Squamous cell carcinoma usually appears in the external ear canal and moves into the middle ear, interfering with sound transmission. It may appear after a chronic suppurative ear infection, but it can begin to grow for no apparent reason at any age. It is most common, however, in middle age. Survival rate for this type of skin cancer, even after treatment with radiation and radical surgery, is only about 30%.

A glomus tumor is relatively slow-growing and develops from clusters of nerve cells that regulate body function. These cells are located in either the jugular vein or the back wall of the middle ear. Patients with this type of tumor have a conductive hearing loss as the tumor grows, filling the middle ear and eroding into the inner ear. More common among women, these tumors can cause a pulselike tinnitus followed by a sensorineural hearing loss, dizziness and facial paralysis. Treatment includes radiation and surgery.

DISEASES RELATED TO HEARING LOSS

In some cases, hearing problems result not from a disease that primarily affects the ear, but as the result of a secondary, underlying condition, such as AIDS, Lyme disease, diabetes, kidney disease or syphilis.

AIDS

Infection with the human immunodeficiency virus (HIV) can result in acquired immune deficiency syndrome (AIDS) or AIDS-related complex. Both AIDS and ARC are associated with neurological complications that include hearing loss; an estimated 75 percent of adult AIDS patients, and 50 percent of ARC patients have abnormalities of the hearing system.

Why this happens is unknown, although direct infection of the nervous system by HIV is well documented. Hearing disorders in AIDS could be caused directly by HIV infection of the cochlea or the central auditory system. On the other hand, many AIDS complications are caused by opportunistic infections rather than the HIV itself. The most common of these infections (cytomegalovirus, or CMV) is known to damage the hearing system in congenital cases of AIDS. More than 90% of AIDS patients also have cytomegalovirus.

Autoimmune Inner Ear Disease (AIED)

This syndrome causes progressive hearing loss and/or dizziness triggered by immune cells that attack the inner ear. Usual symptoms include a relatively rapid reduction of hearing accompanied by tinnitus (ringing in the ears), which occurs over a few months. Alternatively, there may be attacks of hearing loss and tinnitus that resemble Ménière's disease, and attacks of dizziness accompanied by abnormal blood tests for antibodies. About half of patients with AIED also have balance symptoms.

The immune system is complex, and there are several ways that it can damage the inner ear. Several well-known autoimmune diseases such as systemic lupus erythematosis (SLE), Sjoegren's syndrome (dry eye syndrome), Cogan's disease, ulcerative colitis, Wegener's granulomatosis, rheumatoid arthritis, and scleroderma can cause or be associated with AIED. Still, AIED is rare and probably accounts for less than 1% of all cases of hearing impairment or dizziness. About 16% of patients with bilateral Ménière's disease and 6% of persons with Ménière's disease of any variety may be affected by immune dysfunction.

There are several ways that a person's immune system could begin to attack the cells of the inner ear. In one theory, damage to the inner ear triggers substances that provoke additional immune reactions. (This theory might explain the attack/remission cycle of disorders such as Ménière's disease.) In the most commonly believed theory, antibodies or rogue T-cells cause accidental inner ear damage because the ear shares common antigens with a potentially harmful substance, virus or bacteria that the body is fighting against. This is the favored theory of AIED.

There is increasing evidence that genetically controlled aspects of the immune system may boost susceptibility to common hearing disorders such as Ménière's disease. There is also evidence for a genetic vulnerability to ototoxic drugs such as gentamicin.

The diagnosis of AIED is based on careful review of the patient's family history, findings on physical exam, blood tests and the results of hearing and vestibular tests.

Treatment for patients with a classic rapidly progressive bilateral hearing impairment may include steroids (such as prednisone) for four weeks. In most patients who respond to steroids, a chemotherapy drug such as cytoxan or methotrexate can be used over the long term.

Lyme Disease

Lyme disease is the most common disease in the United States that can be caught from ticks or insects. In addition to a host of other symptoms it can cause a hearing loss. When an infected deer tick bites you, it may pass on the disease, although only about 10% of those who are bitten get sick. Most states have reported cases of the disease, but Lyme, Connecticut where the condition was first diagnosed, has the highest rate of infection.

Because the deer population is growing so fast, the number of Lyme disease patients is also escalating.

In the first stage of the disease, as many as 80% of victims develop a red "bull's-eye" rash surrounding the bite site, enlarging gradually over a few weeks. Any rash that is at least two inches in diameter should be considered evidence of Lyme disease. This rash can appear anywhere between three and 32 days after the bite. This may be followed by intermittent flu-like symptoms; during this stage, about 15 to 20% of people develop a hearing loss together with migrainelike headaches and painful arthritis. The hearing loss is evidence of central nervous system involvement, which may also cause facial numbness, pain and weakness in arms and legs, memory loss, stiff neck and severe fatigue.

Diabetes

This metabolic disorder causes a decrease or absence of insulin, the hormone responsible for the absorption of glucose into cells, where it's used for energy. Because diabetes tends to break down blood vessels and peripheral nerves, it can interfere with blood supply to the ear and the internal auditory canal. This can result in a breakdown of cochlear and vestibular nerves and cause a sensorineural hearing loss.

Kidney Disease

Kidney disease requiring renal dialysis and transplantation often results in a type of sensorineural hearing loss that can be caused by a number of factors, including electrolyte imbalance, inadequate dialysis or drug toxicity. These factors can affect the components of the inner ear fluid and alter the normal function of the cochlea.

Syphilis

The inner ear hearing loss that occurs among adults who contract syphilis tends to appear more slowly than it does in children with congenital syphilis, as either a hearing loss or a fluctuation in intensity. Treatment with penicillin and steroids is usually given for some months; if hearing improves, the steroids may be continued indefinitely to stave off a recurrent hearing loss. Although some syphilis-related hearing loss responds to treatment right away, other cases do not, even in the face of continued treatment. Because syphilis causes a sensorineural hearing loss, patients usually understand speech poorly even with the use of hearing aids.

HEREDITARY EAR DISEASES

Deafness may be caused by a wide range of inherited abnormalities. Most causes of genetic deafness are present at birth, and are discussed in Chapter 3. However, one genetic condition known as Paget's disease doesn't usually cause hearing problems until adulthood.

Paget's Disease

This common genetic disease often occurs in middle age and affects the normal process of bone formation, weakening and deforming bones of the skull, pelvis, collarbone and long bones of the leg. Changes in the skull can cause inner ear damage, resulting in tinnitus, vertigo and a sensorineural hearing loss. Many people do not require treatment, but others find that analgesic drugs provide pain relief and normal bone formation. Surgery may be required to repair deformities.

For More Information About Genetics and Deafness

Many large universities and hospitals have clinical genetic services. Ask your doctor or local health department for a list of genetic service providers. Or contact one of these national groups:

American Society of Human Genetics
American Board of Medical Genetics
9650 Rockville Pike
Bethesda MD 20814
(301) 571-1825

Genetic Services Center
Gallaudet University
800 Florida Ave. NE
Washington DC 20002
(202) 651-5258 (voice/TDD)
(800) 451-8834, ext. 5258 (voice/TDD)

March of Dimes Birth Defects Foundation
Professional Education
1275 Mamaroneck Ave.
White Plains NY 10605

National Research Register for Hereditary Hearing Loss
Boys Town National Research Hospital
555 30th St.
Omaha NE 68154
(402) 498-6631 (voice/TDD)

National Society of Genetic Counselors
233 Canterbury Dr.
Wallingford PA 19086
(215) 872-7608

INJURY AND HEARING LOSS

Your hearing can be damaged from a sudden, intense noise (such as a gunshot) or by a head injury that can either injure the delicate hearing mechanism or the brain itself. Since we will discuss hearing loss due to noises in Chapter 4, in this chapter we'll focus on injury-related hearing loss.

While the skull is designed to protect the brain and delicate internal structures such as the inner ear, severe head injury can cause both a sensorineural and conductive deafness in one or both ears. Hitting the front or the back of the head can damage the organ of Corti, or cause a transverse fracture of the temporal bone, leading to sensorineural deafness, vertigo and tinnitus. Fracture of the temporal bone can completely destroy the hearing and balance mechanism on the affected side. This type of deafness is usually permanent, although the dizziness that can accompany it will usually fade away over a period of several weeks. The unsteadiness and swaying toward the affected side may also subside after a few months. Sometimes a transverse fracture of the temporal bone results in an incomplete hearing loss, but this is uncommon.

Head Injury

Severe head injury can cause either a sensorineural or conductive hearing loss in one or both ears.

Sensorineural hearing loss after severe head injury can be associated with a fracture of the temporal bone, which may completely destroy the hearing and balance mechanism on the affected side. This type of deafness is usually permanent, although the dezziness that can accompany it will usually subside over several weeks, and the unsteadiness may fade after several months. Sometimes, a transverse fracture of the temporal bone causes an incomplete hearing loss, but this is uncommon.

It's possible to have hearing damage after a head injury that doesn't fracture the temporal bone, especially from a blow to the back or side of the head. Deafness from this type of injury is usually similar to that which comes from excess noise. An injury like this also often causes dizziness, which is made worse when you change the position of your head. Although there may be hearing loss on the side of the injury, there also may be a mild hearing loss on the opposite side, due to a concussion of the inner ear.

Conductive deafness after injury is caused by blood pooling in the middle ear and external ear canal; occasionally, the ossicular chain (hammer, anvil and stirrup) is disrupted and the eardrum is ruptured. As the blood is absorbed and the eardrum heals, hearing usually returns to its preinjury level. Occasionally, conductive deafness after a head injury can be permanent, but the maximum degree of hearing loss is usually no more than 60 dB. This means that if speech is loud enough, you can not only hear but also understand what is being said. Surgery also can sometimes restore hearing in this type of injury.

Treatment

Hearing loss as a result of such damage to the middle ear can sometimes be corrected; a ruptured eardrum can heal itself in time, and the small bones of the ear may be repaired or replaced. Using the modern technique of microsurgery, ear specialists can repair or rebuild an eardrum in many cases. Using a technique called myringoplasty, surgeons can close a hole in the eardrum, using a tissue graft from elsewhere in the body.

Normally, permanent hearing loss is mild, although the loss may be greater if the ear is very sensitive or the noise was quite loud. Because there is almost always some amount of temporary hearing loss after an acoustic trauma, some time must pass before the amount of permanent damage can be measured.

Air Bags and Hearing Loss

The sudden impact of an air bag hitting a passenger's face may cause hearing problems. According to a team of British researchers, the sound of an air bag inflating can cause noise from 150 to 170 decibels, lasting about 0.1 seconds, a sound which scientists believe may damage hearing in humans.

Researchers base their conclusions on two cases in which drivers suffered hearing loss and ringing of the ears (tinnitus) in low-speed accidents. Ear problems following air bag inflation may be underreported since passengers often don't remember the noise of the inflation, and attribute their loss to injuries suffered in the accident itself.

DRUGS AND DEAFNESS

It's possible to develop a hearing problem after using certain drugs or chemicals that affect hearing and balance by interfering with the function of the inner ear. The cochlea and vestibular system are susceptible to the effects of a range of ototoxic drugs, especially some antibiotics. The negative effect of some ototoxic drugs is increased when taken in combination with other drugs, or when taken for long periods of time. Often, hearing loss caused by these drugs can't be reversed because the drugs damage hair cells, which don't regenerate; they can also harm the auditory nerve.

Often tinnitus (ringing in the ear) is the first symptom, although some damage can occur before *any* symptoms appear. The developing fetus is particularly susceptible to these drugs. However, the actual incidence of drugs and resultant deafness has been hard to establish because of the problems and complexity in studying the ear.

A number of factors place some people at higher risk when taking ototoxic drugs, including age, earlier ear infections, sensorineural hearing loss, impaired kidney or liver function, extreme drug sensitivity, simultaneous use of loop diuretics or drugs that are toxic to the kidneys.

The hallmark warning sign of imminent ear damage is tinnitus, so if you're taking any of the following drugs and you experience ringing in your ears, you should consult the doctor who prescribed the medication right away.

Antibiotics

Some very powerful antibiotics, taken to fight a life-threatening infection, may be associated with hearing loss. While some of these drugs cause a permanent hearing loss, the law requires that you be told if one of these ototoxic drugs is being prescribed.

The most common class of ototoxic antibiotics are the aminoglycosides, which appear to cause hearing problems when dosage is continued for more than 10 days. (The exception to this is streptomycin, which can cause a hearing loss within five days.) Any patient treated for longer than this time should undergo cochlear and vestibular testing before, during and after therapy. Examples of the aminoglycosides include:

- amikacin
- dihydrostreptomycin
- gentamicin
- kanamycin
- neomycin
- netilmicin
- ribostamycin
- streptomycin
- tobramycin

Neomycin is considered to be the most toxic of all drugs to the cochlea, and damage may result in hearing loss that continues irreversibly even after treatment is stopped. Warning signs may include tinnitus or impaired balance, but these symptoms don't always occur.

Other types of antibiotics, including erythromycin, azithromycin and viomycin, also can cause hearing loss. Viomycin and azithromycin can cause permanent hearing loss, but all known cases of erythromycin ototoxicity have been reversed once the drug has been discontinued, and only large doses (more than four grams per day) have been associated with erythromycin toxicity.

Loop Diuretics

These powerful drugs are fast-acting chemicals that help remove excess water from the body by increasing the flow of urine. They are especially powerful when given by injection and are helpful in the emergency treatment of heart failure. While permanent hearing loss is possible, most of the time the hearing loss, vertigo and tinnitus is reversible within 30 minutes and a day after medication is stopped.

In general, doctors try to avoid using loop diuretics with premature infants or patients receiving aminoglycoside antibiotics. These drugs include furosemide ethacrynic acid, lasix, bumetadine, piretamide, azosemide, triflocin and indapamide. Other diuretics (such as dyazide and the thiazides) haven't been found to have ototoxic effects.

Some studies suggest that aspirin may help protect against the damage from antibiotics (which is unusual, since high doses of aspirin may also cause a temporary hearing loss). Scientists at the University of Michigan say lab tests with guinea pigs show that salicylate prevented inner ear hair cell damage, which is exactly the kind of damage that antibiotics cause. Hair cells are important because they allow the inner ear to detect sounds and transmit signals to the brain.

Salicylates (aspirin)

High doses of salicylates (such as about 10 pills of aspirin or drugs with aspirin in them per day) can cause tinnitus and up to a 40 dB hearing loss in both ears. Normally, more than 12 aspirin tablets per day must be taken before there is a danger of hearing loss, although each person's sensitivity to the drug varies. The degree of hearing loss depends on the concentration of the drug in the blood. Both tinnitus and hearing loss are reversed between 24 and 72 hours after the drug is stopped.

Although many drugs can be toxic to the delicate sensory tissue of the ear and can cause permanent hearing loss, aspirin is unusual in that the inner ear hearing loss it causes is reversible.

People who already have nerve deafness may notice that aspirin has a greater effect on hearing at lower frequencies. On the other hand, research reports in 1999 suggest an ingredient in aspirin may prevent a type of deafness caused by antibiotics by preventing inner ear hair cell damage.

Quinine Derivatives

Less than two grams a day may cause a transient tinnitus, hearing loss, vertigo, headache, nausea or vision problems. There have been cases of permanent hearing loss and tinnitus, but usually only when high doses of the drugs were continued after symptoms appeared. Otherwise, symptoms can quickly disappear when the drugs are discontinued. Examples of these drugs include quinine, chloroquine, quinidine and hydroxychloroquine.

Anti-Cancer Drugs

A few of the anti-cancer drugs used in chemotherapy, such as cisplatin, may also cause a hearing loss, but in a life-or-death situation you may face a choice of hearing loss or cancer fatality. Anti-cancer drugs linked to hearing problems include:

- cisplatin
- bleomycin
- vincristine
- nitrogen mustard
- vinblastine

Chemicals

Some environmental chemicals can damage the delicate hearing mechanism within the ear as well. These include:

- trichloroethylene
- xylene
- styrene
- butyl nitrite
- toluene
- hexane
- carbon disulfide
- mercury
- manganese
- tin
- lead
- carbon monoxide

Other Substances

Substances that may temporarily reduce hearing ability or increase tinnitus include alcohol, carbon monoxide, caffeine, oral contraceptives and tobacco (nicotine).

Nicotine interferes with the flow of blood throughout the body by narrowing blood vessels including those to the ear. The chemical can cause tinnitus in addition to hearing loss; in addition, research suggests that smokers have a higher failure rate after reconstruction of the eardrum (myringoplasty).

Deafness from abuse of narcotics has been rarely reported. However, recent studies show that overuse of a combination of the narcotic pain reliever hydrocodone and acentaminophen (a product called Vicodin) can lead to total deafness. This rapid, progressive hearing loss has been treated successfully with a cochlear implant.

EXTERNAL EAR DISEASES

In general, anything that blocks the external ear canal can cause a hearing loss; this may include impacted earwax, a foreign body lodged in the canal, or a narrowing of the canal because of disease.

Impacted earwax blocking the canal can prevent sound from reaching the middle ear, causing a mild conductive hearing loss (especially for higher frequencies). Symptoms are worsened if water enters the ear, causing the ear to swell. Large plugs of earwax must be removed by a doctor; smaller plugs may be removed at home. You can remove hard wax with mineral oil drops; soft wax can be removed with hydrogen peroxide drops or a commercial softener. The drops may be applied overnight and then removed by irrigating the ear with warm water from an ear syringe. Cotton swabs shouldn't be used because of the danger of pushing wax deeper into the ear.

Foreign objects in the ear don't usually cause a serious hearing loss unless they totally block the canal, or perforate the eardrum. Foreign objects that disrupt the labyrinth can cause a sensory hearing loss.

Perichondritis

An infection of the connective tissue covering the cartilage of the external ear is called perichondritis; it may destroy the cartilage and deform the ear, narrowing or closing the ear canal.

Cancer

Cancer is sometimes found in the external ear, and the resulting tumor can destroy the adjacent tissue and spread to nearby lymph nodes.

CHAPTER 3
CHILDREN AND HEARING LOSS

The lack of early detection of hearing problems in children is one of the most serious public health problems in the United States today. The average age at which moderate to severe hearing impairment is detected in children is two to three years of age, but these problems can and should be identified and treated much sooner. If undetected and untreated, hearing loss in children leads to delayed speech and language development and can contribute to emotional, social and academic problems. Ideally, doctors should identify infants with hearing loss before age three months, so that intervention can begin by six months of age.

Because prompt diagnosis of hearing problems could help offset lapses in language development, the American Academy of Pediatrics now recommends that all newborns be checked for hearing loss. Hearing impairment in infants can cause delays in speech, language and cognitive development, according to the academy experts. Often, hearing loss is not diagnosed in children until they are two or three years old and not speaking properly. Yet if hearing is detected early enough, babies can be fitted with hearing aids or be exposed to sign language. Because children learn language by being exposed to it, without experiencing either spoken or sign language, it's hard for these children to develop adequate speech or sign.

Although hearing loss is more frequent than other disorders that are now tested for at birth (occuring in four out of every 1,000 births), screening is only required in 10 states. For example, babies are routinely checked for the metabolic disorder of phenylketonuria (PKU), which occurs in only one out of every 16,000 births.

Newborn screening tests are noninvasive and painless, and usually include either tests of the small hair cells in the cochlea, or the use of ear cuplets and sensors on the baby's head to measure brain response to sound.

In the past, only newborns in certain high-risk categories were tested for hearing problems. These high-risk categories included infections or lack of oxygen at birth, bacterial meningitis, exposure to rubella or herpes, defects of the head or neck (such as cleft palate or malformation of the ear itself), severe jaundice requiring transfusion, family history of childhood hearing loss and low birth weight. Among these high-risk infants, chances of having a congenital hearing problem is between one out of 20 to one out of 50.

Parents are usually the first to suspect a hearing loss, and the earlier a loss is found the better the chances of preventing language and learning delays. Any child who has a history of frequent ear infections and who shows signs of poor hearing, not following directions, poor pronunciation or behavioral problems should have a hearing test. If a parent or doctor suspects a hearing problem, the child's primary care provider may choose to conduct a hearing screening for a preschool age child, but infants and young toddlers will need a referral for special tests. A pediatrician should conduct ongoing exams when a child has middle ear fluid. If present for several months without clearing, consultation with an otolaryngologist should be considered.

If a child care provider or parent has any doubt about slower-than-normal sound and speech-language development in a child, these concerns should be discussed with the child's primary care provider, and hearing testing should be seriously considered. (For more information, brochures are available from the American Speech-Language-Hearing Association at 1-800-638-8255 or through e-mail at *actioncenter@ asha.org.*)

PRENATAL/PERINATAL CAUSES OF HEARING LOSS

Between 7% and 20% of deaf and hard-of-hearing people lost their hearing before birth. The three major threats to the hearing mechanism of a woman's unborn baby are viral diseases, ototoxic drugs (drugs that can harm hearing) and the condition of a woman's uterus during pregnancy.

Infections

The most common causes of prenatal deafness are viral diseases contracted by the mother, and of these, the most dangerous is rubella; other viral diseases that can harm hearing include influenza, mumps, toxoplasmosis, cytomegalovirus (CMV) and herpes simplex. Of course, almost any severe infection can damage the fetal hearing mechanism, especially during the first trimester when the fetus seems to be especially vulnerable. Only the common cold appears to carry no threat at all to the hearing of an unborn child.

Bacterial infections are also a concern. If a mother contracts a bacterial infection before giving birth, she can transmit the infection via the bloodstream to her baby. Other infectious agents that might be in the amniotic fluid can be swallowed by a fetus and then pumped up the eustachian tube into the middle ear, where they can create an ear infection.

German measles (rubella)

A mother who contracts German measles during the first three months of pregnancy may give birth to a child with some degree of hearing loss. Children affected by this type of deafness experience severe but incomplete injury to the organ of Corti, but they are seldom totally deaf. The resulting deafness is likely to be more noticeable in the higher frequencies.

When a pregnant woman contracts rubella, she usually has a mild rash and fever, although often she may have no symptoms and not even realize she has been infected. About a third of children born to mothers who contract rubella are at risk for deafness, especially if rubella occurs in the first few months of pregnancy. In some cases, the child's deafness may be progressive because the virus persists in their system after birth.

It's also possible that the virus in the mother may persist after the initial infection, and subsequently injure an embryo conceived weeks or months after the mother's infection. In fact, injury to a fetus has been recorded as late as the seventh month of pregnancy following a rubella infection.

The first recognized outbreak of rubella epidemic occurred in Australia in 1942 and again in the early 1960s. The rubella virus was isolated in the mid-1960s and by 1968 a successful vaccine was developed. Today the risk of rubella-related deafness is far less likely because a vaccination is available for those women who have never had German measles but who would like to become pregnant. In fact, following the German measles epidemic of the 1960s, many states began to require rubella testing for women when applying for a marriage license.

Toxoplasmosis

This generalized protozoan infection can be contracted by pregnant women and passed on to their unborn babies. Women can become infected after handling the litter of infected cats or (more rarely) by eating contaminated food. Up to 45% of American women of reproductive age carry the organism, although most may not have symptoms. One baby out of every 800 will acquire toxoplasmosis from its mother; toxoplasmosis causes hearing loss in about 17% of children infected in the womb.

Symptoms of toxoplasmosis include fatigue and muscle pain, although the pregnant woman may not have any symptoms at all. A doctor can't confirm the disease unless the mother had a negative toxoplasmosis test early in the pregnancy. The infection in the mother can be treated with medication, but an infection early in pregnancy may cause a miscarriage.

However, even if a mother becomes infected while pregnant, most babies don't develop the infection themselves. Those babies who do don't show evidence of the infection immediately, but many doctors advise treatment anyway.

Cytomegalovirus

Discovered in 1956, the cytomegalovirus belongs to the family of herpes viral infections that may trigger symptoms similar to the common cold but that usually causes no symptoms in healthy people. CMV is the largest, most complex virus to infect humans. This infection is fairly common in pregnant women; if a woman becomes infected for the first time while she is pregnant, she can pass the infection on to her baby.

CMV is now considered a possible cause of many previously unknown cases of nongenetic hearing loss. In fact, some studies suggest that CMV has replaced rubella as the most common viral cause of prenatal deafness. This could be because CMV is extremely common (about 80% of adults have antibodies to this virus in their blood, indicating a previous infection).

About half of all infected children born to mothers infected with this virus during pregnancy will have a bilateral, sensorineural hearing loss of varying severity. Hearing loss in these infants most often is profound, although there are milder losses in some babies.

CMV is acquired by close personal contact with bodily secretions of someone infected with CMV, and is harmless to anyone but a developing fetus or those with weakened immune systems (such as AIDS patients). Babies can get CMV from their mothers in the womb, during birth or in the first few weeks of life. They can get the disease from mothers with a first-time CMV infection during pregnancy, or if the mother has a reactivation of a past infection.

Women with toddlers who attend day care are often infected, since CMV can be transmitted in urine and saliva from child to child. While young children rarely have symptoms, they can excrete the virus in their urine and saliva for months to years. Anyone is exposed to CMV who works in a child care setting or with many diapered infants. The infection may also be transmitted from blood transfusions, since so many people (including blood donors) have CMV without symptoms. While most people are infected before adulthood, very few experience any signs of illness.

Almost all babies infected before birth are perfectly normal—only about 10% of those infected in the womb are sick, and of these, 20% to 30% may die; most survivors will have permanent damage. Infected babies may have problems in many organs, including the brain, eyes, lungs and liver; many will have hearing problems. Recent studies suggest that a small number of seemingly normal CMV-infected babies may develop problems later in life.

There is no cure for congenital CMV because the virus damages the baby before birth, and antiviral drugs can't repair this damage after the birth. If you are pregnant and have other children in day care, experts suggest you take care to wash your hands well after changing diapers and wiping noses. Disposable wipes may be a good idea. If you are pregnant and concerned, you can request a test for CMV antibodies when you begin prenatal care. Babies born to mothers who have already contracted CMV are at less risk of congenital CMV infection.

Other Viruses

Several other viral infections are also linked to hearing loss in the prenatal period, including the herpes simplex II virus, influenza and mumps. There is also a risk of hearing loss when a child contracts mumps after birth.

Bacterial Meningitis

One of the most common causes of acquired sensorineural deafness in newborns is bacterial meningitis, an infection of the coverings of the brain. Most cases of meningitis occur in children under age five; recent studies suggest that about 6% of children with bacterial meningitis sustain a sensorineural hearing loss, although some experts believe the numbers are much higher.

Bacterial meningitis in infants is usually caused by *Escherichia coli (E. coli)* bacteria, which can cause a hearing loss ranging from mild to profound. About half the infants who contract this disease will have a profound hearing loss which is usually permanent. Meningitis can cause a sudden, profound and irreversible deafness in both ears. Often the cochlea is damaged when bacteria is transmitted along the cochlear nerve from the covering of the brain. Prognosis for children who contract bacterial meningitis is poor; about half of those who live will have severe problems, including hearing loss, retardation and seizures. Sometimes children with meningitis get an ear infection with a conductive deafness; this can be cured with antibiotics.

Because this type of deafness is incurable, physicians generally try to prevent or treat meningitis early to head off such complications. Recent studies demonstrated that *Haemophilus influenzae* type B (HIB) meningitis patients who received dexamethasone right away had less hearing loss than children who did not. It is not clear from these studies whether dexamethasone benefits children with other kinds of bacterial meningitis.

Sometimes when deafness is caused by bacterial meningitis, the person retains a limited ability to hear, so that a powerful hearing aid can be of some help to amplify sounds, but not to enable the patient to recognize speech. Tinnitus is not often present, although there may be a brief attack of vertigo. Balance problems may also occur. Mental retardation occurs in about 15% of those children whose deafness is associated with meningitis. If your child has had meningitis, take the baby or child for a hearing test after recovery, and have the child retested periodically for the next 12 months.

In the early 1900s, meningitis was the most common clearly identified cause of acquired total deafness in children. Since then, a preventive vaccine (the Hib vaccine) has cut the risk of the disease. A prescription antibiotic called rifampin can prevent cases of Hib and meningococcal meningitis after exposure. Still, it's possible that a child may survive meningitis but still experience total destruction of the inner ear.

Group B Streptococcus

By 1964, doctors recognized group B strep as a threat to a newborn's health and hearing. Today it is responsible for most of the serious illnesses in babies younger than two months old.

Group B streptococcus is a round bacterium grouped in chains. While there are several different groups of streptococci, group B seems to infect pregnant women and newborns. The bacteria occur in soil and vegetation and are found normally in humans and many animals. However, between 4% to 40% of pregnant women (depending on the region of the country), experience a group B infection in the genital area. About half of these women will give birth to babies affected by Group B strep, but only one in 100 of these newborns will have any symptoms.

Most experts recommend screening all pregnant women for Group B strep at 26 to 34 weeks of pregnancy. Some suggest giving antibiotics to all mothers with a positive group B strep culture during labor and delivery.

Almost all babies (99%) born to mothers with Group B strep present in the vaginal area will be healthy. Most babies born with Group B will survive, but about half will suffer from long-term hearing loss.

Syphilis

Syphilis is caused by a spirochete transmitted from mother to child during pregnancy; it may cause an inner ear hearing loss in the child either during the first two years of life or at puberty. In fact, 35% of affected newborns will eventually go on to experience some degree of hearing loss. This eventual hearing loss is hard to quantify, since the deafness may show up suddenly later in childhood (or even in adulthood). Children tend to experience sudden hearing loss in both ears; if it appears before age 10, the deafness is usually profound.

Syphilitic labyrinthitis is usually caused by congenital syphilis and results in a sudden, flat sensorineural hearing loss or a sudden, increasing fluctuation of sensorineural hearing loss. Fortunately, incidences of congenital syphilis are today very rare. When they do occur, they can be treated with antibiotics.

Other Factors

Rh Factor Incompatibility

If you have Rh-negative blood and you give birth to a child with Rh-positive blood, the cells from your baby trigger the development of antibodies to the Rh-positive blood. While this will not harm your first baby, subsequent pregnancies carry a risk of damaging the hearing mechanism of the fetus when your antibodies attack the red blood cells of any Rh-positive fetus.

The incompatibility can injure the ears or nervous system of your newborn during the first few days of life, either directly or as a result of jaundice. This type of jaundice is caused by abnormal destruction of red blood cells at or shortly after birth. As hemoglobin is broken down, it produces bilirubin, which can cause jaundice as it accumulates in certain areas in the brain. The auditory system is one of the systems that is likely to be injured by this bilirubin buildup.

Massive transfusions for your baby, if done promptly, can ease the problem. A transfusion performed too little or too late may not prevent permanent injury to your baby's hearing mechanisms.

Fortunately, hearing problems for newborns due to Rh-sensitization are becoming rare since the development of Rh (D) immune globulin. When injected into the mother 72 hours before delivery, it prevents 99% of the incidences of sensitization.

Cerebral Palsy

Cerebral palsy is a general term for nonprogressive disorders of movement, posture or speech caused by brain damage during pregnancy, birth or early childhood. Between two and six infants out of every 1,000 develop CP, shortly before or after birth. Of these, between 25% and 30% will have hearing problems.

Cerebral palsy can be caused by a mother's infection that has passed to her unborn baby, or from too much bilirubin in the baby's blood right after birth. In the newborn, cerebral palsy can be caused by a head injury, encephalitis or meningitis.

Kernicterus

Extremely high levels of bilirubin (bile pigments) in a newborn that occurs as a result of jaundice can sometimes lead to a condition called kernicterus. This fairly rare complication of jaundice can damage the cochlear nuclei in the brain, causing hearing loss.

Loss of Oxygen

During birth, anoxia (complete loss of oxygen) and hypoxia (reduced oxygen) are the two most frequent causes of damage to the organ of Corti, the body's hearing organ. Any disturbance of the infant's breathing or circulation can cause a loss of oxygen to the blood and brain. About 6 percent of newborns experience a sensorineural hearing loss ranging from mild to severe if deprived of oxygen at birth. In premature infants, about 5 percent will experience some type of mild-to-severe sensorineural hearing loss.

The complete loss of oxygen, while very rare, can kill cells unless corrected very quickly. Anoxia can be caused by a long labor, heavy sedation of the mother, obstruction of the baby's respiratory passages with mucus, poor lung development, or congenital circulatory or heart defects. The only way to prevent anoxia is to prevent these conditions.

Smoking During Pregnancy

New research suggests that pregnant women who smoke may triple their children's risk of developing an ear infection at birth, perhaps by interfering with the babies' immune systems. Children of women who smoked during pregnancy were far more likely to suffer middle ear infections or ear surgery by age five than those whose mothers didn't smoke.

An Australian study found that children born to women who smoked between one and nine cigarettes each day showed a 60% higher risk for ear infection. The children of women who smoked 10 to 19 cigarettes daily showed a 260% higher risk, and those who smoked more than 20 cigarettes a day had children with a 330% higher risk. The study also found that children born to women who smoked more than a pack a day were three times more likely to undergo ear surgery before their fifth birthday.

Atresia

In about one out of every 30,000 live births, a baby is born with a poorly developed or absent portion of the ear. Atresia of the ear usually occurs during development of the external or the middle ear, and usually affects only one side. Surgery can repair the ear's appearance; if the canal is closed, surgery can restore hearing by creating a passage for sound to reach the inner ear. Complete external and middle-ear atresia in one ear usually causes only a 60 dB hearing loss for speech. Hearing loss after surgery depends on the severity of the ear's malformation, but half the time there is at least a 20 dB improvement.

Cleft Palate

A number of children with cleft palates also have mild to moderate conductive hearing loss because of the cleft condition of the mouth; this loss is usually medically treatable. A hearing assessment is usually given during speech tests to find out if a hearing loss is present.

Down Syndrome

This chromosomal disorder that results in mental retardation and physical deformities also can lead to a hearing loss. People born with this syndrome often have irregularities in the middle and inner ears and are susceptible to middle ear infections that can lead to conductive hearing loss.

Low Birth Weight

Premature infants with a low birth weight (3.3 lbs. or below) are at risk for a sensorineural hearing loss ranging from mild to severe. Approximately 5% of these low-weight infants will have hearing problems. However, full-term babies who don't weigh much aren't at risk for hearing loss.

Ototoxic Drugs

Certain drugs that can affect the hearing mechanism (especially the cochlea) may affect the hearing of a developing fetus if taken by the mother during pregnancy. They are particularly damaging to the developing fetus during the sixth or seventh week of pregnancy.

- *Streptomycin*   When the antibiotic streptomycin is given to a pregnant woman at any time, it can cause a sensorineural hearing loss in the baby ranging from mild problems hearing high-frequency sounds to a severe hearing loss in both ears.
- *Alcohol*   It has been reported that fetal alcohol syndrome may cause a sensorineural or conductive hearing loss in up to 64% of infants born to alcoholic mothers. Fetal alcohol syndrome is a combination of birth defects caused when a pregnant woman drinks too much alcohol. Although small amounts of alcohol can harm a developing fetus, the syndrome appears only if the mother *consistently* abuses alcohol during pregnancy (at least two mixed drinks or two to three bottles of beer or glasses of wine each day).
- *Aminoglycosides*   (kanamycin, neomycin, gentamicin, tobramycin and amikacin) The incidence of prenatal deafness due to this class of drugs is very low for most people. These drugs have been reported to cause hearing loss in infants only when mothers who took them had kidney problems and received diuretics (ethacrynic acid and furosemide) in addition to an aminoglycoside. It has been suggested that there may be a genetic susceptibility to hearing problems associated with this class of drugs.
- *Aspirin*   High doses of aspirin and other salicylates can cause ringing of the ears and a hearing loss of up to 40 decibels, both directly related to the amount of the drug in the bloodstream. Although many drugs can be toxic to the delicate sensory tissue of the ear and can cause permanent hearing loss, aspirin is unusual in that the inner ear hearing

loss it causes is reversible. Both hearing loss and tinnitus will disappear within one to three days after the drug is stopped. Normally, you'd have to take more than 12 aspirin tablets a day before there is a danger of hearing loss, although every person's sensitivity to the drug is different. Patients who already have some degree of sensorineural hearing loss may find that aspirin can have a stronger effect on hearing at lower frequencies. Drugs containing quinine also may cause a similar, reversible hearing loss.

- *Thalidomide*   This sleeping drug was never approved by the FDA for sale in the United States, although today in this country it is under investigation for use in other diseases such as leprosy. In the experience of pregnant women in Europe, this drug caused hearing problems and malformations of the ear (among other serious birth defects) in many newborns during the 1960s.

CHILDHOOD CAUSES OF ACQUIRED DEAFNESS

Almost any of the infectious diseases of childhood also may affect the inner ear. Often in these cases only one ear is damaged, although it's possible for both ears to be affected.

The inner ear may harbor pus-forming infections similar to the infections in the middle ear that occur during the first year or two of life. This can lead to a severe or total loss of hearing. The infection usually reaches the inner ear via the connection between the inner ear and the cranial cavity. If the infection reaches the inner ear, it may destroy the auditory nerve, the organ of Corti, and most of the other bits of the delicate auditory structures.

While far rarer, it's possible for typhoid fever or diphtheria to affect the ear by toxins formed by bacteria. These toxins can destroy the organ of Corti and its associated structures. Formerly a common cause of acquired deafness in the United States, massive immunizations in this country have made these toxins quite rare.

Infection

If your child has a hearing problem that disappears and reappears from time to time, it's probably not psychosomatic. Rather, it may be related to allergies and chronic colds. This type of hearing loss is not easy either to detect or to treat, since sometimes the child appears to have normal hearing and other times there seems to be a real problem. If this is happening to your child, you should mention the problem to your doctor.

Ear Infection

If you have young children, chances are you already know a great deal about ear infections, since these pesky problems are responsible for 30 million pediatrician visits each year in the United States. Almost all American children will have at least one infection by the time they are six years old. Children are most likely to be infected before age two. They are prone to these infections because their eustachian tubes are shorter, straighter, narrower and more horizontal, making it easier for bacteria to enter from the back of the throat. Some children have recurrent attacks through age 10.

Infections of the middle ear (otitis media) occur in the cavity between the eardrum and the inner ear; they can produce pus, fluid and hearing loss. If you have a cold, you may experience swelling and blocking of the eustachian tube, the passage that connects the back of the nose to the middle ear. This tube may become blocked by the infection, or by enlarged adenoids (often associated with infections of the nose and throat). Fluid produced by the inflammation can't drain off through the tube, and instead collects in the middle ear. This fluid accumulation allows bacteria and viruses drawn in from the back of the throat to breed, causing infection.

The most common types of bacteria that cause ear infections normally live in your child's throat, and include *Streptococcus pneumoniae, Haemphilus influenzae* and *Moraxella catarrhalis.* During the winter, both viruses and bacteria may lead to ear infections.

Acute ear infection causes a sudden, severe earache, deafness, tinnitus (ringing in the ear), sense of fullness in the ear and fever. It can be harder to detect an ear infection in a young infant, but you can suspect such a problem if the baby has a low-grade fever, cold with thickened discharge and a poor appetite, and if the baby is irritable, pulls its ears, shakes his head and cries in the middle of the night. There may or may not be fluid draining from the ear.

There are four basic types of ear infections: serous otitis media, otitis media with effusion, acute purulent otitis media and secretory otitis media.

The mildest form is *serous otitis media,* also called "glue ear," in which thin, watery fluid gathers in the middle ear that reduces hearing acuity by interfering with the movement of the ossicular chain of bones. This is the most common cause of hearing problems in children. While doctors aren't sure what causes it, it's believed to be associated with drug treatment of pus-producing ear infections without proper drainage. When antibiotics are prescribed but the fluid is not drained, it remains in the middle ear cavity, making the ear more susceptible to further ear infections and reducing hearing acuity. Usually, the person is unaware of the hearing loss until both ears are affected; by this time, the fluid has become thick and gluey, and can cause a permanent deterioration of the bones of the middle ear.

In *otitis media with effusion,* fluid and infection develop often at the same time as an upper respiratory infection or enlarged adenoids.

This form of infection can lead to the third, most serious type: *acute purulent otitis media.* In this condition, pus fills the middle ear and can cause such pressure that it actually bursts the eardrum. This viral or bacterial infection occurs most often in children.

Occasionally, recurrent infections can change the cells lining the middle ear, which then produce large amounts of thick fluid, resulting in *secretory otitis media.*

A chronic ear infection is usually caused by repeated attacks of acute ear infection, with pus seeping from a perforation in the eardrum together with some degree of deafness. Complications include inflammation of the outer ear (otitis externa) and damage to the bones in the middle ear— sometimes causing total deafness. It may also lead to a cholesteatoma (a matted ball of skin debris that can erode bone and cause further damage to the ear). Rarely, infection can spread inward from an infected ear, causing a brain abscess.

A middle ear infection caused by thick fluid in the middle ear (perhaps caused by improper drug treatment of a draining ear infection) is known as "mucous otitis media." The fluid that collects in the middle ear causes hearing loss, which may vary between a mild high-tone loss to a considerable loss for all tones. In the presence of thick mucus, the hearing loss is most severe. Hearing is restored when the thick fluid is removed by puncturing the eardrum. If the fluid isn't removed, the conductive hearing loss will persist, and the condition may lead to adhesions in the middle ear that firmly fix the tiny bones of the middle ear.

A doctor can diagnose an ear infection by examining the ear with an otoscope. A sample of discharge may be taken to identify the organism responsible for the infection. Usually, a doctor will not try to determine which bacteria are causing the infection, although these tests may be done on a hospitalized or very sick child. These tests require draining the middle ear and culturing the liquid.

Until you can see your doctor, some of the pain can be relieved with nonprescription pain relievers, or by placing a warm cloth or heating pad over the affected ear. Before the development of antibiotics, these infections were the single greatest cause of hearing loss. Today, your doctor can treat acute infections with antibiotics (usually amoxicillin), although there may sometimes be continual production of a sticky fluid in the middle ear. Deafness can occur, but it usually disappears with treatment. Since the mid-1980s, some strains of bacteria have acquired resistance to amoxicillin. If your child has both an ear infection and conjunctivitis, the cause is almost always *H. flu,* and the drug cefixime may be the better antibiotic choice.

Your doctor may also remove pus and skin debris from the affected ear, and prescribe antibiotic drops, if necessary. Ephedrine nose drops can help establish drainage of the ear in children. Your physician may cut into the eardrum (a process called "myringotomy") to relieve pressure during an ear infection.

OtoLAM

Otolam is a new laser technique for treating infants and young children with ear infections by creating a tiny hole in the eardrum to drain fluid and immediately ease pain. The hole stays open for several weeks and ventilates the middle ear without the need for a surgical procedure under general anesthesia to insert tubes. Special ear drops make the procedure painless, and there is no bleeding, post-operative grogginess or any of the side effects usually associated with general anesthesia. Parents can stay with their child during the office procedure, which takes less than five minutes once the ear drops have taken effect.

The holes close up on their own in three to four weeks, but the time the hole remains open can be varied according to the child's specific condition. Three to four weeks of middle ear ventilation prevents fluid from building up again in the middle ear and provides enough time, in most cases, for the underlying infection to clear. In addition to promoting healing, this reduces the likelihood of recurrence.

Although OtoLAM won't replace tubes (especially for children with chronic infections), it may soon be another widely used treatment for ear infections. Studies have not yet found whether OtoLAM is better than tubes. Although the procedure was approved by the FDA in 1996 for treating ear infections, the technology is expensive, and doctors intending to use it will need extensive training.

Ear Infection Vaccine

One day, a vaccine may make ear infections a disease of the past— or at least help reduce the frequency. The vaccine now under development is aimed at preventing one of the most common bacterial causes of ear infections: *Strep pneumoniae* (not the germ that causes strep throat, but a totally different bug usually called "pneumococcus"). New versions of the vaccine are being developed specifically for illness in babies and young children to help prevent more serious infections, such as meningitis and pneumonia, as well as the less threatening ear infections. Unfortunately, there are more than 85 types of this bacteria, and the vaccines are effective only for about four to eight types.

The procedure can be performed on an appropriate child at the first sign of ear infection, limiting repeated courses of antibiotics. It can also prevent an acute episode from progressing to a chronic condition, reducing the risk of hearing loss and other cognitive learning disabilities.

Candidates for OtoLAM include ear infection patients who have not responded to typical antibiotic treatment or a tympanostomy, as well as those for whom the risk of general anesthesia and conventional myringotomy surgery is too high. Clinical studies show OtoLAM to be safe and effective for infants and young children with ear infections.

Complications

The serious—but rare—complications of ear infections include bacterial meningitis and mastoiditis, a serious infection in the hair cells behind the middle ear. Mastoiditis requires high-dose antibiotics and often surgery to clean out pus and drain the ear. Warning signs of mastoiditis include prolonged high fever, severe ear pain, reddening, swelling and tenderness behind the ear and puslike drainage from the ear.

Chronic Ear Infections

While acute ear infections are a fact of life during childhood, chronic infections are more serious, since they can cause permanent damage due to constant irritation. A chronic condition may not cause enough discomfort to bring immediate diagnosis and treatment. Left uncorrected, chronic pus-filled ear infection can cause permanent hearing damage. In some cases, acute infections never fully clear, and a low-level infection spreads to the mastoid bone behind the ear. Once the mastoid bone becomes infected, your doctor may recommend a mastoidectomy (an operation in which the mastoid bone is removed) to prevent spread of the infection.

These chronic conditions are usually treated with antihistamines and decongestants if they are associated with nasal congestion or allergies. Antibiotics are usually prescribed for chronic middle ear infection with effusion or chronic pus-filled middle ear infection. As long as the eardrum is unbroken, eardrops won't help the condition because they can't reach the affected area. If the situation doesn't improve and the adenoids are part of the problem, your doctor may recommend their removal.

Alternatively, your doctor may suggest an ear tube to facilitate drainage. While the ear tube is in place, the ear must remain dry for the entire period of treatment (which can be several months to years). This can be hard for anybody, but it's especially difficult for children. Critics complain that while the procedure is done on an outpatient basis, it still requires brief general anesthesia. It can be very difficult to avoid getting water in the ears while the tube is in place. In rare cases, the tube has caused severe scarring or a permanent hole in the eardrum.

Those in favor of the tube say that the procedure usually decreases the frequency and severity of middle ear infections. Hearing is restored and the operation allows the middle ear to be ventilated, reducing the risk of permanent changes in the lining of cells that might occur with prolonged infection.

Risks for Ear Infections

There are a number of factors that increase a child's likelihood of getting ear infections. You might notice more ear infections if your child is:

- Younger than two years
- Bottle-fed
- Male
- Native American or Hispanic
- Living in crowded conditions
- Attending day care
- Allergic
- Living with household cigarette smoke

Scarlet Fever

Also known as scarlatina, this acute infectious disease is caused by the streptococcus bacterium that can lead to complications such as sinus infections, ear abscesses and mastoiditis. Spread by droplets in the air, scarlet fever gets its name from the reddish flush and rash it causes, in addition to sore throat and high fever. Once a dangerous and common childhood disease, it is today fairly uncommon in the United States. It is believed that the reduced threat of the disease is due to a change in the virulence of the bacteria and has nothing to do with the development of drugs used to treat the condition. If it does occur, it is usually easily treatable if medication is started promptly.

Viral infection

Viruses are common causes of sudden, high-frequency hearing problems. Because viruses are so small (much smaller than bacteria), they are carried to the ear directly from the bloodstream instead of first passing through the cerebrospinal fluid in the cranial cavity. Unlike bacteria, viruses do not stimulate the formation of pus. Still, they are capable of destroying the delicate hearing structures (such as the organ of Corti). The resulting hearing loss can be quite severe, but it does not usually worsen over time.

Chickenpox

This common, mild childhood infectious disorder has been known to cause sudden severe deafness in one ear. Related to the herpes family of viruses, chickenpox is caused by the varicella-zoster virus. After infection, the virus lies dormant within nerve tissues and may erupt as herpes zoster (shingles) later in life. One episode of the viral disease confers lifelong immunity.

Chickenpox appears first as a rash on the body, face, upper arms and legs, under the arms, inside the mouth and sometimes in the bronchial tubes. While children usually have only a slight fever, adults may become quite ill with severe pneumonia and breathing problems. Complications include encephalitis (brain inflammation), which can lead to central hearing loss.

While the incidence of deafness and other complications related to chickenpox is small, the American Academy of Pediatrics recommends that all children receive the vaccine against chickenpox.

Measles

This viral illness causes a rash and fever, and may lead to hearing problems or deafness as a result of complications of ear infections or encephalitis (brain inflammation). While measles usually affects children, an attack may occur at any age.

Measles is spread by airborne droplets with an incubation period of up to 11 days before symptoms appear. The illness can be transmitted during this period and up to one week after symptoms occur. Once very common around the world, today measles appears much less often in developed countries because of the availability of vaccinations.

Encephalitis

This term refers to an inflammation of the brain, which can cause central hearing problems. The hearing loss is usually the result of problems with the brain, not problems with the hearing apparatus, although sometimes there may be a problem with the cochlea.

Encephalitis is usually caused by an infection; viruses are the most common, although the disease can result from many different kinds of organisms, including bacteria, protozoa or worms, or by chemicals. There are two types of viruses that cause encephalitis: viruses (such as rabies) that invade the body and don't cause trouble until they are carried to the brain cells in the blood, and other viruses (such as herpes simplex, herpes zoster and yellow fever) that first harm nonnervous tissue and *then* invade brain cells.

Mumps

This acute viral disease is the most common cause of severe, one-sided deafness, which usually appears suddenly and happens without ear pain or discomfort. The deafness often goes unnoticed for many days (or years) after it occurs. Often, a patient will say he only recently noticed deafness in one ear. Close examination and history reveal that the deafness has in fact been present since an attack of mumps in childhood.

Deafness due to mumps usually causes complete loss of hearing in one ear by irreparably destroying the inner ear without affecting the balance mechanism. If any hearing does remain in the affected ear, the deafness doesn't become progressive. The deafness occurs when the mumps virus spreads to the lining of the brain.

There is no specific treatment for mumps other than painkillers and fluids. In the United States, most children are given a combination measles, mumps and rubella (MMR) vaccination at 15 months of age to protect them against these diseases. The vaccination is given earlier in areas experiencing a measles epidemic.

External blockage

Your child may also experience a hearing loss if there is some type of blockage in the ear canal, caused either by excess wax buildup or by a foreign object lodged in the ear.

Cause of Hearing Loss for Deaf/Hard-of-Hearing Students in the U.S. 1982–83, 1987–88 and 1992–93*

CAUSE	1982–83	1987–88	1992–93
Heredity	6,390	6,063	6,324
Maternal rubella	9,001	2,438	992
Pregnancy complications	1,854	1,367	1,137
Prematurity	2,225	2,244	2,238
Rh Incompatibility	792	274	179
Trauma at birth	1,350	1,151	1,176
Meningitis	4,033	4,156	3,934
Otitis Media	1,667	1,613	1,782
Measles	419	174	132
Mumps	126	48	22
Infection	1,467	1,179	1,062
High fever	1,734	1,364	1,127
Trauma after birth	438	317	340
Cytomegalovirus	not reported	337	638

*Annual survey of hearing-impaired children and youth, Center for Assessment and Demographic Studies, Gallaudet University

If the object is an insect that is still alive, you can try adding a few drops of mineral oil to the ear to immobilize the insect; this may decrease the discomfort until you get to the doctor's office. Blockages should be removed only by an ear specialist, since the eardrum could be damaged if the wax or object is pushed *into* the ear. Your doctor will remove the object by using a small device called an alligator forceps, or by using suction or fluids to flush out the blockage. It's important to have this treated because wax can be a fertile breeding ground for bacteria, fungi, yeasts or viruses (especially if the ear is often submerged in water).

HEREDITARY CAUSES OF DEAFNESS

Deafness may be caused by a wide range of inherited abnormalities. Most causes of genetic deafness are congenital (present at birth) and unchanging. These genetic types of deafness are responsible for about half of all types of deafness in children.

Types of Genetic Hearing Loss

There are about 200 different types of genetic hearing problems ranging in degree from mild to profound. A large percentage of hearing problems that occur at birth or during the first few years of life are hereditary, as are many kinds of progressive hearing loss that occur later in life.

Although some kinds of hearing loss are associated with other physical characteristics or medical problems (changes in the eye or hair color, kidneys, or heart), most types of genetic hearing loss do not involve other types of physical changes.

The ability to hear is one of many different physical traits that are handed down in families.

There are several ways that genes can influence a person's ability to hear. Each child receives half of the genetic material from each parent. All cells in the human body have 23 pairs of chromosomes (a total of 46); because the chromosomes are paired, each segment in one chromosome has a corresponding segment in its partner. The genes (a chemical coding system of the actual units of inheritance) are also paired, one on each chromosome. Each gene provides information for the development and functioning of various organ systems.

There are many different gene locations that affect hearing, and many different varieties of genes. Different forms of deafness may involve different gene locations. "Recessive" genes are genes that must come from both parents before a trait it controls will result. A gene is "dominant" if the trait is expressed when only one gene of the pair is present. The different types of genetic mechanisms that can result in a hearing loss are:

Autosomal Recessive

Deafness genes with an autosomal recessive pattern account for between 75% and 85% of hereditary deafness. (Autosomes are the chromosomes other than the two sex chromosomes.) Both parents usually have normal hearing, but each carries a recessive gene for deafness; when a child inherits both of these recessive deafness genes, the child will be deaf. Usually, there is no family history of deafness. If both parents have this recessive gene, the risk of having a deaf child is one in four (or 25% for each pregnancy). The odds of having a child who does not carry even one of the abnormal genes is also one in four. The remainder (one in two) will carry a recessive gene, like the parents, and one healthy gene, and so will not be deaf.

Autosomal Dominant

This pattern of inheritance accounts for about 20% of hereditary deafness. In this pattern, usually at least one parent is deaf, and the deafness appears in each generation, affecting about the same number of boys and girls. The risk of having another deaf child is 50%. None of the hearing children will be carriers, because if they had the deafness gene, they would be deaf themselves. The children of these hearing children would have no higher risk of having a deaf child.

In the rare case that both parents are deaf from the same type of autosomal dominant gene, they would have a 75% chance of having a deaf child with each pregnancy, and a corresponding 25% chance of having a child without the gene.

With this type of inheritance, the deafness gene is sometimes created from a mutation in a sperm or egg cell without any prior family history. Once the gene has mutated, it will have the same effect on future generations as if it had been passed down through the family. Often, this type of inherited deafness varies so much within a family that it can be hard to be sure of the pattern without careful study. For example, one person might be profoundly deaf, while another is only mildly hard of hearing.

X-Linked Inheritance

This is an unusual cause of deafness in which the abnormal gene is located on the X chromosome. Out of all the chromosome pairs in the human body, one pair determines the sex of the child; a female has two X chromosomes (an XX pattern) and a male has one X and one Y chromosome (an XY pattern). When the 46 chromosome pairs divide in making sperm, half the resulting sperm cells will have an X, half a Y.

In an X-linked genetic hearing disorder, the abnormal gene is located on the X chromosome. Females are usually protected by having another normal gene on their other X chromosome. But the male, having only one X, isn't protected if he receives the abnormal gene. Thus, females are carriers and have a one in two chance of giving the abnormal gene to any one son, who will be deaf, or to a daughter, who will be a carrier. Affected males cannot pass the deafness on to their sons, because they give them only the Y chromosome, but all their daughters will be carriers because their daughters must receive the damaged X chromosome from their fathers.

Chromosomal Disorder

This problem can cause a hearing disorder when the 46 chromosomes are being reduced to 23 in the formation of egg or sperm. The best-known example of a chromosomal disorder is Down syndrome, which is often associated with some degree of hearing loss. These genetic accidents are not usually passed on.

There are about 200 different types of genetic hearing problems, ranging in degree from mild to profound. A large proportion of hearing problems that occur at birth or during the first few years of life are hereditary, as are many kinds of progressive hearing losses that occur later in life.

Although some kinds of hearing loss are associated with other physical characteristics or medical problems (changes in the eye or hair color, kidneys, or heart), most types of genetic hearing problems don't involve other physical changes.

Because hearing problems are so often genetic, it's common to refer a family with a deaf member to a genetic counselor or a genetic team. A medical geneticist can often tell whether someone's hearing problem has been inherited. Genetic counseling for hearing loss always includes a detailed family history, a medical history of the deaf person, and a pregnancy history of the mother of that person. The individual or family is then seen by the medical geneticist for a physical exam to uncover clues in the appearance that might suggest a basis for the hearing problem. In cases where it is possible to determine the cause of the hearing problem and how a gene has passed through the family, the team meets with the individual or the family and explains how the hearing loss was inherited, and what the implications and possibilities are for future generations. This knowledge can be very important since the earlier a child is diagnosed, the better the issues around the deafness can be addressed. If there is more than one person in the family with a hearing loss, the problem is almost always genetic.

Hearing Loss Genes

New research has found mutations in several genes that are linked to deafness. The gene called Connexin 26 may be responsible for as many as 40% of cases of inherited hearing loss. Most of these children are born to par-

ents with normal hearing. About 40% of children with this genetic mutation will have a profound hearing loss. Another gene (GJB2) mutation is
the predominant cause of inherited moderate-to-profound deafness in the
Midwest. Although there are many deafness-causing mutations in the
GJB2 gene, one mutation (called 35delG) causes the most cases of deafness. Couples who have had one child with GJB2-associated deafness
have a 17.5% chance of having a second deaf child.

Hearing Gene

Scientists have also recently discovered a gene that plays a significant role
in the development of cells essential to hearing. This discovery raises
hope for the development of treatments for hearing loss because of disease, trauma and aging. The gene (Math1) sends a signal that triggers certain ear cells to mature into hair cells in the inner ear. Hair cells are
responsible for both hearing and balance, and loss of these cells is a common cause of deafness. Once these cells have been destroyed (either
through trauma, disease or aging), they cannot be re-created. With these
findings, doctors may one day be able to generate new hair cells in those
with hearing loss.

Genetic Diseases That Cause Deafness

There are a number of diseases that can be passed down in families that
will result in hearing loss. These include Paget's disease, Alport's disease,
Cogan's syndrome and Pendred's syndrome.

Alport's Disease

This genetic disease causes kidney inflammation in childhood, followed by
a sensorineural hearing impairment in young adulthood and eye problems
later in life. It's more common among men than women.

There is no clear relationship between the extent of kidney disease
and the onset of deafness. Treatment is supportive, since glucocorticoids
and cytotoxic agents don't help. This disease is not known to recur following transplantation.

Cogan's Syndrome

This inflammation of the cornea, which occurs for no known reason, can
also damage new bone formation around the round window and destroy
the organ of Corti and cochlear nerve cells. It can lead to vertigo, tinnitus
and severe sensorineural hearing loss. Treatment with steroids is often effective in suppressing disease activity; in some patients, drugs may be tapered
off and stopped, while others require maintenance-level treatment.

Pendred's Syndrome

An inherited condition that causes deafness (usually at birth) and development of goiter (enlarged thyroid) in childhood. People with the syndrome have different degrees of hearing loss, but it is severe for more than half of them. The syndrome is probably the most common form of deafness that appears with another condition (in this case, goiter).

Scientists are not sure what causes the problem, but recent research suggests that Pendred's syndrome may be related to a gene mutation that produces a defective form of the protein pendrin. New research suggests that pendrin may be associated with the transportation of iodide in the thyroid. For those with Pendred syndrome, a defect in iodide transport may cause the thyroid to enlarge, although the gland will usually continue to function normally.

Iodide is probably not involved in normal ear function, but pendrin also transports chloride, which is structurally related to iodide. Researchers suspect that problems with transporting chloride may lead to deafness. Concentrations of chloride (along with potassium and sodium) are normally found in the inner ear; if any of these electrolyte concentrations are abnormal, the inner ear may be unable to properly transfer sound waves to the brain.

These new genetic findings could eventually lead to strategies designed to correct the chloride and iodide transport problems caused by the underlying genetic defect.

Refsum's Disease

This rare disorder of lipid metabolism is inherited as a recessive trait and can cause hearing loss and retinitis pigmentosa, among other symptoms. Also known as "heredopathia atactica polyneuritiformis," it is characterized by a high level in blood and tissue of a fatty acid called phytanic acid, a substance derived from phytol (a component of chlorophyll). Humans absorb phytol from milk and the fat of cows and sheep, and most people can break down the phytol and phytanic acid. Those with Refsum's disease can't break it down, and so as they eat food containing phytanic acid the amount in their body gradually rises. While small amounts of phytanic acid are harmless, it becomes toxic as the level rises. In Refsum's patients, it causes three groups of problems:

Congenital: A few abnormalities, such as short fingers and toes, are present at birth in a small group of patients, and rarely cause problems.

Progressive: Deafness, retinitis pigmentosa and inability to smell begin slowly in childhood, and very slowly progress as the person ages. Some evidence suggests that if phytanic acid is controlled, blindness won't progress.

Sudden-onset: Weak, unsteady gait can suddenly appear in a Refsum's patient, but if treated it can improve just as quickly. Caused by nerve damage, the unsteadiness will not improve only if it has gone untreated for a long time.

Refsum's disease was first described in 1946 by Professor Refsum in Oslo, who noticed two Norwegian families with an unusual combination of impaired vision and weak gait. It was not until 1963 that the high phytanic acid level in the blood was discovered. The condition may affect men and women equally, appearing at any time from childhood to middle age, but symptoms usually appear by age 20.

In 1997 the gene for Refsum's disease was identified on chromosome 10. The protein product of the gene (PAHX) is an enzyme that is needed to metabolize phytanic acid. Refsum's disease patients have problems with PAHX.

The main treatment involves dietary changes. First, patients should try to maintain the same weight, since fat stores are used for energy during weight loss, which would release phytanic acid. Patients should avoid eating food containing animal fat from plant-eating animals, including milk products and fat from mutton and beef. This lowers the blood level of phytanic acid. Plasmapheresis (removal and reinfusion of blood plasma) may be necessary. Once hearing and vision problems appear, however, treatment can't usually repair the damage. See also REFSUM'S DISEASE, INFANTILE.

Infantile Refsum's Disease (IRD)

This rare disorder is characterized by the reduction or absence of cell structures that get rid of toxic substances in the body, and by the buildup of phytanic acid in blood and tissue. IRD should not be confused with classical Refsum's disease; the two are different conditions. IRD is one of a group of genetic diseases called leukodystrophies that affects the growth of the fatty covering of nerves in the brain.

In addition to hearing loss, symptoms may include eye problems such as retinitis pigmentosa (a potentially blinding eye disease) and nystagmus (rapid, jerky eye movements), decreased muscle tone, failure to thrive, developmental delays, poor muscle coordination, enlarged liver, low cholesterol levels and abnormalities of the face.

The disorder begins in infancy. There is no cure, although a few physicians around the world are studying the effectiveness of DHA (docosahexaenoic acid) or AA (arachidonic acid). Otherwise, treatment is supportive. The prognosis for patients is poor; death usually occurs in the person's 20s.

Usher Syndrome

This genetic disorder is characterized by hearing loss and a type of progressive vision loss called retinitis pigmentosa. Some individuals also have balance problems. There are three types of Usher syndrome:

- *Type I:* The child is born with a profound hearing loss, early onset of retinitis pigmentosa and balance problems.
- *Type II:* The child is born with a moderate to severe hearing loss, delayed retinitis pigmentosa and no balance problems.
- *Type III:* The child is born with a hearing loss and retinitis pigmentosa that worsens over time together with the possibility of balance problems.

Individuals with Type I Usher syndrome have a profound hearing loss in all frequencies and are considered to be deaf from birth. Many people with this type of Usher syndrome say they get little or no benefit from hearing aids. Those few children who have had cochlear implants can distinguish some sounds (even those related to speech) but still don't understand speech clearly. The vast majority use sign language as their primary mode of communication and are culturally deaf.

Children with Type II Usher syndrome have a moderate hearing loss in the lower frequencies; in the higher frequencies it is severe or profound. The loss does not get worse as the person ages. Only a small amount of additional loss (about 10 dB) occurs over several decades in adulthood. Even within a family, however, there may be some difference in severity from person to person. With hearing aids, these children do well in regular classrooms, usually with preferential seating in the front of the class. These children most commonly use oral speech and language and are culturally hearing, though a few have moderate to profound hearing loss and have gone to schools for the deaf. When vision deteriorates, they lose the ability to read speech from the lips. Since the hearing aid does not fully correct the hearing loss, they may become functionally deaf-blind, particularly in noisy, dark environments such as restaurants or bars in the evening, at dances, or other social events. They may then choose to use FM systems, avoid such environments, or converse in sign language.

Children with Type III Usher syndrome have a progressive hearing loss that gets significantly worse with time. Type III has not been as well defined as the other two types. Only a handful of reports have appeared in the medical literature, and most of the documented Type III cases have occurred in Finland. The primary distinguishing feature in Type III is that the hearing loss gets steadily worse over the years so hard-of-hearing teens become deaf in mid-to-late adulthood.

All children born with any type of Usher syndrome also have retinitis pigmentosa, an eye disease that causes gradual loss of vision. The eye becomes less able to adjust to low light, resulting in night blindness. As RP progresses, the field of vision narrows until only central vision remains ("tunnel vision"). Many people with Usher syndrome will retain at least some central vision for a long time. In Usher syndrome Type II, onset of RP is typically delayed until the 20s or 30s.

Humans need to use three senses in order to keep themselves balanced—vision, proprioception (feeling the position of bodies and limbs) and vestibular (feeling changes in speed and direction). Children with Type I have a vestibular system that doesn't work; they can't feel changes in speed or direction, and as their vision decreases, their visual balance system becomes less reliable. Those with Type II have a normal vestibular system, but their visual system also becomes less reliable as their vision decreases. Scientists don't know much about the vestibular system of persons with Type III. As more information on Type III becomes available, a more clear picture of vestibular function will emerge.

Originally described in 1959, Usher syndrome may account for 10% of all cases of congenital deafness. The condition is one of the rarer autosomal recessive genetic conditions, in which both parents must carry an abnormal gene at the same point on the chromosome in order for a child to be born with the disease. Since each parent carries only one recessive abnormal gene and one dominant healthy gene, they both have normal hearing because the dominant healthy gene on the paired chromosome counteracts the abnormal recessive one.

The presence of the abnormal gene is revealed when one-fourth of the children of a couple with these recessive abnormal genes inherit both abnormal genes, and are born with Usher syndrome. If a child inherits only one Usher-causing gene (the other gene of the pair cannot cause Usher), that person will not have Usher syndrome. But, like the parents, that person will be a carrier of Usher syndrome. If a person who has Usher syndrome marries a person who is not a carrier, none of their children will have the condition. However, all of their children will be carriers. If a person who carries Usher syndrome marries a person who does not, none of their children will have the syndrome. But there is a one in two chance that each child will be a carrier. If two people with Usher syndrome (caused by the same gene) marry, all of their children will have the condition.

Scientists have identified genes causing all three types of Usher syndrome to five different places on the chromosomes.

Although there is no treatment for this condition, regular exams by an opthalmologist are recommended for all deaf children, which can help identify Usher syndrome early (usually before age six).

There are a number of conditions that may be confused with Usher syndrome. Rubella (German measles) used to be one of the most commonly suspected conditions. Other syndromes are characterized by eye symptoms or hearing loss patterns that are different from those in Usher syndrome as well as abnormalities of other body parts.

Waardenburg's Syndrome

Waardenburg's syndrome is a rare genetic syndrome that affects hearing, skin and eye color and facial structure. About half of all patients with this disorder have a nonprogressive sensorineural hearing loss ranging from mild to severe in one or both ears, although only a slight few will be profoundly deaf in both ears. There is a great deal of variation in the sensorineural hearing loss among people with the syndrome; at least half of those with the gene have no hearing problems at all. Only about one out of five have a hearing loss severe enough to require some aid to verbal communication. Some with the gene are totally deaf, and others are deaf in one ear, yet have completely normal hearing in the other ear.

The disorder, which is genetically transmitted to offspring in a dominant manner (only one gene is needed to cause a problem), carries a 50% risk that siblings will be born with a variation of the syndrome. Still, only a few people who have this abnormal form of the gene show all the features of the syndrome, and only a very small number have profound deafness in both ears.

A Dutch opthalmologist, P. J. Waardenburg, was the first to notice that some people with two different-colored eyes often had hearing problems. Dr. Waardenburg went on to study other characteristics of the syndrome, which is now named after him. Researchers believe there may be some connection between hearing and the development of pigmentation during fetal development.

In Waardenburg's syndrome, usually one eye is brown and the other is bright blue, but occasionally patches of brown and blue are mixed in the same eye. As with hearing loss, not everyone who carries the gene has two different-colored eyes. In fact, in some large families there may be only one or two such individuals. In addition to the distinctive eye coloring, those with the WS gene may also have a patch of white hair; other gene carriers become prematurely gray. Not all gene carriers have these distinctive markings.

In addition, people with the syndrome have an unusual type of face; the eyes appear to be more widely spaced than average with eyebrows that grow together in the center. In addition, there may be cleft lip or cleft palate, or a colon problem known as Hirschprung disease in some individuals. These last two features are even less common than the primary features. Other than the hearing loss, most people with WS do not have any particular medical problems.

Since WS is inherited in a dominant fashion, typically families have several generations who have one or more of the features. Many of these family members are unaware that they have the gene because the feature can be so mild. WS may be much more common in the population than previously believed; as many as two to three out of every 100 children in schools for the deaf may have the syndrome. Since most people with the gene have little or no hearing loss, for every child with WS and a severe hearing loss, there are four to five family members who have relatively normal hearing but also have the gene.

Can Your Child Hear?

Your doctor may be highly trained to detect disease, but parents are around their children all the time and often simply sense when something "doesn't feel right" about their child's health. If you suspect your child may have a hearing loss, you could be right.

At the age of 0 to three months, your baby should:

- Look startled if there is a sudden loud noise
- Stir in sleep, wake up, or cry if someone makes a noise
- Recognize the sound of your voice, usually quieting down and becoming calm when your voice is heard

At the age of three to six months, your baby should:

- Respond to your voice
- Move the eyes to search for an interesting sound
- Turn eyes toward you when you call the child's name

At the age of six to 12 months, your baby should:

- Turn toward you when you call his or her name from behind the child
- Turn toward an interesting sound
- Look around when hearing new, interesting sounds
- Understand simple words like "no" and "bye-bye"

If your baby can't do some of these things, contact your pediatrician. The earlier your baby's hearing loss is diagnosed, the better for your child. Insist on a hearing test if you have concerns. Don't hesitate to take your child to a hearing specialist if you aren't satisfied with your pediatrician's response to your concerns.

TESTING IN INFANCY

What happens if you think your newborn may have a hearing problem? Since detecting a hearing problem in newborns is essential so that interventions can begin immediately, medical technology has come up with a way of detecting the *brain's* response to sound that does not require any participation on the part of the child.

If Your Child Can't Hear . . .

A pediatrician should consider a hearing evaluation in the follow-ing situations:

- Children at high risk for hearing problems, such as those with abnormalities of the skull or face, who were born premature or with a history of intrauterine infection, or who have meningitis, genetic conditions related to hearing loss or a family history of deafness
- A child who has a speech or language delay (such as no bab-bling in a six-month-old, no words by 18 months, or no word combinations by age two)
- A child whose parent is concerned about hearing; hearing loss-es at specific frequencies may exist despite normal language development
- A child whose eardrums are hard to see because of wax, or small ear canals (the ears may need to be cleaned and evaluat-ed by an otolaryngologist)

For infants and young children, electrophysical hearing tests work best because they don't require the child to give a conscious response. These tests include electroencephalic (EEG) audiometry, brain stem evoked response audiometry and otoacoustic emissions tests. For the very young, hearing thresholds for pure tones can be deciphered from these methods.

Because it would be too expensive to test *every* newborn in order to locate the few who do have a hearing problem, the parents of infants are given a "high-risk questionnaire" to determine if their child is at risk for hearing problems. This questionnaire consists of a number of factors, including:

- a family history of hearing loss or genetic biochemical abnormality associated with deafness
- blood incompatibility between mother and child
- ototoxic drugs during pregnancy (especially streptomycin and kanamycin)
- unusual bleeding during the first trimester
- admission to the newborn intensive care unit
- low APGAR rating (a well-baby assessment that tests breathing, heart rate, color, muscle tone, and motor reactions)
- maternal infection (such as herpes or cytomegalovirus during pregnancy)

- premature delivery, fetal distress, prolonged labor, difficult delivery or birth injury
- apnea, jaundice, multiple anomalies (whatever the cause)

If the child has one or more of these factors, physicians will recommend an *auditory brain stem response test*. This hearing test measures brain wave activity in response to sound.

Auditory Brain Stem Response Test (ABR)

The ABR is not a direct measure of hearing, but a measure of nerve activity. It's used with children who can't respond in the soundproof booth, since in this test no responses are required from the child.

As the child sleeps (with or without sedation), earphones and electrodes record activity from the hearing nerve. This test, which measures high-pitched sounds better than low-pitched sounds, is often used by hospitals to test newborns.

As nerve impulses pass through the lower levels of your baby's brain from the auditory nerve on their way to higher brain centers, they make connections in the brain stem near the base of the skull. The ABR tests this electrical activity in the brain stem. It can determine how well certain portions of the infant's auditory system in the brain responds to a presented tone or beep. Clicks or tone pips are fed into the ear, and a computer then analyzes brain activity to see if the brain waves change. Rather than a true test of the entire process of hearing, the ABR determines whether auditory signals are reaching the brain.

By repeating the stimulus up to 100 times and averaging the response by computer, the responses can be enhanced while eliminating random background electrical activity. This way, auditory thresholds can be established that are quite close to those that can be obtained in conventional audiometry.

This noninvasive test is useful for the detection of hearing loss in newborns and infants, for the medical diagnosis of auditory disorders (including tumors) and for confirming psychological hearing loss. It can be performed on individuals of any age, including the youngest infant.

Electrocochleogram

This test measures impulses in the cochlear nerve by inserting a thin electrode through the eardrum into the promontory of the basal turn. This indicates how well the cochlea is functioning.

Electrodermal Response Audiometry

This special hearing test procedure measures sweat changes on the hands or feet in response to sound or speech, and records these changes on a graph. The test is one of the nonspecific electrophysiologic tests used to estimate the auditory threshold in infants who can't respond voluntarily to sounds.

Otoacoustic Emissions (OAE) Test

This quick method of testing hearing can be given to the youngest children (even used for screening in the newborn nursery). It's based on the fact that the ear not only hears noise, but also makes noise. By measuring the very faint noises made by the ear, the test can estimate how well the ear itself can hear. An ear that doesn't hear well won't make the expected noises. These noises are much too faint to be heard by the naked ear, but there are machines that can measure these sounds.

CHAPTER 4

NOISE-RELATED HEARING LOSS

If you work in a noisy environment, there's a good chance that eventually you'll damage your hearing. If a noise is loud enough to hurt your ears, it's loud enough to damage the delicate hearing mechanism within your ears.

How loud is too loud? Normal conversation usually takes place at about a 60 dB noise level; a noisy restaurant may raise that level to about 75 dB. Prolonged exposure to noise above 90 dB is enough to damage the hair cells that line the cochlea of the inner ear. To give you an idea of how loud that is, imagine standing on the sidewalk in New York City at rush hour. The decibel level of that noise would be about 80 dB, which is the very edge of the "safe" range. The noise of a motorcycle or snowmobile lies between 85 and 90 dB, and a rock concert is between 80 and 100 dB. If you stand three feet away from a jackhammer without ear protectors, you're most likely damaging your ears from the 120 dB noise level; a jet engine from 100 feet away is 130 dB.

Most people in the United States assume that noise-induced hearing loss is only a problem for senior citizens. However, recent research has uncovered an astonishing loss of hearing among students: 15% of school-age children and 61% of college freshmen tested all showed hearing problems. Conversely, studies have found that natives in the African jungle, exposed to no excess noise at all, show almost no decrease in hearing acuity as they age. The biggest increase in hearing loss is among "baby boomers" now in their 40s and 50s. From 1971 to 1990, hearing problems in this group jumped 26%, almost all due to increased noise.

HOW NOISE-RELATED HEARING LOSS OCCURS

Damage to hearing from too much noise occurs mostly in the cochlea, overloading the tiny, irreplaceable hair cells. In addition, excess noise can reduce enzymes and energy sources in the cochlear fluids and change the structure of the cochlear mechanism, which provides most of the nourishment to the hair cells.

As exposure to noise continues, stress on the hair cells increases. The tiny hairs on top of the cells become fused together, the hair cells disintegrate, and finally the nerve fibers to the hair cells disappear. At this point, since hair cells don't regenerate, damage is permanent.

72

In the case of "acoustic trauma"—a sudden, sharp, very loud noise—the entire mechanical inner ear system vibrates so violently that its attachments are disrupted, membranes in the cochlea may rupture, and hair cells are torn from the basilar membrane. The rupture of the cochlea membranes results in a mixing of ear fluids that poisons any hair cells that weren't destroyed in the initial blast.

Most sounds (other than acoustic trauma) that can produce lasting damage are high-intensity noises that occur over a long period of time—eight hours a day for more than ten years, for example. Such noise-induced hearing loss is quite common, for example, among rock musicians.

Once the hair cells are damaged, a sensorineural hearing loss can result because the hair cell loss affects the workings of the inner ear. Sensorineural hearing loss usually cannot be corrected, because a hair cell, once destroyed, can never be regenerated.

Ototoxic Drugs

It's possible that noise-induced hearing loss can be made much worse by certain ototoxic drugs that, if taken in the presence of excess noise, could harm an ear it would otherwise leave unaffected. (For more information on ototoxic drugs, see Chapter 2).

On-the-Job Hearing Loss

A number of industrial environments produce enough noise to impair hearing. In part, this occurs because although noise above 90 dB can hurt your hearing, a person can work in the presence of noise up to 120 dB before it begins to be painful.

If you work at a job in the presence of 90 dB noise, there might be slight ringing or muffling of noises, but after an evening or weekend away from the noise, these symptoms will probably fade away. A person tested after working all day in the presence of 120 dB noise might show a slight loss of hearing, but after a few days away from the job, a retest would show hearing has returned to normal. This is called a "temporary threshold shift."

However, after several months of this type of exposure, the hearing loss would become permanent. You would probably not notice work-induced hearing loss because the deficits show up first among the high frequencies, which interferes very little with the understanding of speech. Not until the loss worsens and begins to affect the middle frequencies would a hearing loss be noticed. By that time, the loss could be permanent.

You don't become "used" to working around noise; if after some months or years the noise seems less noticeable, it is only because a hearing loss has already taken place.

High-Risk Ototoxic Jobs

If you work in one of the following jobs, you are at risk for hearing loss. They include:

- boilermaking
- weaving
- aircraft maintenance
- blacksmithing
- riveting
- blasting
- machine manufacturing

- metalworking
- loud rock music production

In addition, you could be at risk if you work in any job involving:

- large presses
- high-pressure steam
- large wood saws
- heavy hammering (such as iron or steelworking)

If you work around noisy machinery, you should understand that if it is necessary to raise your voice to be heard by someone less than two feet away, you should wear protective devices. A person working in an environment this noisy should have a hearing test once a year and always wear ear protectors—or find a different job.

Recreational Hearing Loss

Hearing loss due to recreational noise is becoming more and more common. Some of the common activities associated with loud noise and hearing loss include:

- Sitting close to speakers at live music performances
- Frequenting dance clubs or exercise classes with loud music
- Using cassette players and headset stereos at loud levels
- Loud audio systems and car stereos
- Electronic arcade games
- Target shooting, speedboating, motocross, or auto racing
- Firecrackers

The Hazard Zone

TYPICAL DECIBEL	EXAMPLE
0	Lowest sound audible to the human ear
30	Quiet library, soft whisper
40	Living room, quiet office, bedroom away from traffic
50	Light traffic at a distance, refrigerator, gentle breeze
60	Air conditioner at 20 feet, conversation, sewing machine
70	Busy traffic, office tabulator, noisy restaurant. At this decibel level, noise may begin to affect hearing if exposure is constant.

The Hazardous Zone

80	Subway, heavy city traffic, alarm clock at two feet, factory noise. These noises are dangerous if exposure to them lasts for more than eight hours.
90	Truck traffic, noisy home appliances, shop tools, lawn mower. As loudness increases, the "safe" time exposure decreases; damage can occur in less than eight hours.
100	Chain saw, stereo headphones, pneumatic drill. Even two hours of exposure can be dangerous at this decibel level; with each 5 dB increase the safe time is cut *in half*.
120	Rock band concert in front of speakers, sandblasting, thunderclap. The danger is immediate; exposure at 120 dB can injure ears.
140	Gunshot blast, jet plane. *Any* length of exposure time is dangerous; noise at this level may cause actual pain in the ear.
180	Rocket launching pad. Without ear protection, noise at this level causes irreversible damage; hearing loss is inevitable.

Source: American Academy of Otolaryngology; © 1983.

- Power lawnmowers, leaf blowers, chainsaws, and power tools
- Some of the early-model cordless telephones
- Rattles and squeaky toys used too close to an infant's
- Toys imitating firearms
- Musical toys such as trumpets, drums and xylophones

Noise Level Limits

You must wear ear protectors on any job whose noise level tops the following limits, according to OSHA:

DECIBELS	HOURS
90	8
95	4
100	2
110	1/2
115	1/4

Pregnancy and Noise

New research has found that pregnant women who work in noisy environments may be at risk for damage to the hearing of their unborn children. In the past, sound was thought to be muffled by the mother's abdominal tissues and fluids in the uterus before reaching the fetus. But in one recent study of unborn lambs, chronic loud noises and short, loud bursts of noise (such as the sound of a weapon firing) triggered hearing loss while the lamb was in the womb. Not only did the lambs' hearing become less sensitive after chronic loud noise exposure; after birth, the tiny hairs that pick up sounds in the lambs' inner ears were often deformed. Because developing lambs are about the same size as humans, the animals are good models for human pregnancy.

For this reason, experts are now suggesting that pregnant women avoid loud noise if possible, such as rock concerts, jet skiing, snowmobiling and mowing the yard. If a woman has to speak loudly to be understood, the noise level is potentially dangerous to the adult and the unborn child.

However, data are not yet solid enough to recommend that employers bar pregnant women from jobs with high noise exposure. While a few human studies have shown mild hearing loss among children of women who work in noisy places, the studies aren't conclusive since they didn't measure hearing right at birth.

OHSA

The Occupational Health and Safety Act includes a wide range of rules to protect workers in many dangerous occupations. An essential requirement of this act states that any industry in which employees are exposed daily to continuous noise levels of more than 90 dB for eight hours must either reduce the noise or protect the hearing of exposed workers. The 90 dB level specified is the level at which conservation of hearing should begin.

Studies have indicated that hearing loss in the workplace begins once noise exceeds 80 dB, although there is not a significant risk until noise reaches 90 dB. Although studies indicate that continual exposure to 90 dB noise will result in a hearing loss of about 15 dB, it does not mean that everyone who works in this environment at 90 dB will have the same loss; some workers' ears will be injured severely while others may remain healthy. This is because hearing loss is also related to noise environment outside of the job, which can vary a great deal.

At this time, the only way to protect your ears against damage from noise above 80 dB is to wear protective ear devices, such as ear plugs or earmuffs.

Noise Control Laws

Legislation aimed at controlling noise in public is certainly not new. In the first century, Julius Caesar issued an ordinance banning chariots from the streets of Rome during the night. Things haven't improved much since.

In this country, legislation aimed at controlling noise in public was first enacted in 1968 by the U.S. Congress as part of its amendment to the Federal Aviation Act. One year later, Congress included hearing-conservation rules for plants with federal contracts as part of the Walsh-Healy Act.

Unusual in its inclusion of safety provisions for private enterprise, the regulations paved the way for the Occupational Health and Safety Act of 1970 that brought together a host of safety regulations in industry. Included in the action was a section that applied the noise regulations of the Walsh-Healy Act to all workers in all industries.

The law requires industry to define areas in their plants where noise exceeds an equivalent of 90 dB for an eight-hour workday; each time noise level increases by 5 dB, the allowable exposure time is cut in half.

If possible, excessive noise should be lowered; if workers' hearing can't be protected by limiting the exposure or the level of the noise, the law requires the company to provide either protective hearing devices or annual hearing tests to identify those experiencing progressive hearing loss.

This 1970 legislation was followed two years later by the Noise Control Act, which gave the Environmental Protection Agency power over federal regulatory action in noise control. The Labor Department maintains control over the Occupational Safety and Health Administration, and the Federal Aviation Agency retains authority over aircraft noise regulatory action.

HOW TO PROTECT YOUR EARS

There are two types of ear-protecting devices: earplugs (which fit inside the ear canal) and earmuffs, which fit outside the ears. Earplugs and earmuffs worn together provide the most effective protection against noise. The most important thing about any device used to protect the ears from noise is the seal. You can tell if the seal is good enough by talking to yourself—your voice should sound lower, muffled and a bit louder than when you aren't wearing protectors, since you're hearing the sound of your own voice through your skull. Other sounds around you should be much quieter.

Ear protection devices are assigned a "noise reduction rating" (NRR) that describes how well they insulate noise. Devices now on the market range from 0 to 30 NRR; for the best protection, look for a product with a range above 20.

Earplugs

If you want to protect your ears against noise, don't buy premolded earplugs designed for swimming. These work well in keeping your ears dry, but they won't screen out noise well enough. Most of these over-the-counter plugs are usually available in one size only, and ear size varies from one person to the next.

In order to be effective in screening out excess noise, earplugs must fit snugly in the ear canal so that no air can pass through. In addition, because your ears may not be the same size, you'll need earplugs of different dimensions. If your ears happen to be the same size as the plugs sold in the store, you might get a good fit, and you'll certainly save money over the years. Everyone else should buy custom earplugs.

Custom-fit earplugs are made to fit only one person's ears, usually by an audiologist or hearing aid dispenser. These are a good choice especially if you work in a noisy environment or in a high-risk profession. One type of earplug has a valve that allows soft sounds (such as speech) to pass through, but closes for loud sounds.

In fitting the earplugs, the dealer makes an impression of the ear canal and sends the dimensions to a manufacturer, where the soft rubber earplug insert is made. These fitted earplugs should be used only by adults, since the ear canals of children and teenagers change quickly. Earplugs must fit properly in order to shut out sound and must be kept clean to avoid infection. Most types give about 30 dB protection against excess noise.

Flexible Foam Cylinders

These new devices give excellent noise protection (up to 28 NRR) and cost less than a dollar a pair. They're handy because you don't need to have them fitted by a dealer; you just compress the foam-rubber cylinders and put them into your ears yourself, where they re-expand and form an extremely tight seal. The down side—they can't be washed, so they must be regularly replaced.

Earmuffs

Earmuffs can provide even more effective sound protection than can plugs, and are preferable if there is a draining ear or chronic infection. In addition, some people can't wear earplugs comfortably because of the shape of their ear canals. Others don't like the feeling of having their ears plugged up.

Earmuffs completely cover the ear. The earpieces are made of sponge material and are held in place by a tension headband. Earmuff protectors generally cost more than earplugs, but they are harder to lose and some believe they are more comfortable for daily wear. Those who wear glasses, however, may find that the glasses interfere with the earmuff's seal. You can buy earmuffs in sporting-goods stores for about $25 to $30.

Other Protectors

Dry cotton is almost useless in protecting against excess noise. Some types of disposable ear protectors are made of cotton, wax and other specially treated material, and these are only somewhat effective.

Modify Your Environment

If you find yourself working in a noisy environment and the thought of wearing ear protectors makes you cringe, there are a few other ways you can try to muffle some of the noise.

- Wrap noisy machines with insulation.
- Place foam pads under noisy machines (printers, typewriters, meat grinders, food processors, copiers).
- Mount noisy machines on rubber (not concrete).
- Use drapes and carpeting in all work areas if possible.
- Use noise-reduction plastic boxes for encasing computers and printers.

Remember, working in a noisy environment can really affect your ability to hear—and can be psychologically stressful as well. It may seem tedious to wear hearing protectors, but it's simpler and less expensive than hearing aids.

CHAPTER 5
CHOOSING A HEARING AID

Only about 20% of Americans with a hearing loss actually use a hearing aid. In part, this is because many people have trouble accepting hearing loss and are often unwilling to do anything about it.

Part of the problem may be that many people wrongly assume that a hearing aid will solve their hearing problems. When the person realizes that using an aid isn't simply a matter of popping one in the ear, the aid is often abandoned. The key to success with a hearing aid is daily practice coupled with hearing therapy, counseling and a positive attitude.

Some of you may have never thought about a hearing aid, and some may have rejected that idea. Others may have bought an aid only to end up leaving it in a drawer in frustration. Before learning about the different types of aids—and what's new on the horizon—it's a good idea to fully understand what an aid can and can't do.

What a Hearing Aid Can Do

A hearing aid can boost the loudness of sound, which can improve your understanding of speech. You'll be able to hear high-pitched sounds, and they may help you function in social situations. Moreover, the hearing aid can alert others that you do have a hearing problem, which may remind them to make a more concerted effort to communicate with you.

What a Hearing Aid Can't Do

You still won't be able to hear very soft sounds, because if the hearing aid was set to transmit these softest sounds, normal speech would be far too loud. Even with a perfectly working hearing aid, you will probably still have a slight hearing loss.

Hearing aids won't return your hearing to normal levels—but they'll help you take advantage of the hearing you have left by making sounds louder and speech easier to understand for those with certain types of hearing loss.

Basically, an aid modifies the sound traveling into your ear. Once it gets there, if your brain and inner ear distort that sound the aid can't do anything about the distortion. It can only make this distorted sound louder and help you try to figure out the noise.

A hearing aid is just a machine. As a result, it can never duplicate the true sound that people with normal hearing experience. Some consumers say that the sound produced by a hearing aid is mechanical and artificial.

One of the main problems with hearing aids is that they amplify *all* sounds, not just the ones you want to hear. Particularly when the source of sound is far away, such as up on a stage or in a large building, other environmental noises can interfere with good perception. Hearing aids favor sounds in the frequency of speech; this means that sounds that lie outside this range may be altered by a hearing aid.

GETTING A HEARING AID

The first step in obtaining a hearing aid is to have an accurate diagnosis and hearing evaluation done by an otologist, otolaryngologist and audiologist. These specialists can determine whether a hearing aid will help, and what type that will do the most good. This is especially important since aids can be expensive, and are not generally covered by health insurance.

In the early days of hearing aid development you couldn't be sure that the person fitting an aid really knew what he or she was doing. But by the 1970s the states began to require licensing for hearing aid dispensers. Today, in all but four states all hearing aids may be fitted and sold only by licensed specialists, who may be called "dealers," "specialists," "dispensers," "hearing instrument specialists" or "dispensing audiologists." By federal law, hearing aids may not be sold directly to consumers, because they are considered to be medical devices and are regulated by the U.S. Food and Drug Administration. A certified hearing aid audiologist is an audiologist certified by the American Speech-Language-Hearing Association as qualified to dispense hearing aids. The certified hearing aid audiologist must hold a master's degree in audiology, pass a national certifying exam and earn a certificate of clinical competence.

While it's possible to buy an aid through the mail, the best idea is to be fitted only after a hearing test. Since most people with hearing problems hear some frequencies better and others less so, such a test can help the dispenser adjust the aid for maximum benefit.

Your hearing aid dealer will be responsible for making the impression for the earmold and making sure the aid fits properly. The dealer will also explain the general care and use of your aid, and can repair a malfunctioning unit. Generally, the dealer can offer suggestions about using a hearing aid or about possible changes in models and the settings in which they can be used.

Before audiologists moved into the dealership field, hearing aids were sold by people who were not required to have additional training in the field. Most learned the trade by apprenticing to an experienced dealer; for many years, no licensure or registration was required. Some dealers call themselves audiologists, but this title should be used only by those who have earned at least a master's degree in audiology.

Medical Waiver

Today, most states have laws that prohibit anyone from selling a hearing aid before the client has been examined by a physician who can rule out the possibility of a medical problem. (Waivers are permitted for those whose religious beliefs preclude physician visits.)

Hearing Aid Analysis

When an audiologist tells you a hearing aid may be of help, you'll be asked to come for a hearing aid evaluation. During this appointment, further tests will help pinpoint which type of hearing aid will be best for your particular type of hearing loss. Your audiologist will write a report of the results of your test and forward them to your ear specialist. You may obtain a copy of this report if you wish.

Hearing Aid Evaluation

There are several ways to determine what sort of hearing aid you should have:

- *Real ear measurement*   By inserting a tiny microphone inside your ear canal, the audiologist can transmit sounds through the aid via a loudspeaker.
- *Personal judgment*   Your audiologist might ask you to judge at what level of loudness the aid is comfortable.
- *Formulas*   Some audiologists take the results of your hearing tests and apply mathematical formulas to come up with a recommendation.

Next, the audiologist will recommend the type of hearing aid you should buy, making a general suggestion about certain characteristics that might help your situation, or very specific recommendations complete with brand name and serial number. This variation is due to the fact that some people might require specific characteristics that are only available with certain aids. On the other hand, the audiologist might have found that certain companies are more reliable or offer better repair services.

The audiologist should be willing to discuss the different types of hearing aids. A dispensing audiologist can sell you an aid, although you are not under any obligation to buy it from the person who conducted your hearing evaluation.

If your audiologist does *not* sell hearing aids, he or she can give you a list of competent dealers in your area. You may also request such a list even if the audiologist is a dealer. Remember that you have the right to shop around, to compare prices, to ask for a general price quote and discussion of what services are included.

Cost

Prices for hearing evaluations vary from one part of the country to the next, but most range between $35 to $125 and $50 to $100 for a hearing aid evaluation. You can expect to pay less at a university-related clinic.

Basic Hearing Aid Package

Since hearing aids are not cheap—they can range from a very basic $500 to an elaborate $6,000 or more, often not covered by insurance—you'll want to make sure you are getting good value for your money.

Here are some tips on what ought to be included in the total price quote for a hearing aid:

- Cost of the hearing aid
- Cost of the earmold(s)
- Battery pack
- Adjustments to the hearing aid or earmold
- Counseling and orientation
- Return visits (at least two)
- Warranty (at least one year)

Price Comparisons Online

The cost of a hearing aid includes a hearing test, ear impressions for in-the-ear styles, the hearing aid itself and office visits for fittings and follow-ups. Until recently, there has been little price competition. That may change with a new company selling hearing aids on the Internet. Working with a national network of 400 audiologists, company founder Steve McAfee sells discount hearing aids over the Internet at http://www.ahearingaid.com. The New Mexico–based company's Web site lists prices, which are usually several hundred dollars over wholesale, and the buyer pays the audiologist a fee of $500. Consumers can expect to save $800 on an in-the-canal aid that normally retails for about $2,800. It is also possible to compare retail prices on the Web by checking the sites of audiologists.

What to Expect

When you're ready to buy an aid, here's what you can expect:

- Understand the cost of the aid, service and warranties. You will probably pay more for an eyeglass aid.
- The dispenser/dealer will make an impression of your ears from which a personalized earmold will be created.
- Return to the dispenser in about three weeks to try on the earmold and hearing aid.
- You may need more hearing tests after you try on the hearing aid to measure how well you can understand speech.
- The dispenser will teach you how to maintain and use your aid.
- You should receive information about what to do if you develop a sensitivity to the earmold.
- Be sure to ask all the questions you can think of.
- Within several weeks, you should return to the dealer's office to have the aid checked and to discuss your progress in dealing with the device. About 40% of all hearing aids require modification.

Make sure you can return the aid within 30 days for a full refund if it doesn't improve your hearing. Find out about service and warranty when you buy the aid. Within the first month after you purchase a hearing aid, make an appointment for a full hearing examination to determine if the hearing aid is functioning properly.

Hearing Aid Glossary

There are four main characteristics of hearing aids:

- *Distortion:* This is a measure of how well the hearing aid reproduces sound. Any electronic device (such as your TV or radio) distorts sound to some degree.
- *Gain:* This is a measure of the power of your hearing aid and how much it amplifies sound.
- *Frequency range:* This explains how much power your hearing aid has in certain ranges of pitches and how far your aid can amplify the high and low pitches.
- *Maximum power output:* A measure of the loudest sound the hearing aid can produce; this can act as a safety valve against damage to your ear from sudden loud noises.

FDA Regulations on Hearing Aids

The Food and Drug Administration has established regulations on hearing aids to protect the health and safety of those with hearing problems:

- A medical test by a licensed physician (preferably one specializing in ear diseases) within six months before the purchase of a hearing aid
- This doctor's written assessment may be waived by the client (18 years of age or older) on signing a document to this effect. Children, however, *must* be evaluated by a physician.
- Health professionals who dispense hearing aids are required to refer consumers to a physician if any of eight specified ear conditions are evident (ear deformity, drainage, sudden or progressive hearing loss, dizziness, significant earwax, foreign body, pain or discomfort).
- A user's instruction book must be given along with every hearing aid, specifying the importance of medical evaluation, instructions for proper use, repair service information, care information, known side effects and so on.

HEARING AIDS

The first hearing aids were fairly simple cone-shaped instruments ranging from a rolled-up tube to an elaborate "ear trumpet," which gave consumers a slight boost in sound. The first true hearing aid appeared in 1921 after the invention of the vacuum tube, but these devices were cumbersome units with large parts and heavy batteries.

Today, a hearing aid system consists of a small microphone designed to pick up sound waves and convert them into electrical signals in a pattern that represents sound waves. These signals are fed into an amplifier, which boosts the signal and sends it to a receiver. The receiver converts the amplified signals back into sound and transmits them into the ear through the earmold. If the earmold is properly fitted, it carries the amplified sound directly into the ear canal. A poorly-fitting earmold, however, causes whistles and squeals and can be irritating and painful to the wearer. This is why custom-fitted molds are often more desirable than ready-made types.

Although a hearing aid can amplify sound, it doesn't necessarily improve the *clarity* of the sound. Unfortunately, aids can't make hearing completely normal, and they require practice and skill to be used effectively. Still, even profoundly deaf individuals can benefit from powerful behind-the-ear aids.

People with only a mild hearing loss may get enough improvement simply with a tiny unit that fits directly into the ear; those with more severe problems may need a larger, more powerful system. Worn on the body, they are sturdier, easier to regulate and less subject to distortion. Still, most profoundly deaf individuals don't wear body aids.

Modern hearing aids do much more than simply amplify sound; they can also filter background noise, change tonal quality and control the loudness of environmental sounds. Researchers have been able to devise smaller and smaller units that are less visible, which appeals to those who don't want others to know they wear hearing aids.

Earmolds

Part of the hearing aid system, earmolds are plastic inserts that fit into the ear or ear canal, conducting the amplified sound into the ear. They come in many shapes, depending on the type of hearing aid and the physical shape of the person's ear.

For example, earmolds in *canal* and *in-the-ear* aids encase all the hearing aid's components. Earmolds for *behind-the-ear* and *eyeglass* hearing aids are placed in the ear and are connected to the hearing aid by a piece of clear plastic tubing. *Body* aids have an earmold that allows a button-shaped receiver to snap into a metal ring on its back, with a cord connecting the earmold to the rest of the aid.

When a hearing aid is selected and fitted, the audiologist or dispenser will make an impression of the ear to customize the earmold. Earmolds are made of various types of material, including hard plastic or several varieties of soft, pliant materials. Hypoallergenic earmolds are also available.

An earmold should fit snugly into the ear without pain or a "plugged up" feeling; a loose fit could cause feedback or whistling. Modifications can alleviate problems; for example, a hole bored in an earmold can alleviate pressure in the ear canal, and a larger vent can alter the response of the aid so that it's more appropriate in certain types of hearing loss.

TYPES OF HEARING AIDS

People with mild hearing loss may get enough improvement simply with a tiny unit that fits directly into the ear; others with more severe problems may need a larger, more powerful system.

Modern hearing aids do more than simply amplify sound; they can filter background noise, change tonal quality and control the loudness of environmental sounds. Strides in miniaturization have led to smaller, less visible aids.

Today's most sophisticated aids may range up to $6,000; most of these are small enough to fit into a pocket. Most are not usually covered by health insurance.

Digital Aids

These newest type of digital hearing aids represent a major breakthrough in computer-tuned sound, and contain miniature computer chips designed to tailor sound to the ear of the person wearing the device. These are actually tiny computers that have a computer chip inside doing the amplifier work, instead of the traditional analog circuitry.

While most people with hearing problems have trouble with certain tones within the hearing spectrum, most aids amplify all tones equally. Digital aids can be adjusted to screen out background noise and amplify certain tones, depending on the environment. Some of the newest aids break down sound into more than twice as many channels as other aids on the market, providing a more personalized hearing experience. They are set by hearing health care providers using an external computer.

These new aids increase the amount of sound processing possible in the same amount of space, minimizing distortion so that they have a clearer, crisper sound. The newest digital aids have the ability to analyze the sound environment and adapt the amplification accordingly, enhancing speech clarity automatically without the necessity of volume controls. You can choose different acoustic "sound settings" for quiet office workdays, crowded meetings, at-home use and so on.

Nonlinear Single-Channel Aids

More advanced technology produced a nonlinear aid that has more amplification given to soft sounds than for loud sounds. Once sounds reach a certain level, the aid automatically adjusts the volume. This type of aid squeezes a wide range of loudness into a narrower range, which is why they are also called compression hearing aids.

Nonlinear Multichannel Aids

This newer type of aid is designed with a consumer's personal hearing needs in mind, based upon how loud certain sounds need to be interpreted for various frequencies. In hearing aids with only one channel, a loud noise of low frequency (such as sound during a party) would trigger the hearing aid to lower the amplification for all frequencies, which would help keep the sound from being too loud—but would also make some high-frequency sounds (such as consonants) too soft to hear. In that same situation, a multichannel aid would decrease the amplification for low frequencies without changing the amplification for high frequencies. If fitted correctly, they can greatly improve speech clarity (especially in noisy listening environments).

Multiple/Automatic Program Aids

Some hearing aids have several different programs that can be selected by a touch of a button (either on the aid or on a separate remote control) to select amplification best suited to different environments, such as listening in a restaurant, in a one-on-one situation or for music. Other aids have automatic volume regulation so that the consumer doesn't have to bother with volume control. However, some people don't like aids that take away too much control.

In-the-Ear Aids

In-the-ear aids are lightweight devices that fit inside the ear canal with no visible wires or tubes. This aid is created from an impression of your ear canal; the components are then built into the case that is molded from this impression.

There are a number of styles of aids that are encased within a plastic shell and are worn entirely within the ear. These include:

- traditional in-the-canal
- custom in-the-ear (ITE) model, which can completely fill the ear canal
- half-concha, a thinner low-profile model
- helix model, an even smaller model (for high-frequency losses)
- completely-in-the-canal aid, the tiniest style, so small it must be removed from the ear by pulling on a thin cord that rests at the bottom of the bowl of the ear.

It's possible to control tone but not volume, which makes them generally helpful for only mild losses. More than half of all the hearing aids sold today are in-the-ear aids.

These new aids are extremely expensive, but they are invisible and offer acoustic and maintenance advantages. The good thing about an in-the-ear aid is that it won't bump into your glasses, and it can provide more power for the higher frequencies. In addition, many people find these aids are easier to put on and take off than the behind-the-ear style. They are of special interest for older people, who may balk at wearing a hearing aid for psychological reasons. Many people like the in-the-canal aids because they aren't especially noticeable and they more closely mimic natural sound, since the microphone rests deeper in the ear canal. This location also cuts down on wind noise.

However, the small size of these aids makes them harder to handle; the battery is particularly tiny and difficult to insert. To adjust the volume, the wearer must insert a finger down into the ear and adjust the control by touch alone. Because they are custom-fitted to your ear, you can't try on these types of aids before you order them. Some people find the aid is uncomfortable in hot weather, and others believe they tend to break down more often than behind-the-ear styles.

These aids also can be more difficult to fit correctly, and usually require several return visits to the dealer/dispenser. Since the smaller the aid the higher the cost, this version is very expensive indeed because the cost includes miniaturized components.

Keep in mind that this very tiny aid doesn't have as much power as other larger aids, and its small battery means that you'll be buying replacements more often. In addition, while larger aids can make room for a telephone coil to pick up the electric signals over the phone, the in-the-canal aid is just too small to pack in any extras.

Behind-the-Ear Aids

Less popular are the behind-the-ear aids that include a microphone, amplifier, and receiver inside a small curved case worn behind the ear that's connected to the earmold by a short plastic tube. The earmold extends into the ear canal from a quarter to three quarters of an inch. Some models have both tone and volume control plus a telephone pickup device.

This style does not require as much maintenance since the earmolds can handle everyday trauma better than smaller, more delicate models. They are easily interchangeable if you have to take one in for servicing. This type of hearing aid is effective for those whose hearing loss ranges from mild to severe, and they may be helpful for those who have problems handling the smaller aids.

Some people who must wear glasses find that the aids interfere with the fit of the eyeglasses. Others don't have enough space behind their ears for such a device to fit comfortably.

Bone Conduction Aids

Bone conduction aids are designed primarily for people with conductive hearing loss that hasn't been effectively treated with surgery. This type of aid, which allows sound to be heard through the bone behind the ear, is used when the ear canal is closed or drainage from the ear is poor.

Eyeglass Models

This model is much the same as the behind-the-ear aid, except that the case fits into an eyeglass frame instead of resting behind the ear. While this means that the eyeglass frame needs to be slightly larger, modern miniaturized parts can be incorporated into an eyeglass frame that isn't too large. Still, not very many people choose to purchase such an aid. They are useful for those whose hearing loss ranges from mild to severe.

Those who do favor this type believe that this aid is less conspicuous than other models, although there is a tube that travels from the temple of the glasses to the earmold. Bone conduction hearing aids are also available in the eyeglass model.

On the other hand, it can be difficult to fit this type of hearing aid. You must purchase a new set of eyeglass frames (and sometimes lenses) and then work with both the hearing aid dispenser and your optician to get the devices properly adjusted. Because eyeglass models tend to need more repairs than other types of aids, you'll find it quite annoying because when either the eyeglasses or the aid needs repair, you'll have to have a backup set of glasses and hearing aid. You might find the eye-and-ears connection annoying for those times when you might want to wear glasses without fussing with a hearing aid, or vice versa.

CROS or Crossover System

This type of hearing aid system, often used in conjunction with the eyeglass model (above), is used by people with normal hearing in one ear and a moderate-to-severe loss in the other. The CROS (contralateral routing of signal) system features a microphone, amplifier, and controls behind the impaired ear that feeds the amplified signal to the better ear, eliminating "head shadow" (which occurs when the head blocks sound from the better ear). The amplified sound from the hearing aid on the one side is added to the normal sound entering the healthy ear.

The two sides are usually linked by a built-in FM radio signal system, although there are wired models available. This system may help make speech easier to understand for those with a high-frequency loss in both ears. It also allows people to understand from which direction sounds are coming. This type of hearing aid can prevent feedback, which occurs when amplification leaks sound into the microphone located near the receiver.

Bi-CROS (bilateral contralateral routing of signal) systems use two microphones (one above each ear) that sends signals to a single amplifier. Sound then travels to a single receiver, which transfers it to the better ear via a conventional earmold. Bi-CROS aids are usually the eyeglass type, used for those with an unequal hearing loss in both ears, one of which can't be helped by amplification. It's unlike the CROS hearing aid, which uses only one microphone. Sound is picked up by microphones in both ears, transmitted to a single receiver, and transferred to the better ear via a conventional earmold.

A CRIS-CROS hearing aid is designed for someone with severe hearing loss in both ears who may be unable to wear hearing aids at ear level because of feedback problems. Feedback occurs when the amplifier leaks sound back into the microphone because it's too close to the receiver. In this case, a CRIS-CROS aid uses two CROS aids behind the ear, each unit encompassing the microphone for the other side.

On-the-Body Aids

These hearing aids feature a larger microphone, amplifier and power supply inside a case carried inside a pocket or attached to clothing. The external receiver attaches directly to the earmold; its power comes through a flexible wire from the amplifier. Although larger than other aids, on-the-body hearing aids are also more powerful and easier to adjust than smaller devices. Their size and body location—and the problem of noise from clothing—make this aid an unpopular choice, although some are still used for people with profound hearing loss or for very young children.

If you are almost totally deaf, you may find you need that extra boost in power available only from the body aid. Moreover, anyone who has any type of physical disability that interferes with the ability to handle tiny parts can benefit from a body aid. On the other hand, such a large aid is bulky and visible. It is rarely used for cases of age-related hearing loss.

Monaural/Binaural Aids

Monaural hearing aids include any aid that provides sound to just one ear, whereas binaural aids include two complete hearing devices, one in each ear. Some wearers find that the binaural system increases direction sense and helps separate sound from unwanted background noise.

Any type of hearing aid may be worn in both ears if the listener can tolerate two aids and can benefit from amplifying residual hearing in both ears. Although it's sometimes assumed that using an aid in each ear should improve hearing, tests of people wearing these aids don't always support this theory.

HEARING AID FEATURES

You may be interested in investigating some extra hearing aid features, such as telecoil circuitry and tone control, which can be used with certain "assistive listening systems and devices" (see Chapter 6).

The telecoil (or T-coil) is a tiny electrical component that can sense magnetic forces generated by another coil nearby, such as the speaker coil in a telephone or a loop or wire around the room or around a person's neck. The major use for a telecoil has been with the telephone, which allows clearer sound reception for the hard-of-hearing consumer. When a hearing aid's control switch is set to the T-switch, the telecoil is connected and the hearing aid's microphone is disconnected. This allows the aid to receive magnetic signals instead of sound, enabling the wearer to hear only the "important" sound coming from the telecoil while screening out annoying background noise.

T-switches have become important with the advent of assistive listening devices and systems. More and more, public areas such as churches, theaters, meeting rooms, have been fitted with assistive listening systems to help people with hearing problems. Where such a system is in place, the hearing aid wearer can turn on the T-mode to receive sound from the induction loop. Or, where certain public places feature FM or infrared systems, the wearer may use a special receiver to connect with the hearing aid in the T-mode. In much the same way, assistive listening devices use the T-switch to improve hearing of TV and radio.

Not all hearing aids have a telecoil (including most canal or in-the-ear aids). Most behind-the-ear and all body aids do have telecoils. Because there are no regulations or standards regarding telecoils, they can vary as much as 30 dB in maximum sound output.

Compression Circuits

If you've ever had problems with a hearing aid in a crowded environment, this could be for you. These circuits can provide easier listening in the presence of noise for almost anyone by cutting their power when your surroundings get loud.

Noise Reduction Circuits

Also called "automatic signal processing," these circuits can sense rising noise levels and automatically adjust themselves to reduce the effects of these sounds. The more sophisticated the circuit, the more expensive.

High-Frequency Aids

This model extends into the high pitches for much clearer speech comprehension and easier listening to music and noise.

Implantable Aids

Unlike the cochlear implant, which we will discuss at the end of this chapter, implantable aids are surgically placed within the ear canal in the hope of overcoming many of the drawbacks of conventional in-the-ear hearing aids. There has been considerable research in the past 10 years into this type of aid. The implantable aid effectively removes the feedback problem and should provide greater comfort. These aids should be more acceptable to those who need amplification but who cannot (or choose not to) use currently available hearing aids.

Tips on Conserving Batteries

- Allow your batteries to dry out overnight by opening the battery compartment of the hearing aid.
- Don't carry batteries in the same pocket as loose change; the coins will drain the batteries.
- Keep extra batteries on hand and change them as soon as you notice the sound getting weaker or distorted.
- Dispose of batteries carefully so pets and children don't swallow them.

IF YOU HAVE A PROBLEM WITH YOUR AID . . .

In some ways, your hearing aid is as delicate an instrument as the human hearing mechanism. It won't last forever (with excellent care, most only last about five years) and the many tiny components can break. For example, if your aid sounds weak and scratchy, or it whistles, buzzes, or clicks off and on, this is *not* simply typical hearing aid behavior that you have to endure.

If your aid is having problems and you can't fix it yourself—and you should never try to open the actual hearing aid case—then it must be returned to the hearing aid dealer or dispensing audiologist. These experts can fix many problems in the office, but sometimes the aids must be sent back to the factory for several weeks. If so, you can borrow an aid from the dealer.

Painful Aids

While many people with hearing problems say everything seems loud after they receive a hearing aid, this is because they have lived for so long with a hearing deficit they have forgotten how loud "normal" sound can be. If you have worn your hearing aid for several weeks and you experience pain or discomfort, you should return to your dealer/dispenser for a readjustment.

You may notice that your earmold feels a bit uncomfortable at first, which is normal. However, if you experience redness, irritation, soreness or swelling, you should go back to the dealer and have the earmold adjusted.

Excess Wax

Many people complain that they have much more earwax after they get a hearing aid. It is true that wearing an earmold seems to boost the production of earwax. Actually, people who don't wear hearing aids have wax that falls out of their ears naturally. When you wear an earmold, the wax can't fall out on its own, and you actually retain earwax. You may need to visit a doctor to have this excess earwax removed.

Caring for Your Hearing Aid

A hearing aid should last about five years, with proper care. You can lower your maintenance and repair costs considerably by following these tips:

- Heat and cold can damage a hearing aid. Don't wear it under a hair dryer or store it near a heat source, and keep it off a windowsill where it can be exposed to sunlight. Don't wear it for more than a few minutes in very cold weather.
- Avoid wearing the aid in the rain or when sweating a great deal, although drops of rain aren't as harmful as mist and vapor—so keep it out of steamy bathrooms and kitchens. Don't inadvertently spray it with hair spray. *Never wear the aid while bathing.*
- Keep the aid in a plastic bag with a silica gel overnight, to help absorb moisture.
- Turn the aid off and remove the battery when you're not using it.
- Don't handle the hearing aid roughly, and try to avoid knocking it onto the floor.
- Wash the ear mold with soapy water occasionally, but never immerse the mechanical parts of the hearing aid.
- Protect it from dust, since small particles can clog up the microphone openings.
- Watch out for wax buildup in the small holes of the earmold. If you produce lots of wax, ask your dispenser about a wax guard, a small screen that can catch wax before it becomes wedged into the hearing aid.
- Clean the battery compartment and connections with a pencil eraser.
- Replace the tubing on behind-the-ear aids when it becomes yellowed or brittle.
- Replace cracked wiring on body hearing aids right away.
- Keep spare batteries with you, and store extras in a cool, dry place.
- Insert only dry, room-temperature batteries into the aid.
- Don't keep more than a month's supply of batteries at one time.
- Take your hearing aid to your dealer/dispenser for a checkup and cleaning once a year.

Acoustic Feedback

A loud squeal from your aid means that there is sound escaping from an ill-fitting earpiece, which is then being amplified. A hearing aid can deliver much louder sound without squeal if the earpiece fits well, but even so, some sound inevitably escapes through the back of the receiver. A very sensitive instrument with high maximum output may squeal too easily. It's possible to lessen squeal in a number of ways:

- Make sure the earpiece fits well in your ear.
- Reduce the volume of the hearing aid.
- Move the microphone farther away from the receiver.
- Adjust the tone control.

For More Information

The National Hearing Aid Society operates a help line for anyone who suspects a hearing loss and is uncertain what to do, or who needs information about hearing loss and hearing aids. The help line may be used by consumers to locate qualified, competent hearing aid specialists and answer questions about hearing devices, dispensing, and service.

Callers can obtain a consumer information kit, which includes a regional edition of the membership directory of the Hearing Aid Society, plus a 22-page booklet covering such topics as how hearing works, signs of hearing loss and types of hearing aids.

The group can also provide information on assistive listening devices, requirements for entering the hearing aid profession, statistics on hearing loss and hearing instruments and so on. The help line does not provide medical advice, recommend specific products, or quote prices.

Although financial assistance is not available through the help line, the help line can provide a list of possible financial resources. All services and materials provided are free. Callers may use the help line numbers 1–800–521–5247; in Michigan, 1–313–478–2610 Monday through Friday, 9 A.M. to 4:30 P.M. EST.

COCHLEAR IMPLANTS

A hearing aid won't help people with dysfunctional hair cells, designed to convert vibration to nerve impulses. In this case, a cochlear implant may be helpful. This device converts sound to electrical impulses transmitted directly through wires to the auditory nerve. Although sounds may not be clear, the implant can enhance sound and improve speech comprehension.

A cochlear implant is surgically implanted in the mastoid bone to stimulate the hearing nerve and enable a hard-of-hearing person to perceive some sound; the implant does not restore normal hearing. It is designed to help people with a sensorineural hearing loss ("nerve deafness"). Cochlear implants are profoundly different from hearing aids and other assistive listening devices, which simply make sounds louder. Sounds provided by even the most powerful and effective hearing aids may not offer much useful benefit to someone with a profound hearing loss in both ears. A cochlear implant, on the other hand, is a medical device designed to bypass damaged parts of the inner ear and electronically stimulate the nerve of hearing.

The first research on cochlear implants was conducted in France more than 30 years ago. Since then, cochlear implant technology has evolved from a device with a single electrode (or channel) to systems that transmit more sound information through multiple channels. Since the beginning, more than 14,000 people worldwide have received cochlear implants.

Cochlear implants are designed to bypass the hair cells that aren't functioning and directly stimulate the auditory nerve. There are a number of different cochlear implants currently available, but all implant systems consist of a microphone, a signal processor, a transmitter and receiver and one or more electrodes that are implanted in or around the cochlea. The implant consists of internal and external components. The internal parts of the device are surgically implanted completely under the skin, and include a receiver/stimulator positioned under the skin in a shallow bed made in the bone behind the ear. The receiver/stimulator is attached to 22 tiny electrode bands, arranged along a flexible tubing that is inserted approximately one inch into the cochlea (the snail-shaped section of the inner ear containing the hearing nerve endings).

The external components worn outside the body include a speech processor about the size of a calculator, weighing about 3 ounces; a headset, including a transmitting coil (a ring about an inch wide) that is held in place over the implanted receiver behind the ear by small magnets; and a microphone worn like a behind-the-ear hearing aid. The recipient wears the external microphone behind the ear as a magnet holds the transmitter to the side of the head near the microphone. Each is connected to the speech processor by a thin cord. The speech processor can be worn anywhere (on a belt, in a pocket). Many recipients are so good at disguising the implant system that others aren't aware of it.

As sound enters the microphone, it is sent to the speech processor via the thin cable that connects the headpiece to the speech processor. The speech processor converts the sound into a special signal using sophisticated software programs. The special signal is sent back up the same cable to the headpiece and transmitted across the skin via radio waves to the implanted device. The signal then travels down to the electrodes in the inner ear, stimulating the auditory nerve, which transmits the electrical signal to the brain, where it is interpreted as sound.

Cochlear implants have significantly improved the communication skills of more adults who have lost their ability to hear after they learned to speak. More typically, speechreading ability improves. Researchers estimate that approximately 250,000 to 500,000 people in the United States could benefit from a cochlear implant.

The simplest version has a single channel (electrode), but multichannel implants with more than 20 electrodes (each implanted farther along the cochlear duct) have considerably enhanced performance. These electrodes are used with a device that encodes frequencies, providing some pitch discrimination. Implants may transmit only certain features of the speech signal (feature-extraction), or the input signal may be transmitted to the electrodes without extraction-specific speech cues.

Although early expectations were limited to hopes that patients would be able to hear enough sound to increase speech-reading ability, many patients can now understand spoken words without speech-reading. Unfortunately, it isn't yet possible to predict who will benefit from a cochlear implant to that extent, nor how well one will work for any particular person. When tested, people with similar devices score from 0% to 90% on speech comprehension.

However, there are some risks involved in the operation. Besides the usual danger inherent in any surgery, the implant destroys residual hearing. There is also risk of skin infection at the surgical site, and possible damage to the facial nerve or vestibular system. However, incidence of damage to date has been slight.

Cochlear implants remain a somewhat controversial choice in the treatment of hearing problems. As yet, it is unclear how much help the implants can provide to hearing or learning spoken or sign language with children deaf from birth, and with those who lost their hearing before acquiring speech or language. Experts stress the implant is not for everyone, and research on its value is continuing. New research suggests that patients with some hearing before surgery do better than those who are profoundly deaf.

Also, new research with implants used in pre- and post-lingually deafened children suggests that they can achieve some awareness of sound with this device. Recently, research suggests some children deaf since birth can understand some words when using the multichannel implant system. The long-term changes due to implant and tissue interaction are unknown. New research suggests that a patient with 10% residual hearing who has been deaf 15 years has a 95% certainty of a word perception score above 25% after surgery.

Good candidates for implant surgery include those whose cochlea is completely ineffective but whose hearing nerve endings still respond to direct stimulation. In these cases, sound activating the implanted electrode stimulates the hearing nerve, and the person can hear noise that is usually described as different from the original sound. This difference occurs because the implant can't match the normal complex process of the ear as it converts sound into nerve impulses. Candidates for a cochlear implant include adults and children who meet the following general criteria:

Adults (18 years of age and older)

- Severe-to-profound sensorineural hearing loss in both ears
- Hearing loss acquired after learning oral speech and language
- Limited benefit from appropriate hearing aids; in other words, a score of 40% or less on sentence recognition tests in the best-aided listening condition
- No medical contraindications
- A desire to be part of the hearing world

Children

- Profound sensorineural hearing loss in both ears
- age two or above
- Little or no useful benefit from hearing aids
- No medical contraindications
- High motivation and appropriate expectations (both child and family)
- Placement in an educational program that emphasizes development of auditory skills after the implant has been fitted

Extensive testing is needed to determine if a patient might benefit from the cochlear implant, since the implant is designed only for those who receive little benefit from hearing aids. Candidates are usually at least two years old. Becoming a cochlear implant patient involves an evaluation, including otologic, audiologic, radiographic and psychological tests.

The first visit usually includes basic hearing tests, hearing aid testing and an examination by a doctor. An examination must be performed to assure there is no active infection or other problem within the middle or inner ear that would interfere with the surgical placement of the implant. Extensive hearing tests must be performed to determine the degree of hearing with and without a hearing aid. Special tests are performed to evaluate benefits from hearing aids. A special hearing test determines patient performance and capabilities with a hearing aid. Speech tests are required for all children and some adults. An electrical test is done that involves a stimulation of the inner ear to ensure the hearing nerve is intact and able to carry impulses to the brain. This test usually takes about an hour, and is only performed on adults. Other tests include a CT scan to show the condition of the cochlea and a psychological evaluation used to make sure the patient understands the process, to evaluate expectations and to evaluate children for any other factors (such as learning disabilities) that may affect performance of the implant.

Cochlear implant surgery is performed under general anesthesia. An incision is made behind the ear so that the mastoid bone leading to the middle ear can be opened. The operation takes from one and a half to five hours, depending on the specific cochlear implant being used, with a hospital stay from one night to several days.

The patient returns to the implant clinic one to two months after surgery to be fitted with the external portions of the device (signal processor, microphone, transmitter) and to learn how to care for and use the system. Cochlear implants differ in the amount of time required to fit them and the amount of training they require. In addition, patients are usually required to continue returning to the clinic at regular intervals for checkup and assessment.

The total cost of the cochlear implant varies, depending on the area of the country in which the surgery is done, but it is much more expensive than a hearing aid. Total costs (evaluation, surgery, device, rehabilitation) may range from between $15,000 to more than $40,000.

Because cochlear implants are medical devices, they are regulated by the Food and Drug Administration (FDA). Each new type of implant must be studied at cochlear implant clinics before it is approved by the FDA for general use. Whether a device is approved or still under investigation may make a difference as to who can receive the implant, how often return visits to the clinic are required and whether insurance companies will pay for the procedure. It will also make a difference in how much is known about the safety and benefits of a particular device. Each manufacturer of cochlear implants provides brochures and other patient information.

Research into new and better implants is continuing with the development of the first of a new generation of implants called the Nucleus 24RCS. It is expected that this new implant will significantly improve patients' ability to distinguish words and other sounds.

In addition, the new device is smaller, so that it will look better than earlier models and lessens the surgical risk to small children receiving implants. This is important, since infants are currently implanted with the same larger device given to adults, requiring special surgical techniques to avoid complications such as tissue death and infection.

The Nucleus 24RCS is a hybrid of the Nucleus 24M that combines the original device with a "curly electrode," a type of electrode that is wrapped around the acoustic nerve fibers; it is this proximity that allows patients to distinguish words and other sounds more easily. Being close to the nerve fibers also lessens the amount of power needed, so that the batteries last longer.

In other new research, Johns Hopkins University scientists discovered that profoundly deaf children who got a cochlear implant are more apt to be fully mainstreamed in schools and to use fewer school support services than similarly deaf children without an implant. The Johns Hopkins study is the first one in the United States to examine the use of special education help (such as speech therapy, interpreters and tutoring) in students with a cochlear implant. The implant appears to give children a significant educational advantage, offering the possibility for the development of verbal language. The results, however, largely depend on the type of rehabilitation the child receives.

FDA Requirements for Cochlear Implants

The FDA regulates medical devices to ensure their safety and effectiveness, and has set a number of requirements for anyone considering a cochlear implant. They require that implant candidates must:

- be severely to profoundly deaf;
- experience no significant benefit from hearing aids;
- be at least two years old (the age at which specialists can verify the severity of a child's deafness).

In addition, candidates should:

- be strong enough to withstand general anesthesia;
- be highly motivated and realistic about benefits;
- have an unscarred cochlea;
- have no current ear infection.

CHAPTER 6
ASSISTIVE DEVICES

If you have hearing problems, you're probably well aware of those times when it's especially hard to understand conversation or certain sounds. Maybe you miss hearing your alarm clock, or you have trouble understanding speech in a large hall. Some people have trouble with telephones.

Modern technology has come up with an astonishing array of assistive devices aimed at those with hearing problems. Today, you can take advantage of a variety of assistive listening systems, devices, communication aids and alerting devices. You may even want to get a "hearing dog" trained to react to sounds.

ALERTING DEVICES

If you can still hear some sounds, you may not need anything fancier than a loud windup alarm clock. Alternatively, you could try using a timer set to regulate lights on and off at specific times. Others may be interested in some of the wide range of alerting devices—compensatory devices that alert people to a sound (such as a doorbell, crying baby, telephone, timer) by activating a visual light signal.

Visual Alarms

Some of the most common assistive devices are those that alert you to a particular sound, such as a doorbell, timer, crying baby or telephone by activating a light signal. Visual alarms usually feature one or more flashing lights, turned on either through direct wiring or by using a signal transmitted through the building's wiring system. Some can even alert you to different sounds by using a different light pattern for each sound. Other lights can be set to go off when someone knocks at the door. Very bright strobe lights can be set to go off if the phone rings or a smoke alarm is triggered. Other devices can alert you that your car's turn signal has been left on while you're driving. Ordinary clock radios or electronic alarms can be adapted to flash one or several lights.

Vibrator Alarms

Ordinary clock radios or electronic alarms may also be adapted to turn on a small vibrator under the mattress or pillow. A doorbell can be hooked to this vibrating system; other devices vibrate a wristband to alert you to a ringing phone or other sounds.

Phone Ring Alternatives

If you can't seem to hear the phone ringing when you're in another part of the house and you don't care for alerting light devices, you do have alternatives:

- Make sure the phone is turned up to full volume (the adjustment knob is usually underneath the phone or on the side of a wall model).
- Have the phone company install a louder ringing device in the phone.
- Get a ring at a lower pitch.
- Have the phone company install extra ringing devices in other parts of the house.
- Add another phone and jack.
- Get a cordless phone and carry it with you around the house.

ASSISTIVE LISTENING DEVICES

Even with the most powerful hearing aid, you may find you still can't hear well in a large auditorium. Background noise will often interfere with comprehension, lessening your ability to pick up specific sounds.

Because of this, many large public meeting rooms are often equipped with one of a number of different alternative listening device systems, including induction systems, infrared systems, audio loop systems, direct audio input and extension microphones (including AM and FM transmission systems).

Many public places advertise their systems; all you have to do is ask which part of the room you should sit in. If you don't have a hearing aid with a T-switch to take advantage of these systems, you might be able to borrow a specially-equipped receiver.

There are many types of devices, including those that offer input to the ear, extension microphones and telephone and TV devices.

Induction Device

It's possible to generate a magnetic field capable of transmitting sound from a coil connected to a sound source that transmits sound to a specifically-equipped hearing aid. This coil can be a loop of wire worn around the neck, embedded in a small flat plastic device hooked over the ear, or placed in the receiver of a telephone. A second coil that picks up this magnetic signal is built into many hearing aids. Called a telecoil (or T-coil), it is activated by using the special "T-switch" on hearing aids.

The advantage of the T-coil is that it enables the microphone in the hearing aid to be turned off, so background noise doesn't interfere with sound from the induction system. For hearing aids without a T-switch, special receivers are available that have a telecoil that can pick up and amplify the inducted sound.

An induction loop system refers to a loop of wire placed around an entire room that is connected to a microphone and an amplifier. The system's microphone picks up sound and changes it into electrical energy that is then amplified and sent through the coil of a wire (or induction loop) strung around the room. The electrical energy flowing through the wire coil creates a magnetic field that can be picked up by anyone sitting within the loop who is wearing a hearing aid with a T-coil. The T-coil acts as antenna that picks up the electromagnetic energy and delivers it to the hearing aid's receiver, where the energy is converted into sound.

Direct Audio Input (DAI)

This device makes it possible to transfer sound directly to a hearing aid, taking advantage of the aid's amplification and eliminating through-the-air noise. With some aids, the DAI signal can be heard while in the T-mode, turning off the microphone and further eliminating background noise. The hearing aid, however, must be equipped to accept a DAI attachment.

Extension Microphones

An extension microphone is used to move the microphone closer to the sound source rather than to rely solely on the microphone built into the hearing aid. Because microphone sensitivity drops rapidly with distance, an extension improves the signal and tends to minimize background noise.

There are several types of extension microphones. "Hard-wired" devices consist solely of an additional microphone which is connected via cable to the hearing aid either by earphones, induction loop or DAI. Most devices need an amplifier worn in the pocket, on the belt, or held in the hand, but there are palm-sized models combining a microphone with amplifier. Super directional models can accurately pick up a voice six to ten feet away if there isn't too much background noise.

For people who need less amplification and don't wear a hearing aid, there are amplified microphones attached to a battery-powered pocket amplifier. The amplifier can be connected to the ear by an earphone or built-in speaker held close to the ear. As with the hard-wired microphone, this device's cable can be as long as necessary.

Personal FM wireless systems are considered to be the ultimate in extension microphones. This transmitter can broadcast 150 to 300 feet without connecting cables and can provide for another microphone in addition to the one built in. Receivers can use earphones, induction couplers, or DAI, but have no built-in speaker. Each unit is about the size of a cigarette package and can be useful in public auditoriums if the receiver frequency matches the one being broadcast.

The transmitter can be connected directly to the sound source, such as a TV or microphone; the sound is carried on a specific FM radio frequency through the air until it reaches the FM receiver tuned to the same frequency. The receiver changes the signal, and the electrical energy is sent to the ear through a headset or hearing aid. If a hearing aid with a T-coil is used, it can connect to a necklace loop attached to the receiver. FM systems can be very helpful for people with a profound hearing loss.

AM Listening Systems

A person with a hearing problem can listen via an individual AM receiver headset or a portable radio to sounds transmitted on an AM radio. The AM transmitter can also be connected to a public address system. Unfortunately, this system is open to the same interference that disrupts regular AM radio broadcasts.

FM Listening Systems

The frequency modulation (FM) system includes both a transmitter and receiver; it picks up sound and transmits it over a specific FM frequency for a distance up to 300 feet to a person wearing a special receiver. The FCC has set aside the FM frequencies between 72 and 76 megahertz for such use by both public and private systems.

The transmitter can be connected directly to the source of the sound, such as a TV set or a microphone; the sound is carried on a specific FM radio frequency through the air until it reaches an FM receiver tuned to the same frequency. The receiver changes the signal, and the electrical energy is sent to the ear, either through a headset or a hearing aid. If a hearing aid with a telecoil is used, it can connect to a necklace loop attached to the receiver.

Alternatively, a hearing aid with direct audio input capability can be linked to the FM systems with a special attachment called a boot, which fits on the bottom of a behind-the-ear aid and connects to the receiver by a wire. With characteristically good sound quality, the FM system can be very helpful for those with severe or profound hearing problems.

Infrared Systems

Some large group rooms and public places are equipped with a PA system that is plugged into an infrared light emitter that transmits sound via invisible light waves. An infrared transmitter can be connected directly to a sound source or a microphone; the transmitter then uses harmless infrared light to transmit sound to portable infrared receivers, available with headphones or "stethoscopes," which then change the signal into electrical energy and back into sound.

Although a person without a serious hearing loss may use the headphones without a hearing aid, someone with a greater hearing loss may connect a hearing aid directly to an infrared receiver or use the aid's telecoil capability together with a neck loop or silhouette inductor. With a neck loop, the infrared receiver sends the electrical signal to the loop, where it creates an electromagnetic signal picked up by the hearing aid. This signal is converted into electrical energy and then converted into sound at the aid's receiver.

Unlike FM transmission, light waves do not pass through walls and are not affected by neighboring radio frequency signals. However, infrared transmission may be affected by intense sunlight. Infrared devices are most helpful if you have a mild to moderately severe hearing loss.

TELEPHONE DEVICES

The telephone is often one of the biggest obstacles to communication for a deaf person because the sound is frequently distorted, and visual cues are impossible.

The hearing aid telecoil (T-coil) was developed in America to take advantage of a defect in telephone design—the fact that the magnetic signal "leaks" out of the phone. This noise "leak" can be picked up by a hearing aid equipped with a T-switch. In the United States, all telephones sold must be labeled "hearing aid compatible" and all public phones, by law, must meet these requirements.

Some telephone attachments can minimize the feedback that occurs when the telephone receiver is held against a hearing aid. For a less expensive approach, a plastic foam-filled cap designed for telephone comfort can be slipped over the receiver instead. Using a T-switch on the hearing aid with a compatible phone will also eliminate feedback.

An amplifying headset can be used that utilizes an amplifier built into the receiver with adjustments for volume control. One modular portable model may be substituted for unamplified handsets of similar modular units when away from home.

There are two types of attachable portable amplifiers. One type increases the audio signal either by slipping over the handset receiver or by plugging into the modular fitting at the base of the phone. The second type slips over the receiver and converts the audio signal into a strong magnetic signal that is then picked up by the T-switch of a hearing aid. There is also an attachable amplifier that combines both types.

TELECOMMUNICATIONS DEVICE FOR THE DEAF (TDD)

This mechanical device allows people to type phone messages over the telephone network. The "TDD" term is generic, and replaces the earlier term TTY, which referred specifically to teletypewriter machines. A TDD is basically a typewriter connected to a telephone line by a modular plug or acoustic modem. The conversation is displayed on a screen above the keyboard. Some TDDs have a printer, which provides a permanent record on special paper of all messages transmitted and received. A TDD is required at both ends of the phone line in order to communicate.

The TDD was invented in 1964 by Robert Weitbrecht, a deaf physicist and licensed ham radio operator, together with James Marsters, a deaf orthodontist. The two wanted to investigate the possible ways a hard-of-hearing person might communicate by using a TTY with a radio or telephone. Working together in California, the two decided a telephone system would be more logical since many hard-of-hearing people already had telephones in their homes. A radio system, they reasoned, would require the deaf person to get a license from the FCC.

In some states, phone companies lend or sell TDDs at subsidized prices, and more and more public agencies are installing them. In addition, relay services are available to connect TDD users and voice calls through an interpreter. By law as of 1991, every state must have a TDD relay service in place.

TDDs and computers use different codes for the letters of the alphabet and other characters, and therefore cannot normally communicate, although you can equip your personal computer with a modem to make it function like a TDD. (A modem is a device that allows a computer to use a telephone line to transmit information to other computers with compatible modems).

Most TDDs with built-in modems can understand only transmissions in the Baudot code. Personal computers use the ASCII code, and modems designed for use with a computer accommodate only that code. However, there are several modems available that have the ability to communicate in both Baudot and ASCII codes.

Today there are a wide variety of other TDD products. Some come in small, lightweight, portable sizes; some have built-in answering machines that respond only to TDD calls. There is also an answering machine that can respond to both voice and TDD calls.

In 1989, IBM introduced the Phone-Communicator, a system that allows a person with a TDD to communicate over phone lines with anyone owning an IBM compatible personal computer. The Phone-Communicator includes an automatic answer mode capable of recording messages from touchtone telephones and TDD callers.

The popularity of email and Internet communication may make the TDD less essential for communication in the deaf community.

Wireless TTY

This revolutionary new wireless service allows deaf and hard-of-hearing individuals to engage in near real-time telephone conversations while mobile and separated from traditional TTY (TDD) machines. Developed by reachNET, a Baltimore-based wireless technology company, "wireless TTY" gives the deaf community the same freedom and convenience that hearing individuals enjoy when using mobile telephones. Until now, wireless technologies for the deaf community have been restricted to two-way messaging and paging services. With wireless TTY, a deaf person can now make near real-time TTY calls anytime.

ReachNET is offering its Wireless TTY application via BellSouth Wireless Data's nationwide network, which covers more than 93% of the U.S. urban business population located in 492 Metropolitan Statistical Areas (MSAs) and non-MSAs with a total population of 200 million people.

Using the Wireless TTY application over the BellSouth network, individuals can place and receive calls to and from other TTY machines, and relay services or e-mail via the RIM Inter@ctive Pager 950, a compact handheld device that features a full keyboard and can be worn on a belt or slipped into a pocket. Once the two parties connect, they can engage in near real-time conversations.

Combining the features of a personal computer, pager, and cellular telephone, Wireless TTY provides a range of functions, including near real-time TTY service, e-mail, outgoing fax, two-way paging, an electronic address book and a vibrating alert.

ReachNET uses the latest technology to ensure the highest levels of service, including encryption technology that guards against eavesdropping, cloning and theft. The RIM Inter@ctive Pager 950 is manufactured by Research In Motion Limited, an Ontario, Canada-based company that develops leading-edge, wireless communications products.

Contact: ReachNET Web site at http://www.reachnet.net or by calling toll-free 1–888–RNET–008 or 1–877–RNET–TTY.

TDD Distribution Programs

Many states have programs that provide eligible deaf and hard-of-hearing people access to telephone communication. Usually they are administered by the state agency responsible for deaf programs. Once applicants are screened for medical and financial eligibility, they may be given a TDD at no charge, or allowed to buy one at substantially reduced rates.

Message Relay Service

In this one-way message service, an operator relays a message from a hearing person without a TDD to a deaf person who has a device (or vice versa). This is different from a "relay service" in which both hearing and deaf parties are on the line at the same time, with an operator acting as a go-between.

National Directory of TDD Numbers

You can buy a national directory of residential numbers of TDD users in each state together with a business section of listings by states in such categories as auxiliary (hearing and speech services), health (including mental health), human resources (including social services), interest groups (including associations and organizations) that can lead you to the professional mental health services you are seeking.

Copies are available for $20 plus $4 shipping/handling from: Telecommunications for the Deaf, Inc. (TDI) 8716 Colesville Road, #300, Silver Spring, MD 20910.

Devices for Professionals

Many professionals who don't use hearing aids require some amplification in special situations. A doctor with a mild hearing loss, for example, may benefit from an electronic stethoscope—and these are also available for patients with a hearing loss who need to hear heart sounds or to take blood pressures.

A nurse in a convalescent home who provides services to hearing-impaired people may find a portable amplifier useful to establish quick communication with non–hearing aid users. These devices include an old-fashioned speaking tube, horn or a handheld electronic communicator.

Autocuers

This speech processor breaks units of speech down into "cues." The equipment consists of special eyeglasses and a small boxlike speech processing microcomputer. Cues are activated by tiny light-emitting diodes, which show up in digital form on the eyeglasses worn by the deaf person. To use an autocuer, the deaf person reads the lips of the speaker as well as the cues on the eyeglasses in order to get the entire message. Cues and lips can be lined up and read at the same time by moving the head.

Tactile Feedback Device

This device provides a substitute for sounds the deaf person can't hear by converting sounds into a pattern of sensations on the skin. It's generally used in speech therapy, although it may also be used to help speech-read.

One typical device uses electrodes incorporated into a belt to stimulate the skin with electrical pulses that feel like finger taps; different sounds produce different patterns of stimulation. By learning what these sounds "feel" like, a person can learn them and eventually put these sounds together in words and sentences. Unfortunately, it's hard to produce enough distinct patterns with the electrodes to represent the large variety of sounds in speech.

TELEVISION DEVICES

An estimated 20 million Americans have enough of a hearing loss that they can't fully understand TV programs. Many of these individuals either choose ways to improve sound, or use some type of captioning for TV programs.

If a listening jack is provided on the TV set, you can simply plug in earphones. Other devices use a cable to connect a TV listening jack to the microphone jack of a portable amplifier. An extension microphone could be mounted near the TV speaker if there is no listening jack on the TV. A small portable radio that receives both UHF and VHF audio TV broadcasts (with better sound quality) can be placed nearby; the radio's speaker or its earphone can be used.

For people with a T-switch on their hearing aids, the audio induction loop will eliminate background noise. An amplifier that converts the TV audio signal to an induction signal is needed, and either a necklace loop or a loop system around the wall or under your chair can be used. Loop or wire can be permanently installed, avoiding a cable stretched across the room.

Infrared systems pick up the TV sound with a microphone and then transmit it by invisible infrared light (the same technique used for TV remote control units). A viewer wears a stethoscope type or clip-on receiver; sound is transmitted to the ear via earphone, neckloop or DAI.

Captioned TV

Captions are subtitles that appear on certain programs when a signal triggers a TeleCaption decoding device; captions enable even profoundly deaf people to understand TV programs and movies. Captions are made by translating the audio portion of a TV program into typed dialogue that usually appears across the bottom of the screen. American TV signals are made up of 525 lines, which include both the picture and a black bar made up of 21 lines, called the "vertical blanking interval." Digital information encoded on one or more of these 21 lines within the black bar can be transmitted to TV receivers, where they can be decoded and displayed on the TV screen. The 21st line is the bottom line of the vertical blanking system, and is used in this country for closed captioning.

Today, captions are produced at the headquarters of the National Captioning Institute in Falls Church, Va. and at the Caption Center at WGBH-TV in Boston. Since it first aired closed captions, the NCI's output has grown from an initial 16 hours of programming a week to almost 400 hours.

A free service of TV and cable networks and home video programs, captioning is funded by corporations, foundations, producers, networks and program sponsors. Private support of the service has increased since 1982, when all federal funding of the program stopped. The NCI Caption Club was formed in 1983 to accept contributions toward expanding the number of closed-captioned programs.

Published TV schedules usually mark captioned programs with a "C" or "CC"—and the TeleCaption decoder itself provides a Program Listing Update Service (PLUS), which is a daily listing of captioned programs and sponsors.

Caption-Capable TV Sets

In the past, a special decoder on top of the TV set was needed to receive and translate closed captions within TV programs. However, federal legislation passed in 1990 required all TV sets with screens 13 inches or larger manufactured for sale in the United States to include built-in closed caption decoders. Called the Television Decoder Act of 1990, the law required built-in decoder circuitry in most new television receivers as of 1993, and charged the FCC with developing standards for the new decoders. The FCC turned to the Electronic Industries Association (EIA) to determine the caption features that could be implemented and how decoders could be improved.

During an EIA-suggested transition period, all new features need to be backward compatible to work with the set-top decoders sold since 1980. As a result, features such as new placement options and an extended character set are being phased in gradually. The EIA estimates more than 20 million new televisions with built-in decoders are sold each year. That means every home in America will have at least one decoder-equipped television by 2000. The original caption decoders (TeleCaption I) went on sale in 1980. These models were sold as stand-alone decoders or were built into television sets. Five years later, the National Captioning Institute introduced the TeleCaption II. This same basic decoder design was also used in subsequent set-top models TeleCaption 3000, TeleCaption 4000 and TeleCaption VR 100. However, set-top decoder sales never reached more than about 350,000 homes. There was a huge difference between the number of decoders sold and the potential audience for captioning—22 million deaf and hard-of-hearing viewers. Many viewers who could benefit from captioning didn't buy a decoder either because of cost, installation problems or because consumers were unaware of the service. These factors, combined with the potential educational benefits of captioning for millions of children and adults struggling with literacy or learning English as a second language, were the reason Congress passed the Television Decoder Circuitry Act of 1990.

Several companies still manufacture set-top decoders. Since the FCC only regulates receivers, these decoders are not necessarily FCC compliant, and the decoders might not respond correctly to new features. The Caption Center regularly tests new set-top decoders to determine if they are compatible with the new features. (For a list of professional or consumer-grade decoder manufacturers, contact The Caption Center.)

Since many older set-top decoders aren't compatible with many of the features outlined in the FCC rules, a transition schedule was designed to phase in the various new caption features. All caption providers should adhere to this schedule. The TeleCaption I decoder (pre-1985) will be the first to become obsolete. Caption agencies send special compatibility codes for the TeleCaption II (TC 3000, 4000 and VR 100), but these decoders won't be able to display relocatable roll-up or mid-screen placement. In 2002 these compatibility codes will be phased out, and the TeleCaption II generation will no longer function correctly.

Captioning in six colors (cyan, yellow, green, magenta, red and blue) has been a part of the basic decoder specification from the beginning, but set-top decoders never implemented this feature. Today, codes for color captions don't adversely affect older decoders; all the captions simply display as white text on a black background. (Receivers with built-in Tele-Caption I decoders marketed by Sears in the early '80s were able to display color captions, although very few of these units are still in service.)

Almost all modern receivers containing FCC-compliant decoders implement the color feature. Caption text may be white or in one of the seven colors, as determined by the caption service provider. The color of the background (usually black) is determined by the receiver manufacturer.

The TeleCaption II generation of decoders included some new features that were incompatible with the original TeleCaption I. The most important of these is paint-on style. When the TeleCaption I decoder receives paint-on style, it ignores the paint-on caption and displays no caption at all. It remains in this state until it receives a pop-on or roll-up caption, which are the most common types of captions. Also added in 1985 were 11 new characters (Ç, Ñ, °, à, è, â, ê, î, ô, û and the transparent space), which don't display correctly on the TeleCaption I. These characters don't make the TeleCaption I stop working; they just appear as incorrect characters. In mid-1994, caption service providers began using features that were not completely compatible with the TeleCaption I.

Captioned Media Program

Today captions appear not just on TV programs, but on most movie videos as well. The Captioned Media Program is a free loan service of theatrical and educational films and videos captioned for deaf viewers that was set up in 1958 by the Department of Education. The program also provides money for several closed-captioned TV programs, including the live-captioned news on the ABC, NBC and CBS networks. The program grew out of a private, nonprofit corporation established by the Junior League of Hartford and the convention of American Instructors of the Deaf that was designed to caption films for deaf viewers. Because the expense and size of the job soon became too much for the small company, Congress passed PL 85-905, which established Captioned Films for the Deaf (now the Captioned Media Program) as a government service.

All videos are open captions, and there are more than 4,000 titles in the library with more than 300 added each year. Educational videos include all school subjects from preschool through college, together with appropriate lesson guides. General interest videos include movie classics, travel, hobbies and recreation.

Deaf individuals, parents and teachers may borrow videos by filling out an application form (also available on-line). Videos may be ordered through the mail or from the Internet free of charge; prepaid return labels are included.

For more information contact: Captioned Media Program, 1447 E. Main St., Spartanburg, SC (29307; (800) 237–6213 or TDD: (800) 237–6819; http://www.cfv.org.

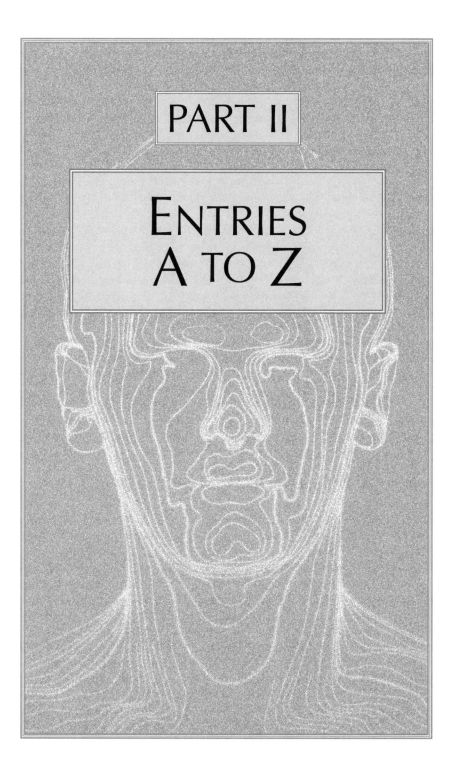

PART II

ENTRIES
A TO Z

A

ABLEDATA An information and referral project that maintains a database of more than 25,000 assistive technology products. The project also produces fact sheets on types of devices and other aspects of assistive technology. Contact: ABLEDATA at 8455 Colesville Road, Suite 935, Silver Spring, MD 20910; telephone (voice): (800) 227–0216 or (301) 608–8998; (TDD) (301) 608–8912; website: http://www.abledata.com

Academy of Dispensing Audiologists A professional association formed in 1977 to support the dispensing of hearing aids by AUDIOLOGISTS with advanced degrees in rehabilitative practice. The ADA holds an annual meeting in the fall together with seminars providing information on all aspects of hearing aid dispensing. They publish a quarterly magazine (*Feedback*) for professionals but do not offer information for consumers.

acoupedic method See AUDITORY-ORAL METHOD.

Acoustical Society of America The premier scientific society in acoustics, dedicated to increasing the knowledge of acoustics and its practical applications. Founded in 1929, this group holds regular meetings to discuss research, and publishes the *Journal of the Acoustical Society of America*. The society holds two meetings a year to discuss current research.

Acoustic Neuroma Association A professional association that provides information and support to patients with an ACOUSTIC NEUROMA or other problems affecting the cranial nerves. Founded by a patient in 1981, the nonprofit group provides information on patient rehabilitation to health care professionals, promotes research on acoustic neuroma and provides information to the public on symptoms, diagnosis and treatment.

The association publishes a quarterly newsletter, distributes a patient information booklet, presents a twice-yearly national symposium, provides access to a network of local support groups, compiles a registry of statistical data on acoustic neuroma treatment and maintains a website for patient information and discussion. Contact address: PO Box 12402, Atlanta, GA 30355; telephone 404–237–8023; website: http://132.183.175.10/ana/m.

acoustic reflex A reflex contraction of a small muscle in the middle ear that stiffens the chain of ossicles (hammer, anvil, stirrup) to protect the inner ear.

acoustics The science concerning the properties, production, control, transmission, reception and effects of sound. Thus subdivision of physics, has two major branches: architectural acoustics and environmental acoustics.

Architectural acoustics involves the study of how sound waves operate in closed spaces and how to create the best acoustical conditions for a variety of purposes (such as sound transmission in concert halls and theaters). Environmental acoustics focuses on noise pollution and its control, including improved insulation, room partitions and so forth.

Other minor branches include musical acoustics (the operation and design of musical instruments and the study of how musical sounds affect listeners), engineering acoustics (development of high-fidelity sound recording and reproduction), ultrasonics (acoustical phenomena with vibration rates above the audible range of 20,000 hertz), underwater sound, mechanical vibration and shock and speech communication.

acoustic spectrum The distribution of the intensity levels of various frequency components of a sound.

acupuncture Acupuncture has been used to treat SENSORINEURAL HEARING LOSS and Ménière's disease.

adenoidectomy The surgical removal of the ADENOIDS, the twin lymph nodes at the back of the nose above the tonsils. This operation is usually performed on a child with abnormally large adenoids that are causing recurrent middle ear or sinus infections which could lead to hearing loss. Often, an adenoidectomy is performed at the same time as a tonsillectomy.

There are few aftereffects of the operation, and the patient can usually begin to eat normal meals one day afterward.

adenoids The two lymph nodes above the tonsils at the back of the nose that are partly responsible for protecting the body's upper respiratory tract against infection. Although they tend to enlarge during childhood when these types of infections are common, adenoids usually shrink after about age five and disappear by adolescence.

However, they sometimes continue to grow, obstructing the eustachian tube and causing hearing problems. In addition, secretions behind the nose that are obstructed by oversized adenoids can lead to infections of the nose (rhinitis) that can spread to the middle ear.

Occasional infections can be treated with antibiotics, but surgery to remove the adenoids (ADENOIDECTOMY) may be needed if infections become chronic.

AIDS.Net   A special computer bulletin board established by DEAFTEK. USA, a nonprofit group providing electronic mail service for deaf and hard-of-hearing people. AIDS.Net is an information-sharing network about AIDS established after a conference on AIDS and deafness held in 1988 in Toronto.

Information for the bulletin is provided by agencies and professionals serving deaf people. Currently, members in the United States, Canada and England are participating in AIDS.Net. Subscribers are also free to ask questions of experts provided by the bulletin board. CONTACT: International Communications Ltd., PO Box 2431, Framingham, MA 01701; telephone 508–620–1777 (voice/TDD).

Alberti, Salomon (1540–1600)   This 16th century German physician and professor at the University of Wittenborg was the first to call attention to people hard of hearing—those who can hear loud sounds and are not deaf—and attributed deafness to "some lack" in the development of the fetus. He claims to have discovered the cochlea, and knew about the modiolus.

Alexander Graham Bell Association for the Deaf   A private, non-profit organization serving as an information center, publisher and advocate of effective ways of teaching deaf and hard-of-hearing persons to improve their abilities to speak, speechread, use residual hearing and process spoken and written language. It also aims to empower those with hearing problems to function independently.

Since its inception in 1890 as the American Association to Promote the Teaching of Speech to the Deaf, the association has had one primary purpose: to promote the use of speech, SPEECHREADING and residual hearing by hard-of-hearing people.

Most of the first members of the group were articulation teachers who used the VISIBLE SPEECH method, a system of written symbols representing the anatomical formation of speech sounds, invented by Alexander Melville Bell (Alexander Graham's father). Since then, the association has grown into an international organization serving 4,500 members in 38 countries. Its members fall into four categories: professionals in the deafness field, parents of hard-of-hearing children, deaf adults who can speak and speechread and others who believe in the importance of oral communication.

Although it began as an active proponent of speech for deaf people, the organization has gradually expanded its interests to include research, family support and financial assistance to help deaf students attend classes with hearing peers. It also sponsors workshops and biennial conventions and publishes the *Volta Review,* a professional journal published six times a year; *Newsounds,* a newsletter published 10 times a year; and *Our Kids Magazine.* In addition, the association sells books of interest to members through mail-order catalogs and presents books on various oral topics for teachers, parents and deaf and hard-of-hearing adults.

Three distinct sections within the organization focus on the needs of three specific groups: deaf adults (Oral Deaf Adults Section), parents (International Parents Organization) and teachers (International Organization for the Education of the Hearing Impaired).

Oral Deaf Adults Section   This voluntary, nonprofit service section was formed in 1964 to help improve the education, employment and social opportunities of deaf people. Members receive a newsletter, a membership directory and scholarship support and have access to programs designed to help parents of children with hearing problems.

International Parents Organization   This section provides special help to families of children with hearing problems who are interested in promoting aural/oral education. Membership is open to any member of the association and includes a magazine, *Our Kids Magazine,* family workshops, educational scholarships and a family support network throughout the United States and Canada.

International Organization for the Education of the Hearing Impaired
This special section, formed in 1967, promotes excellence in aural/oral education for deaf children and adults. The aims of this group include the development of effective oral education and communication programs, research into oral communication and an information exchange among educators. (See also BELL, ALEXANDER GRAHAM; VOLTA BUREAU.)

Contact: Alexander Graham Bell Association for the Deaf, 3417 Volta Place NW, Washington, DC 20007; telephone (voice and TDD): 202–337–5220; website http://www.agbell.org.

Ambrosi, Gustinus (1893–1975)   Born in Eisenstadt, Austria, this talented musician and sculptor was best known for his classic sculptures in bronze and marble.

A child prodigy on the violin, he lost his hearing at the age of six after a bout of meningitis and smashed his treasured instrument when he realized he could no longer hear. However, as Ambrosi grew to adulthood he began to consider his deafness a blessing in disguise.

Finding he was no longer able to continue in music, Ambrosi studied woodcarving at the age of eight and became an apprentice at 14 with a sculpting firm in Prague. Within five years he had won two major art prizes, and in 1908 Emperor Fran Joseph gave him lifetime use of an atelier.

Considered a Renaissance man, Ambrosi was a gifted poet, graphic artist and philosopher, although he was known primarily for his lifelike busts.

When old age began to interfere with his ability to sculpt, Ambrosi committed suicide on July 1, 1975 in Vienna.

American Academy of Audiology   A professional membership organization of AUDIOLOGISTS that provides an annual national meeting to exchange research and information about hearing science and hearing aids. The group does not provide consumer outreach.

American Academy of Otolaryngology–Head and Neck Surgery The largest professional organization in this field, representing physicians who specialize in the treatment and surgery of the ear, nose and throat and related structures of the head and neck. It provides continuing medical education and various professional publications and also presents the interests of otolaryngologists to legislators. Its annual convention includes an intensive continuing education program offering a wide range of courses in the latest research and advanced techniques in cosmetic facial reconstruction, cancer surgery, patient management and treatment of allergic, sinus, laryngeal, thyroid and esophageal disorders.

The association publishes leaflets related to ear problems and a monthly journal, *Otolaryngology-Head and Neck Surgery* and also provides physician referrals. (See also OTOLARYNGOLOGIST.) Contact: American Academy of Otolaryngology–Head and Neck Surgery, One Prince St., Alexandria, VA 22316; telephone: 703–836–4444; TDD: (703) 519–1585; http://www.entnet.org.

American Annals of the Deaf   The oldest professional educational journal in the United States, *American Annals of the Deaf* is published jointly five times a year by the Convention of American Instructors of the Deaf (CAID) and the Conference of Educational Administrators Serving the Deaf (CEASD).

The journal, which was first published in 1847 by the faculty of the American School for the Deaf in Hartford, Connecticut, has passed through many different editorial hands. Its primary focus is to publish information of broad interest to those concerned with the education of deaf people. This information includes statistics on deafness, research into the psychology and sociology of deafness, conference reports and philosophical discussions. In addition, the publication includes an annual directory of services for the deaf. Contact: *American Annals of the Deaf,* Gallaudet University, 800 Florida Ave. NE, Washington, DC 20002.

American Association for the Promotion of the Teaching of Speech to the Deaf   The original name of the ALEXANDER GRAHAM BELL ASSOCIATION FOR THE DEAF, this group—founded in 1890—first changed its name to the Volta Speech Association for the Deaf in 1948 and then changed to its present name in 1953.

American Association of the Deaf-Blind   An organization that promotes better opportunities and services for deaf-blind people and assures that a comprehensive, coordinated system of services is accessible to all deaf-blind people, enabling them to achieve their maximum potential through increased independence, productivity, and integration into the community. The biannual conventions provide a week of workshops, meetings, tours and recreational activities. The group also publishes *The Deaf-Blind American*. Contact: American Association of the Deaf-Blind, 814 Thayer Ave., Room 302, Silver Spring, MD 20910–4500; telephone (TDD): 301–588–6545; email: aadb@erols.com

American Athletic Association of the Deaf (AAAD)   Founded in 1945, this group was established to encourage athletic graduates of deaf schools to continue in sports competition. It promotes intramural competition among deaf athletic clubs, supervises regional tournaments and, since 1957, gives financial support to deaf athletes wishing to participate in the WORLD GAMES FOR THE DEAF.

From the early 1900s, deaf athletes discussed the possibility of having a national basketball tournament for deaf people. In 1945 the first competition for the National Basketball Champion of the Deaf was held in Akron, Ohio, pitting top players from teams in Akron, Buffalo, Philadelphia, Kansas City and Los Angeles. (Buffalo won the tournament.) At the same time, members from the deaf clubs all over the country voted to make the tournament an annual event and formed the American Athletic Union of the Deaf to oversee its organization. The AAUD later changed its name to the American Athletic Association of the Deaf to avoid its being confused with the Amateur Athletic Union of the United States.

After the AAAD became affiliated with the Comité International des Sports des Sourds, sponsor of the World Games of the Deaf, the AAAD was able to hold three World Games for the Deaf in the United States: summer games in Washington, D.C. (1965) and in Los Angeles (1985) and winter games in Lake Placid, N.Y. (1975).

The AAAD, which administers more than 150 clubs in eight regions, sponsors annual basketball and softball tournaments, names an annual Athlete of the Year and hosts an AAAD Hall of Fame to honor outstanding deaf athletes, coaches and sports figures. In addition, AAAD is affiliated with four national athletic organizations (skating, ice hockey, tennis and volleyball), the U.S. Olympic Committee's Handicap in Sports Committee and the Amateur Softball Association. Contact: American Athletic Association of the Deaf, Inc., 3607 Washington Blvd. #4, Ogden, UT 84403; TDD 801–393–7916; email: AAADEAF@aol.com.

American Coalition of Citizens with Disabilities   This national nonprofit group, founded in 1974 by the directors of about 150 disabilities groups, was the only one of its kind directed by disabled people. Although no longer in existence, at one time it promoted the human and civil rights of America's 30 million disabled people on local, state and national levels, encouraged research and training and provided information and referral programs.

The coalition also published the *ACCD Newsnet,* which covered disability-related issues and books related to disabilities.

American Deafness and Rehabilitation Association (ADARA)   A nonprofit, interdisciplinary group that promotes efforts to improve and expand rehabilitation services for deaf people, encourage research in deafness and promote the recruitment and training of professionals to work and communicate with deaf individuals.

Formerly called the Professional Rehabilitation Workers with the Adult Deaf (PRWAD), the organization was founded at a national conference of the Rehabilitation Services Administration in 1966. At that time, there was no national group serving those who worked with deaf people (the Convention of American Instructors of the Deaf was only interested in education and teachers, and the National Rehabilitation Association had no section for those who worked with deaf clients). The PRWAD welcomed rehabilitation counselors, psychologists, social workers and other professionals whose clientele were mostly deaf people.

After several years of debate, the name was changed to its present form during the group's 1978 convention, placing "deafness" before "rehabilitation."

Today, ADARA works closely with other organizations to develop legislation serving the needs of deaf people and publishes the quarterly *Journal of the American Deafness and Rehabilitation Association* as well as various monographs sold as separate publications. The association also organizes national and regional conferences, workshops, training seminars and continuing education programs.

Although ADARA does not conduct research itself, its conferences and publications provide scientists with information and bibliographical support. The biennial conference provides a forum for professionals to learn about developments in the field, special problem areas and new treatments and advances. Several states have chapters that continue the work of the national group at the local level.

ADARA has grown from a group of about 300 in 1967 to more than 2,000 members in 1991. Separate sections within the organization address DEAF-BLINDNESS, mental health counseling, social work, and vocational and psychological assessment. Contact: American Deafness and Rehabilitation Association, PO Box 27, Roland, AR 72135; telephone (voice and TDD) 650–372–0620.

American Hearing Research Foundation A nonprofit agency that promotes and finances medical research into the causes and treatments of deafness, hearing problems and balance disorders, encourages collaboration between clinical and laboratory research and works to broaden teaching and professional aims. Contact: American Hearing Research Foundation, 55 E. Washington St. Suite 2022, Chicago, IL 60602; telephone: 312–726–9695.

American Humane Association A national federation of local, state and regional animal care and control agencies that started the first formal hearing ear dog training program in 1976 and helped create other training programs across the country.

Today, American Humane's Center for Hearing Dog Information assists local hearing dog training programs through publications and training aids and helps deaf individuals obtain dogs of their own. (See also CENTER FOR HEARING EAR DOGS; HEARING EAR DOGS.) Contact: American Humane Association, P.O. Box 1266, Denver, CO 80201; telephone: 303–695–0811 (voice); 303–695–4531 (TDD).

American Laryngological, Rhinological and Otological Society A national society of OTOLARYNGOLOGISTS and head and neck surgeons that provides continuing educational opportunities for its members through its meetings. Four section meetings and an annual meeting are held each year.

American manual alphabet See FINGERSPELLING.

American Ministries to the Deaf An evangelical organization whose aim is to proclaim the gospel of Jesus Christ among deaf people around the world. Contact: American Ministries to the Deaf, 7564 Brown's Mill Road, Kaufman Station, Chambersburg, PA 17201; telephone (voice and TDD): 717–375–2610.

American Otological Society A professional organization whose mission is to advance and promote medical and surgical OTOLOGY, including the rehabilitation of hearing impairment, and to encourage and promote research in otology and related disciplines.

American School for the Deaf The oldest school for deaf students in the United States. It offers a wide range of programs guided by the TOTAL COMMUNICATION philosophy—a philosophy implying acceptance of all methods of communication (speech, speechreading, aural, oral, American Sign Language and other manual communication systems).

The school began as a joint collaboration between THOMAS HOPKINS GALLAUDET, a young Andover, Massachusetts divinity student, and Dr. MASON

FITCH COGSWELL, a surgeon and professor at Yale Medical School. When Dr. Cogswell saw Gallaudet's success at teaching Cogswell's young deaf daughter, he was inspired with the idea of reaching other hard-of-hearing students around the country. Gallaudet was sent to Europe by Cogswell and the Hartford, Connecticut city fathers to study both the French and English methods of teaching deaf students.

However, when Gallaudet arrived in England, he discovered that the founder of the English method demanded payment in turn for sharing his knowledge of deaf education. Unable to pay, Gallaudet continued on to France.

In Paris, Gallaudet worked closely with ABBÉ ROCH AMBROISE CUCURRON SICARD, director of the French Institute for the Deaf (now the Institut National des Jeunes Sourds) and his two assistants, JEAN MASSIEU and LAURENT CLERC. Eventually, Gallaudet returned to the United States with Clerc to set up a school for deaf students in Hartford.

The American School for the Deaf (originally known as the American Asylum for the Education and Instruction of Deaf and Dumb Persons) opened its doors April 15, 1817, with a class of seven students.

Immediately successful, it became the first recipient of state aid to elementary and secondary education in the United States when the state government awarded the school a legislative grant in 1819.

Since then, almost 5,000 students have graduated from this school, which has evolved from a small educational institution for deaf children to a multifaceted organization offering more than 75 different programs and services to the deaf community and the general public, including:

- Parent-Child Counseling Program—a home-based early intervention program serving families of hard-of-hearing infants and children through school age.
- PACES program—comprehensive and highly structured psychoeducational and dormitory life for emotionally and behaviorally disordered hard-of-hearing children and adolescents.
- Adult Vocational Services—New England's center for vocational rehabilitation services for hard-of-hearing individuals seeking job training and skills necessary for employment. The comprehensive resource center serves deaf people who need help preparing for, finding and keeping jobs.
- Community Audiological Services—a comprehensive hearing health care service including hearing tests; hearing aid evaluations, dispensing, fitting and repair; earmold impressions; and electroacoustical analysis of hearing aids and amplifications equipment.
- Camp Isola Bella—a recreational residential summer camp for deaf children between ages 6 and 18, located in the southern Berkshire hills of Salisbury, Connecticut.

Other services at the American School for the Deaf include preschool and kindergarten programs; academic and vocational instruction; residential opportunities; extracurricular, cultural and social activities (scouting, athletics, Junior Achievement, student body government); professional consultation and training; and summer recreation and education programs. Contact: American School for the Deaf, 139 N. Main St., West Hartford, CT 06107; telephone (voice and TDD): 203–727–1300.

American Sign Language (ASL) A visual-gestural language used as a primary means of communication by a very large portion of the deaf population in the United States (estimates suggest between 100,000 to 500,000 people). Often called the language of deaf people, ASL has a unique grammar and syntax and is unrelated to English, although it reflects English influences. It also includes FINGERSPELLING (the manual alphabet) to spell out words, including proper names and technical phrases. Some deaf individuals use sign exclusively, others use ASL in combination with SIGNED ENGLISH.

For many years, ASL was not considered a language at all. Critics claimed it lacked grammatical structure and warned that it relegated deaf people to an isolated subculture. Because ASL was considered "grammatically incorrect" by many educators, its usage was forbidden in schools and educational programs for deaf children. Thus, for years ASL was considered a suppressed language, despite its wide use by deaf children and adults from one generation to the next.

However, on the basis of new research, linguists today believe ASL is indeed a language—a visual language that requires many nonmanual features, including facial expressions and body language. It is passed on from parents to children, and children whose parents are deaf and fluent signers learn ASL as a first language.

Many linguists believe that it is only when sign language differs completely from English that it may properly be called AMERICAN SIGN LANGUAGE, although some use ASL as a catch-all term to describe a whole range of manual communication.

At one extreme of the sign language continuum is FINGERSPELLING, in which handshapes are used to spell out each word of the English language while speaking or moving lips. This method (also called the Rochester method or visible English) is occasionally used in a few schools, but it is an unpopular method of communication and can be tiring to use and interpret.

Farther along on the continuum are MANUALLY CODED ENGLISH systems, which use fingerspelling but also include signs and markers. The most common forms of this system are SIGNED ENGLISH and SIGNING EXACT ENGLISH, which base their signs on ASL but include other aspects of the English language.

They often use the first letter of the word (also called initialization) with the basic movement of the sign to give hints to the intended word. These systems also include markers for prefixes, suffixes, plural endings and tenses, together with signs for articles, infinitives and all forms of the verb "to be." Although this system is often used in schools, it is not used by deaf adults except for some initial signs and endings that have found their way into popular usage.

In the middle of the sign language continuum is a system called PID-GIN SIGN ENGLISH (PSE), the system used most often by hearing people learning to communicate with deaf people.

PSE combines the English language with the vocabulary and non-manual features of ASL and is the preferred method of communication by many deaf people. Signs for definite and indefinite articles are omitted, and only one sign is used for the verb "to be" unlike the manually coded English systems.

Finally, American Sign Language, when used in its true sense to mean the patterns used by deaf persons when they communicate in sign in a non-English style, is at the other end of the sign language continuum.

Studies have shown that signs used this way are indeed a recognizable language with its own grammatical pattern, and nonmanual behaviors are an important part of this system. Neither articles nor speech are used, although fingerspelling is used for proper names.

In the United States, variations in ASL can often be traced to different residential schools and educational programs for different deaf communities. For example, the segregation of black deaf students in the South resulted in a variation of ASL used by the majority of the white population. It featured different words and even some different grammatical structures.

The acceptance and resultant surge in the use of ASL by both deaf and hearing people is reflected in the increase of ASL classes, videos and instructional books. Today, ASL has been incorporated with Signed English, speech, speechreading and other modes of communication in many educational programs for deaf students from elementary to postsecondary levels.

Still, there is some resistance to the use of ASL, especially in education where many school officials acknowledge the language but do not officially recognize it as a teaching tool. Despite research to the contrary, these school administrators believe teaching is ASL will interfere with the development of English skills.

In fact, there is still disagreement among deaf people themselves about ASL. Some find a source of pride and an example of cultural identity in the language, but others feel more ambivalent about its use in the wider hearing society. (See also SIGN LANGUAGE; SIGN LANGUAGE INTERPRETERS; SIMULTANEOUS COMMUNICATION; TOTAL COMMUNICATION.)

American Sign Language Teachers Association A national professional organization of AMERICAN SIGN LANGUAGE and deaf studies teachers (formerly known as the Sign Instructors Guidance Network, or SIGN). SIGN was originally formed in 1975 by the NATIONAL ASSOCIATION OF THE DEAF Communicative Skills Program (CSP) to meet the increasing demand for qualified ASL teachers. To promote high quality instruction, teacher evaluations were held in conjunction with biennial NAD conventions and other ASL-related conferences since 1976. Local SIGN chapters were established in 1985, and by 1992 members of SIGN overwhelmingly endorsed a proposal to rename the organization to the American Sign Language Teachers Association (ASLTA).

By 1999, ASLTA had expanded to 25 local chapters. It publishes a newsletter, advocates for legislation recognizing ASL as a language and promotes the hiring of certified teachers of ASL. ASLTA has more than 800 members, including more than 200 certified teachers of ASL. The organization aims to provide an effective avenue for ASL and deaf studies teachers to exchange information on language and culture, instructional methods, materials and evaluation techniques. Contact: American Sign Language Teachers Association at http:www.aslta.org.

American Society for Deaf Children (ASDC) An organization providing advocacy, information and support to more than 20,000 parents, professionals and families with deaf or hard-of-hearing children. The organization was founded in 1967 by members of the CONVENTION OF AMERICAN INSTRUCTORS OF THE DEAF and promotes TOTAL COMMUNICATION as a way of life for deaf children and their families.

ASDC is the only national, independent, nonprofit organization whose sole purpose is to provide support, encouragement and information about deafness to families of deaf and hard-of-hearing children. The fundamental goal of ASDC is to improve education for deaf and hard-of-hearing students and to involve parents in the decision-making process.

Its "Two Years of Love" program includes a range of personalized services presented to a family with a deaf child—ASDC membership and a monthly shipment of books, toys, letters and journals.

In addition, the group provides a speakers' bureau, sponsors task forces, holds regional meetings and a biennial convention, and publishes various brochures, position papers and a quarterly newsletter, *The Endeavor.*

Parent groups can become affiliate members of ASDC, and organizations, agencies and educational institutions can become organization-affiliate members. Contact: American Society for Deaf Children, 1820 Tribute Road, Ste., A, Sacramento, CA 95815; telephone (voice and TDD): 800–942–ASDC; email ASDC@aol.com

American Speech-Language-Hearing Association (ASHA)   The national professional and scientific organization founded in 1925 for speech language pathologists and audiologists concerned with communication disorders. The group provides information and a toll-free helpline number (800–897–8682) for individuals with questions about speech, language or hearing problems.

With more than 40,000 members, ASHA maintains high standards of professional competence, develops good clinical service programs, stimulates research and offers continuing communication about speech and hearing.

New members must hold a graduate degree (or equivalent) in speech-language pathology, speech and hearing science, audiology or allied disciplines. Members in independent clinical practice must meet specific requirements in order to receive the Certificate of Clinical Competence.

Publications include three quarterly publications, *Journal of Speech and Hearing Disorders, Journal of Speech and Hearing Research* and *Language, Speech and Hearing Services in Schools* in addition to monographs, reports and directories. (See also JOURNALS IN THE FIELD OF DEAFNESS.) Contact: American Speech-Language-Hearing Association, 10801 Rockville Pike, Rockville, MD 20852; telephone (voice and TDD): 800–638–8255; email: irc@asha.org.

Americans with Disabilities Act   This law signed in 1990 guarantees a number of rights to all handicapped Americans in four important areas: employment, transportation, public services and telecommunications.

Specifically, the law applies to deaf people as follows:

- A job can't be denied a deaf person if that person is qualified for the job. Businesses must make "reasonable accommodation" for deaf employees—including TDD (TELECOMMUNICATIONS DEVICE FOR THE DEAF) availability and interpreters.
- Medium- and large-sized hospitals, libraries, museums, hotels, restaurants, stores, parks and zoos must make interpreters and TDDs accessible for deaf patrons.
- By 1993, the United States must have developed a TDD relay system for all its deaf citizens, which will allow deaf people to call anyone anywhere at anytime.
- All public service announcements produced or funded by the federal government must be closed captioned. In hotels and hospitals, closed captioning must be made available on request in hotels with TVs in at least five rooms; all hospitals that provide TVs must provide access to closed captions.

American Tinnitus Association   This nonprofit group founded in 1971 provides education and information about TINNITUS to patients and professionals in addition to raising money for research.

Founded by Dr. Charles Unice, who suffers with severe tinnitus himself, the organization offers a wide range of services, including information
and a resource center, referral to a worldwide network of tinnitus clinics,
local self-help groups and activities, professional workshops and seminars,
counseling and guidelines for organizing tinnitus self-help groups and
publishes a newsletter about tinnitus. Contact: American Tinnitus Association, P.O. Box 5, Portland, OR 97207; telephone: 503–248–9985; email:
tinnitus@ata.org.

Ameslan   See AMERICAN SIGN LANGUAGE.

amplitude   One of three measurements detecting the vibration of a
sound wave (the other two are wavelength and frequency). Amplitude is
the vertical vibration that reflects the intensity of sound.

aphasia   A disturbance in the ability to speak, write and/or comprehend
and read, aphasia is caused by damage to the brain rather than by a problem with hearing or sight. Most often, head injury or a stroke in the dominant cerebral hemisphere—especially the Wernicke's and Broca's areas
important for language—causes the brain damage that results in aphasia.

Some recovery can be expected following head injury or stroke with
speech therapy. In general, the more severe the aphasia, the less chance
for recovery.

Architectural and Transportation Barriers Compliance Board   This
independent federal agency is responsible for enforcing the ARCHITECTURAL
BARRIERS ACT of 1968, which prohibits architectural barriers to the handicapped in federally-funded buildings and public transportation systems.
(These buildings cannot have barriers to people in wheelchairs or using
crutches or who are blind or deaf. Buildings and transportation systems
covered by this act must meet the minimum standards for accessibility
established by the American National Standards Institute.)

Any person who believes there has been a violation of the act in a
building built with federal funds can file a written complaint with the
board describing the problem and giving the name and address of the
building.

The board, which investigates every complaint it receives, first seeks
voluntary compliance in a friendly, informal way if a violation is found. If
no informal resolution is possible, the board's executive director may
begin legal action by filing a citation before an administrative law judge,
who then calls a hearing. (The person bringing the complaint does not
need to appear at the hearing and will remain anonymous unless specific
permission to reveal the name is given in writing.)

After the hearing the judge makes the final decision. If the judge's decision supports the board's findings, the judge may issue an order requiring correction of the problem within a specific amount of time.

The board also has a range of other responsibilities, including the development of advisory standards and provision of technical assistance to groups covered in the civil rights section of the Rehabilitation Act of 1973. (See also LEGAL RIGHTS.)

Architectural Barriers Act   Also known as Public Law 90–480, this 1968 law requires federally-funded buildings and public transportation systems to be accessible to handicapped persons. This law applies to those with vision and hearing problems in addition to those in wheelchairs or with other physical handicaps.

The act also sets minimum standards for the design and construction of buildings under the supervision of the General Services Administration, the Department of Housing and Urban Development, the Defense Department and the U.S. Postal Service. These four agencies issued joint standards (the Uniform Federal Accessibility Standards) that include specifications for visual warning alarms, a permanently installed or portable listening system for hard-of-hearing people and at least one volume control on public telephones.

In order to enforce the act, Congress created the ARCHITECTURAL AND TRANSPORTATION BARRIERS COMPLIANCE BOARD in its Rehabilitation Act of 1973 (section 502), giving the board power to conduct investigations and issue orders of compliance. Those who don't comply can face withholding of federal funds. (See also LEGAL RIGHTS.)

Aristotle (384 B.C.–324 B.C.)   Ancient Greek philosopher who coined the term "deaf and dumb." "Men that are deaf are in all cases also dumb," he wrote, "that is, they can make vocal sounds, but they cannot speak." Although Aristotle's use of the term "dumb" meant speechless, it came to take on other, more negative connotations (such as stupid or unable to comprehend). The negative connotations of this word have deeply influenced the rights of deaf people from Aristotle's time up to this day.

ASL Access   A nonprofit organization providing videos about AMERICAN SIGN LANGUAGE to public libraries. The video topics include information about ASL, ASL literature, deaf history and informational videos in ASL. Contact: ASL Access, 4217 Adrienne Dr., Alexandria, VA 22309 or http://www.aslaccess.org

Association of Late-Deafened Adults   This group serves as a resource and information center for late-deafened people and works to increase public awareness of the special needs of ADVENTITIOUS DEAFNESS. It offers a publication, *ALDA NEWS*. Contact: Association of Late-deafened Adults, 10310 Main St. 274, Fairfax, VA 22030; telephone: (TDD): 404–289–1596.

auditory adaptation   A perceived decline in loudness of a sustained acoustic signal commonly found in people with lesions of the cochlea or auditory (eighth cranial) nerve. People with normal hearing, when presented with the same sustained signal, experience no "tone decay" or decrease in loudness over time.

It is also possible to differentiate between lesions of the cochlea and the auditory nerve, since auditory nerve lesions cause a more rapid and extensive tone decay.

Auditory adaptation is measured by Békésy audiometry or conventional tone-decay tests.

auditory agnosia   A defect, loss or failure in development of the ability to comprehend spoken words caused by disease, injury or malformation of the hearing centers of the brain. A person with auditory agnosia may or may not respond to an audiometric test or may give very different results at different times.

auditory analgesia   The control of pain by listening to music or WHITE NOISE through earphones, with the volume under control by the patient.

Because most subjects become less sensitive or insensitive to certain kinds of pain when listening to very loud noise or music, auditory analgesia is sometimes used in dental and obstetrical situations.

auditory aphasia   See AUDITORY AGNOSIA.

auditory feedback   The ability to hear one's own speech, in which the output is fed back to the ear, producing a self-monitoring regulation of speech.

auditory-global method   See AUDITORY-ORAL METHOD.

auditory-oral method   A method of teaching speech to deaf and hard-of-hearing children. Proponents believe that using residual hearing in the most efficient way to develop speech. Therefore, children are encouraged to perceive speech of others through audition alone. This method is also referred to as acoupedic, aural-oral, auditory approach, unisensory-auditory and auditory-global. (See also MULTISENSORY TEACHING APPROACH; SPEECH TRAINING.)

auditory training   The process of teaching a person with a hearing loss to take full advantage of any sound cues that can still be heard. Like

SPEECHREADING, auditory training can help people with hearing losses become aware of cues they might not notice otherwise. The form of auditory training used depends on when the person lost hearing and the type of hearing loss.

Auditory training helps children born deaf learn how to understand the weak or distorted sounds they can still hear; it can also help people with acquired hearing loss learn to pay attention to the act of listening and to separate background noise from speech. It also helps those with HEARING AIDS adjust to the task of using the device.

A person's need for auditory training depends on the ability to understand speech with or without a hearing aid. Often, auditory training is combined with speechreading training in a total AUDITORY REHABILITATION program.

aural-oral method   See AUDITORY-ORAL METHOD.

Australia   As many as 750,000 Australians, 5% of the population, have problems with hearing. Of those, 168,000 have trouble understanding speech even with a hearing aid.

Most of these deaf or hard-of-hearing Australians are elderly and began to lose their hearing after finishing school. Only about 40,000 were born with hearing problems or lost hearing early in life. In addition, conductive hearing loss is particularly high among the aborigines, since most native Australian children have chronic suppurative OTITIS MEDIA. Australia has the lowest prevalence rate of deafness among those developed countries for which statistics were available (35 per 100,000).

Education   Because the educational system in Australia is administered at the state level, most families with children who cannot hear have access to some guidance and counseling during the child's early years. All states have a kindergarten/preschool service for children with hearing problems, generally with large centers in cities and satellite programs in rural areas. The preschools are usually special schools for deaf students, but children may also attend regular preschools if they wish.

As deaf children enter elementary school, services become more fragmented from state to state, although most states do have elementary day schools for deaf students. (When deaf education began in Australia at the end of the 19th century, there were large state residential schools, but by the end of World War II their enrollment dropped; today most deaf students commute to special schools.)

At the high school level, deaf students are generally taught academic subjects by elementary teachers; secondary teachers trained in deafness generally teach vocational studies. Because of the differing pattern of services among states, the educational level of deaf students in Australia ranges from superior to below normal.

There are no specialist higher-education services for Australians. Although deaf high school graduates have the ability to go on to universities, very few do so.

Communication   Because most deaf people in Australia lose their hearing late in life, they reply on HEARING AIDS and SPEECHREADING to communicate. Most schools and services supplement their oral-aural curriculum with a manual system, which is usually a mixture of signs, FINGER-SPELLING and SIGNED ENGLISH. Occasionally, cued speech is used.

AUSTRALIAN SIGN LANGUAGE is a direct descendant of BRITISH SIGN LANGUAGE, introduced by the founders of two large state schools for deaf students. Although Catholic schools for deaf students at first used Irish Sign Language, today these Catholic schools rely on the oral method and use cued speech. There are few people left in Australia who use Irish-Australian Sign Language.

Because Australian Sign Language, like all sign languages, has a grammar alien to English, Australian educators believed it was less useful in schools and have tried to employ Signed English by adding various fingerspelled markers for grammar (tense, plurals and so forth) to Australian Sign Language. Australian aborigines developed an extended communication sign system of their own, and this is now used with deaf aboriginal children.

The National Acoustic Laboratories provide free hearing aids to all military personnel, senior citizens and Australians under age 21 (which allows most school-age children with hearing problems to be properly fitted with hearing aids). The labs are the second-largest provider of hearing aids in the world, and were founded in 1948 to produce hearing aids for the deafened veterans of World War II and children deafened by the rubella outbreaks in the early 1940s.

Organizations for the deaf include the Australian Association of Teachers of the Deaf, the Association of Welfare Workers with the Deaf and the Federation of Australian Deaf Societies.

Australian Sign Language   The sign language used by most deaf Australians incorporates the British two-handed system together with some use of the Irish and American one-handed alphabets.

The British two-handed system was brought to Australia in 1860 when the first two schools for deaf students were established; subsequent Irish Catholic schools introduced IRISH SIGN LANGUAGE.

A *Dictionary of Australasian Signs* was published in 1982 and includes the signs used in Australian schools in English word order.

Although there are no accurate census figures, estimates suggest that about 9,000 deaf Australians use Australian Sign Language.

B

Barry five slate system   A printed system to help deaf children learn to speak, read and write syntactically correct sentences.

Devised in 1899 by Katherine Barry, this system is similar to the five sentence parts system of ABBE ROCH AMBROISE CUCURRON SICARD. Barry's method utilized five large slates, each with one column, to help children categorize the parts of speech in sentences. Each slate contained one part of speech: subject, verb, object of the verb, preposition and object of the preposition.

Beethoven, Ludwig van (1770–1827)   A German musical genius widely regarded as one of the greatest composers who ever lived, Beethoven's life was marked by a heroic struggle against encroaching deafness. Some of his most important works were composed during the last 10 years of his life, when he was completely unable to hear.

During the first part of his life, his art stayed within the bounds of 18th-century technique. However, he experienced a change in direction as he gradually realized he was becoming deaf. The first symptoms appeared in 1800 before he was 30, and by 1802, when he could no longer deny that his hearing disorder was both permanent and progressive, he considered suicide. "But only Art held back," he wrote, "for it seemed unthinkable for me to leave the world forever before I had produced all that I felt called upon to produce."

As his hearing became worse, his piano playing degenerated, although he continued to appear in public from time to time. By 1819 he was totally deaf, and friends communicated to him using "conversation books" in which they wrote down questions and he replied orally.

By 1824, Beethoven finished his last large-scale work—the Ninth Symphony—with the aid of a type of audiophone. Holding a "sound stick" in his teeth with one end touching the piano, Beethoven would feel sound vibrations traveling through the stick to his teeth, the bones of his skull and into his inner ear.

At the end of the premiere of the Ninth Symphony, Beethoven, as conductor, stood alone in front of his orchestra. Totally deafened, he was unable to hear the thunderous applause and stood unaware until one of the soloists made him turn to face the audience.

Beginnings for Parents of Children Who Are Deaf or Hard-of-Hearing   A nonprofit agency established to provide emotional support and objective information to parents of deaf and hard-of-hearing children. The mission of the organization is to help parents be informed so that they can be knowledgeable decision makers. Beginnings can help parents work with schools to get appropriate services for a child, give information on assistive listening devices and provide referrals to other organizations.

Békésy, Georg von (1899–1972)   The inventor of the modern theory of BASILAR MEMBRANE resonance, this Hungarian-born communications engineer wanted to understand the difference between the quality of the human ear and the telephone system. While director of the Hungarian Telephone System Research Laboratory, he studied long-distance communication problems and became interested in the human hearing mechanism.

He studied the inner ear by building mechanical models of the COCHLEA. From this work, he developed his traveling-wave theory, which describes how a sound impulse sends a wave sweeping along the basilar membrane, increasing its amplitude until it reaches a maximum when it falls off sharply until the wave dies out. The point of greatest amplitude is the point at which the frequency of the sound is detected by the ear. He developed highly sensitive instruments that made it possible to understand the hearing process, differentiate between types of deafness and choose proper treatment.

Von Békésy also found that high-frequency tones were perceived near the base (or entrance) of the cochlea and lower frequencies toward its end. He also discovered that location of nerve receptors are most important in determining pitch and loudness. For this theory, Békésy received the Nobel Prize in physiology and medicine in 1961.

Belgian Sign Language (BSL)   The sign language of Belgium includes many regional dialects. Although the country has two official languages (Dutch in the north and French in the south), sign languages in these two areas are quite similar, possibly because the deaf schools in Brussels have included students from both sections of the country.

Belgian Sign Language began in schools for deaf students and was based on signs from the old French Sign Language. Although this country has been traditionally oralist, support for BSL and both the manual codes of Signed Dutch/Signed French (used in communicating between deaf and hearing people) has been growing.

Belgium   The deaf population in Belgium reflects the deep communication divisions between the Flemish and French-speaking natives. The provision of services for deaf Belgians, therefore, depends on the difference between the two groups.

The total number of deaf students in the country is unknown, but there are about 1,500 pupils in special schools for deaf children. Because early diagnosis is stressed in Belgium, most deaf children are diagnosed by the age of one. It is one of the few countries in which deafness rates are declining, reporting 60 per 100,000 for 1950 and 51 per 100,000 in 1974. The differences may reflect a sampling error, however.

Education/Communication   For many years, as in most of Europe, Belgian teachers stressed the oral method of education. Manual communication, although not repressed, was not encouraged. Gradually, Belgian educators have decided that an exclusively oral education does not benefit all students; now many promote a combination of oral and manual communication in order to acquire a command of spoken language.

Cued speech is very popular, as is a Belgian invention called AKA (alphabet of assisted kinemes, or lip movements), which is used to complement spoken language in order to make speechreading easier. In addition, the total communication method using Signed French together with speech is used as an alternative to cued speech or in combination with it. Signed French is based on signs of BELGIAN SIGN LANGUAGE.

Mainstreamed students must learn through speechreading, hearing aids or written material, since there are no sign language, cued speech-interpreters or deaf teachers to help deaf students in schools for hearing students.

Services   Special education is free in Belgium, and the national health service helps pay for hearing aids. All Belgian families receive allowances for children, which are doubled for deaf children.

Little has been done to make television or telephone accessible to deaf consumers, although the national French-speaking television network provides sign interpretation five days a week. There is no systematic captioning system.

Bell, Alexander Graham (1847–1922)   This Scottish-born American inventor dedicated his life to improving methods of communication for deaf students, and was instrumental in instituting the oral method of deaf instruction at almost every school in the United States.

Born in Edinburgh, the son of Melville and Eliza Bell, Alec (as he was then known) was a brilliant child whose interest in inventions would preoccupy him for the rest of his life. With his father, he was also interested in speech disorders and elocution, in part because his mother had severe hearing problems since her childhood. However, she could speak well, used an EAR TRUMPET (a mechanical device to improve hearing), and played the piano.

Bell's father was a pioneer of the "VISIBLE SPEECH" system, in which he tried to develop a universal language for mankind. This system described oral sounds through written symbols and was created in order to improve elocution. Although the system was not originally designed to be used in teaching deaf students, a British teacher recognized its potential and began working with young Alec Bell. With the success of his first experience in teaching deaf students with visible speech, Bell accepted an invitation to teach the method at the Boston School for Deaf Mutes in 1870.

Three years later, Bell was hired as a private teacher for 15-year-old Mabel Hubbard; in 1877 the two were married, forming a union that lasted for 45 years. This remarkable woman was one of the strongest influences on Bell and helped shape his theories of education for deaf children.

In New England, Bell taught instructors at leading schools of deaf students the visible speech system but discovered that, in the long run, the symbols were too abstract for the teacher to apply, and the system fell into disuse.

During this time in New England, Bell began to promote his belief in day schools, instead of the residential facilities then common for deaf students. His first day school was started in 1878 in Scotland with three pupils. Back in the United States, Bell opened a day school in Washington, D.C. in the same building as a kindergarten class for hearing students; his hope was that the two groups would mix.

Bell was an ardent supporter of the ORAL APPROACH, and as he grew older, he focused his efforts on promoting oralism and founding schools to teach deaf students to speak. He was considered the champion of oral education in America and believed it was an educator's job to help deaf students speak English and read lips. He objected strongly to SIGN LANGUAGE because he believed it would prevent students from achieving integration into the hearing world.

Although some proponents of the MANUAL APPROACH argued that sign was the natural language of deaf people, Bell disagreed. He agreed that sign language was of great benefit in developing the intellect, but integration into society was far more important to him than developing the mind. Bell strongly believed that all deaf children could be taught to speak and read lips.

Because of his strong opinions against sign language—he considered a signing deaf adult a "failure"—many deaf adults hated him. They saw his attempts to eliminate sign language as an attack on their culture and identity.

Bell was also a supporter of eugenics, the science of improving hereditary characteristics through controlled mating, and opposed marriages between deaf people because he believed it would eventually create a race of deaf people. After studying statistics of deaf families, he concluded that deafness was often inherited and that those who inherited deafness should only marry hearing people. He wanted to have marriages between people with inherited deafness outlawed but gave up this idea when he decided that such legislation was unrealistic. He advocated that deaf students should not be segregated in schools, that deaf teachers should no longer be hired to teach deaf students and, of course, that sign language should be abolished.

It is not surprising that most of these ideas made him even more unpopular among the deaf population, at least among those who had adjusted to their inability to hear and considered themselves normal. But Bell, dreaming of a utopian society and brought up in a family that prized oral communication, saw deafness as a problem for society, not as an individual condition.

Bell also gave financial support to the cause of oral education. On May 8, 1893, young HELEN KELLER attended groundbreaking ceremonies for Bell's VOLTA BUREAU, an international information center promoting the oral education of deaf people. In 1890 he used his share of royalties from the invention of the Graphophone (a type of tape recorder) to finance the American Association to Promote the Teaching of Speech to the Deaf (ASPTSD) (now called the ALEXANDER GRAHAM BELL ASSOCIATION FOR THE DEAF). Today this association is a leader in the support of oral education, organizing meetings and conventions, lobbying and publishing a journal, the *Volta Review*, in its efforts.

Bell had an extraordinary impact on the educational methods used to teach deaf students in this country. When Bell formed the ASPTSD, only about 40% of deaf students were taught to speak. At the time of his death 30 years later, that number had risen to more than 80%.

Berthier, Jean-Ferdinand (1803–1886)   A political leader of the French deaf "nation," Berthier was born in Louhans, France, and became the most outstanding advocate for deaf people in 19-century France.

A firm believer in promoting public understanding of deafness, he also supported "natural sign language" and thought it helped students learn written French.

Berthier attended the famous Institut National de Jeunes Sourds in Paris and was the first deaf man to receive the Legion of Honor medal. He spent his life fighting negative attitudes toward deaf people, testifying before parliament to revamp laws dealing with (and ignoring) deaf people, and researching the history and heritage of deaf people. (See also INSTITUT NATIONAL DES JEUNES SOURDS.)

Better Hearing Institute   A nonprofit educational organization that offers general information about hearing loss and help available through medicine, surgery, amplification and rehabilitation. It also distributes films, technical information, news and human-interest features, and maintains a Hearing Help-on-Line website at http://www.betterhearing.org.

Founded in 1973, the organization is supported entirely by private donations. Contact: Better Hearing Institute, P.O. Box 1840, Washington, D.C.; telephone: 703–642–0580 or 800–EAR–WELL.

Bilingual, Hearing- and Speech-Impaired Court Interpreter Act

This law, enacted by Congress in 1979, amends the 1978 Court Interpreters Act and requires the court to appoint a qualified interpreter for deaf, speech-impaired or non-English speakers in any criminal or civil action initiated by the federal government.

The director of the administrative office of the U.S. Courts determines the qualifications required of court-appointed interpreters. Each district court must maintain a list of certified oral and manual interpreters for deaf people, obtained in consultation with the NATIONAL ASSOCIATION OF THE DEAF and the REGISTRY OF INTERPRETERS FOR THE DEAF. The interpreter's services are paid for by the federal government.

However, an interpreter is *not* provided for a deaf person who initiates a lawsuit. Although many states will provide an interpreter for a deaf defendant in a criminal trial, few offer one at the time of arrest or in a civil case.

Bonet, Juan Pablo (1579–1623)

The author of the first published book of oral teaching methods for deaf people. Bonet was born on July 1, 1579, in a little town in Spain, Torres de Berrellen. After serving in the army and learning Italian and French, he was hired as secretary by the duke of Frias. The duke's second son, Luis, was deaf, and Manuel Ramirez de Carrion was employed to teach Luis, using the methods developed by PEDRO PONCE DE LEÓN. Bonet spent some time watching Ramirez and took over the education of Luis when Ramirez left.

After about three years, Bonet published *Simplification of the Alphabet and the Art of Teaching Mutes to Speak,* in which he explained the Ramirez-de León technique. The text was not his own method, but by writing down the system, Bonet was able to interest a wide variety of European teachers in the possibility of oral education for deaf children.

Bonet believed in teaching reading and spelling, speech instruction and fingerspelling. However, he did not support the teaching of speechreading.

Bove, Linda (b. 1945)

One of the most influential deaf women in the performing arts, this totally deaf actress may be best known for the character she plays in public television's *Sesame Street.*

In addition, Bove is a founding member of both the NATIONAL THEATRE OF THE DEAF and the Little Theatre of the Deaf, and remains the national theatre's ambassador-at-large.

Bove was born congenitally deaf in Garfield, New Jersey to deaf parents and graduated from Gallaudet University, where she had been active in drama. She toured internationally with the National Theatre of the Deaf, and in 1973 she played "Melissa Halley," a deaf character on the television soap opera *Search for Tomorrow;* other TV appearances include *The Dick Cavett Show, Happy Days* and *A Child's Christmas in Wales.* She first appeared in public television's *Sesame Street* in 1971; by 1976 she was a permanent member of the cast, portraying a deaf member of the neighborhood.

Boys Town Research Registry for Hereditary Hearing Loss   The registry matches families and individuals with hearing loss with collaborating research projects involving hereditary deafness. Participants provide demographic, genetic, audiologic and medical information to assist making that match. Information is kept confidential. The registry's publication, *Hereditary Deafness Newsletter of America,* is written for families and non-genetic clinical and research professionals.

Bragg, Bernard (b. 1928)   A cofounder of the NATIONAL THEATRE OF THE DEAF, Bernard Bragg is an actor, mime, director and lecturer known for his development of "sign-mime," a variation of sign language that features graceful, poetic body movement and motion to highlight dialogue.

Born deaf to deaf parents in Brooklyn, Bragg graduated as class valedictorian from the New York School for the Deaf and went on to Gallaudet University where he excelled in dramatics as an actor and director, and received the Teegarden Award for poetry upon graduation. His father, Wolf Bragg, was a talented actor who had performed in a deaf amateur theatrical group. At that time, there was no deaf professional theater.

Armed with a master's degree in education, Bragg taught for 15 years at a California school for deaf students, where he also performed for Marcel Marceau. The celebrated French mime then invited Bragg to study with him in Paris; after Bragg's return to California, he began performing in small clubs in San Francisco and was named one of the best small club performers by *Life* magazine.

Internationally, Bragg has served as artist-in-residence with the Moscow Theatre of Sign Language and mime and served on the U.S. Intelligence Agency's Overseas Speaker's Program in 1977, traveling all over the world conducting workshops in sign for both deaf and hearing audiences.

He currently serves as artist-in-residence at Gallaudet University.

Braidwood, Thomas (1715–1806)   A pioneer Scottish educator of deaf people best known for his refusal to pass on his methods in oral instruction to anyone outside his own family. This reticence was responsible for the early emphasis on manual education of deaf students in the United States.

Thomas Braidwood taught his first deaf pupil in 1760 and was so pleased with his success in helping the boy speak and understand language that he decided to concentrate on teaching deaf students.

His first school, the Academy For the Deaf and Dumb, opened in Edinburgh in the early 1760's. By 1779, the academy had 20 pupils who were taught to speak, read and write. Although his exact methods were not divulged, it was known that he based his method on the articulation theories of educator Thomas Wallis. This was an oral method, but the use of natural signs and the manual alphabet was not forbidden.

In response to an offer from King George III to set up a school for deaf students in London, Braidwood opened Grove House in 1792 and then a separate school for needy deaf children, where Braidwood's nephew Joseph Watson was headmaster.

Braidwood's schools were successful, but the oath of secrecy kept by the Braidwood family had important consequences for the future of deaf education in the United States. THOMAS HOPKINS GALLAUDET, who had studied the manual communication system in France developed by ABBÉ ROCH AMBROISE CUCURRON SICARD, came to Britain to learn the oral method from Braidwood.

When he got to London, he found that the three English schools for deaf students were all controlled by the Braidwood family, who were unwilling to share their methods freely, as was the custom at the time.

Consequently, Gallaudet returned to Paris to study the French manual system, which he subsequently introduced into the United States. This method became the basis of deaf education and communication in U.S. schools for deaf children.

Brazil   Deaf citizens in Brazil receive limited funds from the state and federal government for diagnosis, treatment, education and rehabilitation. Free diagnosis of simple cases of deafness and routine prescription of hearing aids are provided by the government through its own otolaryngologists and through agreements with private clinics. The state mandates minimal educational and treatment provisions and helps finance the training of teachers for deaf students. Numerous private charitable groups also serve deaf Brazilians. Many large cities maintain good private clinics and professionals, but the treatment cost is often beyond the reach of many Brazilians.

Although there are no exact figures, estimates suggest that there are up to a half million profoundly deaf Brazilians out of a total population of 120 million people. More than half of the deaf students who receive assistance attend school in special classes, one-fourth are in integrated classes, and one-fifth attend special schools.

The predominant philosophy in the schools and programs for deaf citizens throughout the country is to integrate deaf people into the hearing world by developing speech and speechreading skills and utilizing residual hearing. The use of sign language was discouraged between 1950 and 1970, but today its use is spreading slowly across the country.

Brazilian Sign Language   A number of dialects make up Brazilian Sign Language, but communication among people is surprisingly easy for so large a country.

Although Brazilian schools for deaf students became completely oral after the Milan Congress in 1880, there has been more interest in Brazilian Sign Language since the 1970s, and at least one school has adopted the educational philosophy of TOTAL COMMUNICATION.

Brazilian Sign Language is similar to both American and European sign languages, and its one-handed manual alphabet is quite similar to the French system. In Brazilian Sign Language, fingerspelling is used for proper names, fingerspelled signs, technical terms and negative emphasis. The system utilizes hand and body movements, facial expressions, eye gaze, pauses and changes in the rhythm of signing to indicate grammatical and structural meanings, and the space around the body provides an important frame of reference, indicating spatial agreement between verbs and subjects/objects, reference for directional verbs, and so forth.

Breunig, H. Latham (b. 1910)   A chemist, statistician and leading proponent of oral education, Breunig founded the Oral Deaf Adults Section of the ALEXANDER GRAHAM BELL ASSOCIATION FOR THE DEAF. Along with two others, he set up Teletypewriters for the Deaf, Inc., to acquire and recondition surplus teletypewriters donated by American Telephone and Telegraph.

Born in Indianapolis, he lost part of his hearing when he was three years old, a condition exacerbated by an attack of scarlet fever at age five. Two years after that, a skull fracture left him with a 115 dB loss. He attended the Clarke School for the Deaf in Northampton, Massachusetts where he met his future wife, and then attended a public school, where he worked on the school newspaper, became an Eagle Scout and was accepted into the National Honor Society.

He received a degree in chemistry from Wabash College in Indiana and completed his Ph.D. at Johns Hopkins University. While a full-time researcher with the pharmaceutical firm of Eli Lilly, Breunig was active in national organizations for deaf people and was director of the Indianapolis Speech and Hearing Center for 21 years. Committed to the idea that deaf people need to be able to communicate with the hearing world in order to take advantage of opportunities, he attributed his own success in business and as a professional chemist to his ability to speak and speechread.

Brewster, John Jr. (1766–1854)   Considered one of New England's most accomplished folk artists, he was also one of the most successful traveling artists of his day.

Brewster was born deaf to hearing parents, Dr. John and Mary Brewster, in Hampton, Connecticut. Able to communicate in sign language and adept at an early age in art, he obtained several commissions for portraits of family and friends despite a lack of formal training.

Brewster faced great difficulties as an independent artist forced to communicate constantly with strangers in inns or homes. He traveled by horseback in Massachusetts and Maine and was gifted at capturing a model's personality in his portraits.

When the Connecticut Asylum for the Education and Instruction of Deaf and Dumb Persons opened in Hartford (now the American School for the Deaf), Brewster, at the age of 54, was one of its first six pupils. During the three years he lived at the school, he was able to support himself through painting. He left the school in 1820 to continue painting. His paintings hang today in museums in Maine, Massachusetts and New York.

Bridgman, Laura Dewey (1829–1889)   The first deaf and blind person to be educated in the United States, Laura Bridgman was born in Hanover, New Hampshire to a successful farm family. Always a delicate child, at age two she contracted scarlet fever, which destroyed her sight and hearing and left her ill for two years. During this time, she forgot the few words she had learned to speak before her illness, and she retreated into silence.

Bridgman was introduced in 1837 to Samuel Gridley Howe, the founder of the Perkins Institute for the Blind in Boston. Although Laura could barely communicate with her family (she understood shoves and pats on the head), Howe was convinced she was extremely bright and would benefit from instruction.

Her parents brought her to Perkins in 1837, where Howe constantly worked with her to establish a form of communication using labels with raised letters pasted on common objects. When she finally learned that the labels actually represented objects, the greatest obstacle to meaningful communication had been crossed. At Perkins, she studied a variety of subjects, such as fingerspelling, handsewing and how to use a sewing machine.

Although she never learned to talk, she could make about 50 sounds, which she used as names for people she knew. At the age of 23, she was sent home where it was assumed she would be happy with household chores. But the sudden loss of noise and activity affected her poorly; she became bedridden and near death until she was returned to Perkins, where she remained for the rest of her life.

British Sign Language   This highly complex system is the language of the deaf community throughout Great Britain and Northern Ireland, although there are regional dialects. As in many natural sign languages,

BSL has a topic-comment structure: for example, "Drink—you want more?" instead of "Do you want another drink?" It includes an inflection system, with which it is possible to show person or number by the way signs move.

As in AMERICAN SIGN LANGUAGE, BSL and English are quite different, although the two-handed BSL manual alphabet is based on the English alphabet.

There are no exact figures on the number of people who use BSL, but estimates suggest that as many as 30,000 profoundly deaf people in the United Kingdom use BSL and were educated through its use. It includes a two-handed fingerspelling system that was first published in 1680.

Although the use of BSL was widespread by the mid-19th century in combination with English, it fell out of favor as oralism reached popularity in Britain. Today, BSL is becoming increasingly well accepted and is a topic of research and study by linguists.

Bulwer, John   This 17th-century English physician was very interested in manual communication as an orator but later became involved in its uses as a tool to educate deaf students.

Bulwer believed it was possible for deafmutes to learn speechreading and speech, although he believed that sign language and manual alphabets were more practical. His *Philocophus, or the Deafe and Dumbe Man's Friend,* published in 1648, was the first major English book on deafness. In it, he discussed the anatomy and physiology of speech and the etiology of deafness. He also explored the elements of phonetics, describing specific movements of each speech sound and insisting that speech is *movement* rather than *position.*

However, Bulwer was not a teacher of the deaf and never applied any of his theories. Although he hoped to establish a school for the deaf to teach communication methods to hard-of-hearing students, he never accomplished his goal.

C

Canada As in the United States, about one in ten Canadian citizens have some type of hearing problem. Nearly 4,000 children with hearing problems are in special programs, almost half of these students are profoundly deaf. These numbers, however, are estimates since there has been no national deaf census and the figures do not include native Canadians in the far north, among whom hearing loss is reportedly endemic. According to 1941 statistics, Canada's prevalence rate of deafness is 63 per 100,000 (an average rate), although much lower than the United States's rate of 100).

The result is a small and widely scattered minority population served only by a small number of professionals, in a country with a decentralized method of administering social services. This decentralization, in which the provinces fiercely maintain sole right to administer social services for its people, virtually guarantees a crazy-quilt pattern of services for deaf people across the country. Most important, education for Canada's deaf students has no uniform, comprehensive standards or administration.

Although deaf Canadians have made strides in civil rights, including the rights to legal interpreter services and to become adoptive parents, they have not been as successful in effecting improvements in postsecondary education, audiological service delivery and research.

Canada's history has been closely linked to England and France, but the country has allied itself with the United States in its development of educational services for its deaf citizens.

The first school for deaf Canadians was opened in 1831 in Champlain, Quebec by Ronald McDonald, who had spent a year at the American School for the Deaf at Hartford training under Thomas Gallaudet and Laurent Clerc. All schools gradually evolved from reliance on a manual to an oral educational philosophy.

American signs and AMERICAN SIGN LANGUAGE (ASL) have remained the preferred method of communication, although the small French deaf community within the country uses French-Canadian Sign Language. Across the country, there are regional differences in sign.

A bilingual dictionary of the basic vocabulary of sign language used in Canada is being compiled by the Canadian Coordinating Council on Deafness and will include the signs used in French Canada.

Because most Canadians prefer sign language, many disagree with the school-based English sign systems used as part of Total Communication in many educational programs. Many Canadians support a bilingual approach to learning language, with ASL as the first language and English signs as an added benefit to a student's curriculum.

Approximately 80% of Canadians have access to a telecommunication device for the deaf (TDD), and message relay centers operate in large cities.

Captioned television became available with the development in 1982 of the Canadian Captioning Development Agency, which captions a wide variety of Canadian programs in English and French. For a time, the agency also captioned French language telecasts around the world since there was no closed captioning system available to the French.

The Canadian Coordinating Council on Deafness and the Canadian Association of the Deaf are major national organizations with affiliated groups throughout the provinces. Contact: Alberta Association of the Deaf, 10004–105 St., Alberta, Canada T5J 1C4.

Canadian Sign Language   Just as the culture of Canada has evolved along two lines, French and English, so has the language of the deaf community. Canada's deaf community speaks two completely different sign languages: Canadian Sign Language (CSL)—used primarily by deaf people in the English Canadian community—and Langue des Signes Quebecoise (LSQ)—used primarily by deaf French Canadians.

As in many sign languages around the world, much investigation is still being done into the structural properties of the communication methods. It appears, however, that CSL may share certain properties with British Sign Language, and LSQ may be similar to the sign language used in France (Langue des Signes Française [LSF], also called French Sign Language). There is also some evidence that CSL shares some structural similarities with American Sign Language. Still, research also suggests that both CSL and LSQ have different structures from English and French.

Although the Canadian constitution stipulates that English and French are equal official languages, it is extremely rare for a deaf student to be taught both CSL and LSQ.

As with many other sign languages, CSL and LSQ depend on systematic changes in movement, space and facial expression as linguistic devices to change meaning.

CASE   See CONCEPTUALLY ACCURATE SIGNED ENGLISH.

cauliflower ear   A deformity of the shape of the outer ear (pinna) caused by blows or friction that are sharp enough to start bleeding within the soft cartilage of the ear itself. It is most commonly found in boxers and can be prevented by using a protective helmet.

After a severe blow to the ear, swelling can be reduced by applying an ice pack, and blood can be drained from the ear with a needle and syringe. Repeated injuries to the ear, however, will distort its shape in a way that can only be repaired through plastic surgery.

Center for Bicultural Studies, Inc.   This group promotes public education about the interaction between deaf and hearing cultures and fosters public acceptance, understanding and use of AMERICAN SIGN LANGUAGE and other natural signed languages. It disseminates information on deaf culture and American Sign Language, sponsors forums, public discussions and video projects and publishes the *TBC News*. Contact: Center for Bicultural Studies, Inc., 5506 Kenilworth Ave., Suite 105, Riverdale MD 20737; telephone: 301–277–3945.

Center for Hearing Dog Information   A national advocacy resource and referral center for hearing ear dog programs sponsored by the American Humane Association. The center publishes a Hearing Dog Program Directory, which outlines hearing dog programs and also lists support dog training programs (dogs who assist the physically disabled) and agencies that train dog guides for the blind.

Individuals with a severe to profound hearing loss who can demonstrate a need for such a dog can qualify. Only a few programs place children with dogs because children often cannot maintain the necessary control over an animal. (See also HEARING EAR DOGS.) Contact: Center for Hearing Dog Information, 9725 E. Hampden Ave., Denver, CO 80231; telephone: 303–695–0811 (voice); 303–695–4531 (TDD).

China, People's Republic of   There are about three million deaf citizens in China, but services for these people are in woefully short supply. Only about 33,000 of them currently attend schools for deaf students.

The first school for deaf students opened in 1887 at Dengchou, and by 1948 there were 23 such schools, most of which were private. When the People's Republic of China was founded in 1949, the new government mandated major changes in the education of deaf children.

First, the government took control of all schools for deaf students, limited class size to 15 pupils, established a Bureau of the Deaf and Blind to administer education and began research in oral teaching methods. Since then, education for deaf children has grown to more than 30 schools with more than 9,000 staff for 33,000 students.

Students can attend combined schools for deaf and blind children, schools for deaf students only or special classes in regular schools. Still, the school enrollment rate of deaf children is very low, and the system of education is considered poor.

Deaf Chinese citizens are given the same rights as every other member of society and, in cities, receive government-paid medical care and pensions. The government has special rules for its deaf criminals: Since 1980, Chinese law states that if a deaf person violates a criminal law, he or she can be exempt from punishment or only lightly punished.

Although there were no unified language communication methods for deaf Chinese in the past, research into communication did not begin until the founding of the People's Republic. In 1963 the government adopted the Chinese Fingerspelling Alphabet Scheme, based on the Chinese pronunciation scheme and consisting of 30 separate fingershapes.

The primary association for deaf Chinese is the Chinese Association for the Blind and the Deaf, which is headquartered in Beijing and is a member of the World Federation of the Deaf.

Chinese Sign Language   The standard communication mode for the people of mainland China, Chinese Sign Language (CSL) includes 3,000 signs with 41 recurrent handshapes. Although there are three million deaf Chinese, it is unknown how many use CSL.

In general, CSL places the verb last, with the modified followed by the modifier: "Girl sleep not." It has a manual alphabet with 26 letters and four digraphic consonants used to fingerspell words. It is used primarily in schools; deaf Chinese signers rarely use fingerspelling.

Ideograms are still the main type of writing found in China, and 22 of these ideograms are used in CSL. Not surprisingly, given the isolated nature of mainland China, very few of its signs have come from foreign shores.

Chomsky, Noam (b. 1928)   This American linguist is one of the founders of generative grammar, an original system of linguistic analysis. He believes there is a universal pattern in all languages and linguists should study a native speaker's unconscious knowledge of his own language and not the speaker's actual production of language.

Unlike structuralists, who collect samples of language and then classify them, Chomsky developed transformational grammar—a set of rules that can generate structural descriptions for all the grammatical sentences of a language. He then tested results against actual language samples. Transformational grammar has continued to evolve since Chomsky first introduced it in 1957.

Chomsky, whose father was a Hebrew scholar who studied historical LINGUISTICS, teaches modern languages and linguistics at the Massachusetts Institute of Technology.

classifiers   Handshapes that represent or describe certain types of classes of objects or occurrences (for example, upright index fingers brought together to indicate two people meeting).

Clerc, Laurent (1785–1869) This leader in education for deaf people was born in LaBalme les Grottes, the son of a family noted in local politics. Deafened at age one after an infection following a facial burn, Clerc was taken to the famous Royal National Institute for the Deaf in Paris (now the INSTITUT NATIONAL DES JEUNES SOURDS), where he studied with the brilliant deaf instructor JEAN MASSIEU; by the age of 20 he had completed his education and was teaching classes at the institute.

At the school, Clerc met THOMAS HOPKINS GALLAUDET, who had come to learn the manual alphabet developed there. Gallaudet convinced Clerc to return with him to the United States for three years to help establish a school for deaf students.

It was on the ocean voyage to this country that Gallaudet taught Clerc English and Clerc completed Gallaudet's training in manual communication. Once in the United States, Gallaudet and Clerc raised $5,000 at presentations and special programs they conducted throughout New England, an amount that was later matched by the Connecticut general assembly.

With this money, the AMERICAN SCHOOL FOR THE DEAF opened its doors in 1817 in Hartford, Connecticut with seven pupils. The next year, Clerc married one of these, Eliza Boardman, and decided to remain in America. He returned to France to visit only three times.

Although Clerc could not speak, he had great political influence and could write fluently in French and English. With these skills, he was able to convince Americans that deaf children could be educated and that sign language was the best type of communication to use while teaching them. At the age of 73, Clerc retired after 50 years of teaching. He died on July 18, 1869, and was buried beside his wife in Hartford.

cochlea A snail-shaped part of the ear located behind the oval window. The cochlea contains fluid, thousands of microscopic hair cells tuned to various frequencies and more than 20 types of cells. This complex inner ear organ contains the ORGAN OF CORTI, which lies between two fluid channels—the scala vestibuli and the scala tympani.

The sodium-rich PERILYMPH fluid of the scala vestibuli is separated from the potassium-rich ENDOLYMPH fluid of the membranous cochlea by the paper-thin REISSNER'S MEMBRANE. Because these two fluids are separated, they maintain a vital difference in electrical charge imperative for the correct function of the cochlea's sensory cells.

The entire membranous part of the cochlea is surrounded by bone, into which there are two entrances: the round and oval windows.

Sound, traveling through the middle ear, reaches the STAPES (the third bone of the ossicles), which is attached to the oval window by a ligament that allows it to move, transferring sound vibrations to the scala vestibuli.

This fluid brushes the tiny hair cells (or sensory cells) where separate pitches are registered, generating an electrical current that telegraphs sound through acoustic nerves to the brain. Once in the brain, the current is then interpreted as sound.

There are two types of hair cells; about 12,000 outer hair cells and about 3,500 inner hair cells lying close to the core of the cochlea. These hair cells are part of the organ of Corti, which lies on the BASILAR MEMBRANE, both part of the membranous cochlea.

When the hair cells of the cochlea die, there is no way to revive or replace them. These cells can die from a variety of causes, including excess noise and the aging process. The hair cells responsible for registering high notes almost always fail first, perhaps because they are located in a more exposed area.

Cogswell, Alice (1805–1830)   The inspiration behind the establishment of the first permanent school for deaf students in the United States, Alice Cogswell was born in 1805 in Hartford, Connecticut, the third daughter of Dr. MASON FITCH COGSWELL and his wife, Mary.

When Alice was two years old, she contracted cerebrospinal meningitis and lost her hearing before she had completely learned to speak. Whatever speech she had at that point was almost gone by the time she was four, and she could hear very little. Although bright and eager to learn, she fell behind other children her age in spite of the efforts of her family to teach her.

Fortunately for Alice, her neighbors were the THOMAS HOPKINS GALLAUDET family. Alice played with Gallaudet's children and communicated with them using her own code of gestures.

One day, when Gallaudet spelled "hat" for Alice on the ground, using his hat as an illustration, Alice immediately understood that objects had written names and demanded to learn the names of other objects. This was the beginning of real communication between Gallaudet and a deaf child and the start of a lifelong interest for Gallaudet.

When Gallaudet subsequently opened the American Asylum for the Deaf and Dumb in 1817 (now the American School for the Deaf), Alice was first in line to attend, carrying a slate with her to communicate with those who did not know sign language.

Alice, who believed she could not live without her father, died 13 days after he had succumbed to pneumonia in 1830. She was 25 years old.

Cogswell, Mason Fitch (1761–1830)   Cofounder of the AMERICAN SCHOOL FOR THE DEAF, this Connecticut surgeon and Yale University professor first became interested in deafness when his daughter Alice became deaf at the age of two from cerebrospinal meningitis, a childhood illness associated with a prolonged high fever.

Cogswell's neighbor was young THOMAS HOPKINS GALLAUDET, who noticed Alice's struggles to communicate with neighbors and began to teach her. Unable to find a school for the deaf in 18th-century America and inspired by Gallaudet's success, Cogswell sent Gallaudet to Europe to learn how to teach deaf children. When Gallaudet returned with a French expert in deaf education, Cogswell—together with Gallaudet and 10 Hartford city fathers—founded the American School for the Deaf in Hartford. (See also CLERC, LAURENT; COGSWELL, ALICE.)

Coiter, Volcher (1534–1600)   A Dutch physician who first traced the path of sound waves from the ear canal through the EARDRUM and middle ear bones into the COCHLEA.

A student of anatomy for many years in some of the most celebrated universities of Italy, Coiter also served as personal physician to Count Palatine Ludwig VI.

He is best known for his book, *De auditus instrumento,* published in 1566 and the first devoted entirely to the ear. The book contained 17 chapters dealing with the various parts of the organ of hearing from anatomical and physiological points of view. His theories were generally accepted by his contemporaries.

Comité International des Sports des Sourds (CISS)   This group was organized in 1924 by representatives from six nations (Belgium, Czechoslovakia, France, Great Britain, the Netherlands and Poland) and is similar to the International Olympic Committee in that it regulates olympic-style competition for deaf athletes.

Formerly named the Comité International des Sports Silencieux, CISS is made up of many national sports federations of deaf people and is supervised by an executive committee made up of one deaf person from each of eight different countries. All business at its international meetings and congress is conducted in GESTUNO (international sign language), and no interpreters are used.

It is staffed by volunteers and earns money through dues, fines and competition fees. Officers of CISS are chosen by the executive committee from among federation members. (See also WORLD GAMES FOR THE DEAF.)

Conceptually Accurate Signed English (CASE)   Another term for PIDGIN SIGN ENGLISH or SIGN ENGLISH.

Conference of Educational Administrators Serving the Deaf (CEASD)
A nonprofit organization committed to improved management in programs for deaf students and educational options for deaf people.

The organization was founded in 1869 as the Conference of Superintendents and Principals of American Schools for the Deaf. The dream of EDWARD MINER GALLAUDET, then president of the Columbia Institution for the Deaf and Dumb (now GALLAUDET UNIVERSITY), was to unite school principals behind his philosophy of communication in the classroom.

Today, the group tries to promote a continuum of educational opportunities for deaf people in North America and to encourage efficient management of schools and programs for deaf people.

The organization holds annual meetings for its members, who must have administrative roles in educational programs for deaf students. In odd-numbered years, its meeting is held at the same time as the CONVENTION OF AMERICAN INSTRUCTORS OF THE DEAF. At these shared meetings, CEASD dedicates one day for its own business, sharing the convention schedule's presentations for the rest of the meeting.

In addition, CEASD (together with the ALEXANDER GRAHAM BELL ASSOCIATION FOR THE DEAF and the Convention of American Instructors of the Deaf) provides certification programs for teachers of deaf students through a confederation called the COUNCIL ON EDUCATION OF THE DEAF.

Conference headquarters are located in Silver Spring, Maryland at Halex House (the building owned by the NATIONAL ASSOCIATION OF THE DEAF). Both CEASD's office and executive director are shared with the Convention of American Instructors of the Deaf. It also shares administrative responsibility with the convention for its journal, AMERICAN ANNALS OF THE DEAF. Contact: President Barry Griffing, P.O. Box 5545, Tucson AZ 85703; telephone (voice and TDD): 602–628–5261. For journal information contact *American Annals of the Deaf,* Gallaudet University, 800 Florida Avenue NE, Washington DC 20002.

Convention of American Instructors of the Deaf   Founded in 1850, the convention is one of the oldest American professional organizations interested in education for deaf students.

Its initial meeting in New York, organized by instructors at the New York Institution for the Deaf, marked the first time that a convention for deaf educators was held anywhere in the world. Among other things, conference attendees adopted the *American Annals of the Deaf* as their official publication. Today, the convention and the CONFERENCE OF EDUCATIONAL ADMINISTRATORS SERVING THE DEAF manage the journal as equal partners.

The purpose of the convention is to promote the education of deaf students "along the broadest and most advanced lines." The organization is located in Silver Spring, Maryland in Halex House, owned by the NATIONAL ASSOCIATION OF THE DEAF, and shares its office and executive director with the Conference of Educational Administrators Serving the Deaf. Contact:

Convention of American Instructors of the Deaf, P.O. Box 2025, Austin TX 78768; telephone (voice and TDD): 512–441–2225.

Corti, Alfonso (1822–1888)   With the aid of a powerful compound microscope, Corti traced the BASILAR MEMBRANE attached to the lamina and detected thousands of tiny hair cells that rest on the membrane.

Now known collectively as the "organ of corti, these cells make up the actual hearing organ and are linked to the brain through the auditory nerve.

cosmetic surgical reconstruction   A procedure performed to correct a malformation of the external ear (also called PINNA or auricle). The most common cosmetic reconstruction of the external ear is to treat excessively protruding ears caused by hypertrophic development of the conchal cartilage or insufficient folding of the antehelix ridge. In the worst cases, the ears can extend at a 90 degree angle from the scalp.

If cosmetic surgery is to be performed, it is usually done while the child is young. In the operation, a surgeon cuts the skin behind the ear, excises a portion of the exposed cartilage and moves the antehelix closer to the mastoid bone, holding it in place with stitches.

Cosmetic surgery is also beneficial in the treatment of macrotia (an overdeveloped external ear), which can affect one or both ears.

It is also possible to totally reconstruct the ear. Generally, there is a rudimentary ear already present, which is cut in half horizontally to form the new ear. A piece of tubular skin graft or rib cartilage is placed between the two halves, inserted under the skin over the mastoid bone.

cotton swabs   Despite frequent warnings against their use in the ear, these small sticks tipped with cotton are often used to dislodge EARWAX within the ear canal. In actuality, the swabs can push the wax farther into the ear canal, potentially damaging the eardrum. A punctured eardrum with a hole larger than 1.5 mm will produce a conductive hearing loss by interfering with the eardrum's vibration. Larger holes can cause even greater hearing loss; for example, perforation of less than 20% of the eardrum causes a 15 dB hearing loss. Destruction of the entire eardrum can result in a maximum of 45 dB loss. Swabs such as these are particularly dangerous when used to clean the ears of infants, whose uncontrolled movements can force the swab deep into the ear with disastrous results.

An infant's outer ear may be cleaned with a wet washcloth, but nothing should ever be placed into the ear canal. Accumulated earwax in danger of blocking hearing may be removed by a physician; however, most earwax is normal and is a natural way for the ear to protect itself.

Council on Education of the Deaf   Founded in 1960, this group, representing more than 10,000 teachers, sets standards for teachers of deaf students, conducts evaluations of teacher training programs and issues certificates for teachers of deaf students. There are about 15,000 teachers serving more than 46,000 deaf and hard-of-hearing students in classes throughout the United States and Canada.

The council coordinates the efforts of three groups involved in deaf education: the CONFERENCE OF EDUCATIONAL ADMINISTRATORS SERVING THE DEAF, the CONVENTION OF AMERICAN INSTRUCTORS OF THE DEAF and the ALEXANDER GRAHAM BELL ASSOCIATION FOR THE DEAF.

The professional certification of teachers of deaf students had first been studied separately by the Alexander Graham Bell Association and the Conference of Educational Administrators Serving the Deaf. The two plans that had been developed by these organizations were administered separately, as a teacher registry (Bell) and as a certification program (CAID) until 1935, when they were joined into a single program.

Council on Professional Standards   The primary certification and accreditation board of the AMERICAN SPEECH-LANGUAGE-HEARING ASSOCIATION (ASHA) located at the association's headquarters in Rockville, MD. Originally established as a certification board in 1959 as the American Board of Examiners in Speech Pathology and Audiology, the group was renamed in 1980 to better describe its larger role as both a certifying and accrediting organization. The council concerns itself not only with the certification of individuals, but with the accreditation of college and university programs and the clinical programs which employ speech-language pathologists and audiologists. Contact: Council on Professional Standards, c/o American Speech-Language-Hearing Association, 10801 Rockville Pike, Rockville MD 20852; telephone (voice and TDD): 301–897–5700.

Court Interpreter's Act   This 1978 act of Congress ensures that people with hearing problems will be given an interpreter if they are involved as the defendant in proceedings brought by the federal government in a district court. It was later amended and broadened by the 1979 BILINGUAL, HEARING- AND SPEECH-IMPAIRED COURT INTERPRETER ACT. The law requires that either an oral or manual interpreter must be provided at public expense whenever a defendant has a hearing problem that inhibits the ability to communicate or understand testimony.

Before the act was passed, interpreters were allowed but not required, and the decision to have an interpreter was left up to the individual judge. In many occasions, however, judges did not ask for an interpreter, and individuals with hearing problems did not receive communication assistance. Because of this, subsequent appellate court rulings stipulated that without the ability to communicate with lawyers and confront witnesses, hard-of-hearing people are deprived of their constitutional right to due process under the law.

The act requires that the clerk of each U.S. district court maintain a current list of all court-certified interpreters within that court's jurisdiction. The director of the administrative office of U.S. courts is responsible for outlining qualifications for interpreters.

An interpreter may be appointed at the request of the judge, the hard-of-hearing person's attorney or the person himself. Hard-of-hearing people may waive the right to a court-appointed interpreter and use their own interpreters, who will still be paid by the court. The interpreter can interpret simultaneously, consecutively or in summary (although the latter is not recommended).

In court actions outside of federal court, a hard-of-hearing defendant or witness may ask for help from the court clerk in locating an interpreter, but the interpreter may not necessarily be provided at public expense. The presiding judge will determine who should pay for the interpreter.

Further, privileged communications between defendant and attorney through the interpreter are confidential, and the interpreter cannot be required to testify about them. (See also INTERPRETERS AND THE LAW.)

cued speech   This method of communication was developed in 1966 by Dr. Orin Cornett as a speechreading support system that, in English, uses eight hand configurations and four hand positions near the mouth to supplement visible speech. As such, it's closer to an oral than a manual approach.

The hand cue signals a visual difference between sounds that look alike on the lips, such as "p" and "b." These cues enable the deaf person to see the phonetic equivalent of what others hear.

Each cue (hand placement or configuration) identifies a special group of two to four speech sounds. The combination of cues and mouth movements makes all the essential speech sounds appear different from each other, so that the spoken message is clarified.

The hand configurations and locations are called cues, not cued speech, which is the combination of the cues with speech (the cues are not readable alone).

Each hand configuration identifies a group of consonants; vowel sounds are shown by position of the hand in one of four ways, all within a few inches of the mouth (the side of the face, throat, chin and corner of the mouth).

Cued speech can also be used to indicate approximate voice pitch for each syllable uttered, which is important in tonal languages (such as Thai, Cantonese and Mandarin). For example, in Cantonese, the syllable "ma" can mean "mother," "scold," "horse" or "right?" depending on the pitch.

Tone cueing is also helpful in speech therapy. In order to cue tone, a person changes the inclination of the cueing hand to indicate changes in pitch.

Cued speech has been adapted to many languages, and audiocassette lessons designed for self-instruction by hearing persons are available. (See Appendix 13.) The system is generally the same in all languages.

Cued speech was developed primarily because some congenitally deaf persons do not become good readers because they don't have an easy way to learn spoken language as young deaf children, according to Dr. Cornett. Proponents believe cued speech makes spoken language visually clear and solves the communication problem and also helps youngsters learn a spoken language more easily. It is an easily learned system, taking only about 12 to 20 hours to master. It is most successful when used consistently from early childhood.

Initial research suggests that cued speech does help make the spoken language clear, but the long-term effectiveness of the language is not known. One of the recent advances used in conjunction with cued speech is the AUTOCUER, a device invented by Dr. Cornett, which contains a miniature computerized speech processor that automatically analyzes speech input and produces cue-equivalents through light signals.

There was a great deal of initial interest in cued speech after it was introduced in the 1960s, but it was overshadowed by the spread of TOTAL COMMUNICATION at about the same time. Cued speech tries to clear up some of the problems with speechreading. However, it has not been widely adopted in schools, and is not widely popular among the deaf population. It is popular in Australia and Canada, however. (See also NATIONAL CUED SPEECH ASSOCIATION.)

D

dactylology   A term that generally refers to FINGERSPELLING, although it has been used sometimes to include signs.

Dalgarno, George (1626?–1687)   This 17th-century Scottish theoretician's interest in techniques for teaching deaf students grew out of his fascination with the idea of a universal language for all people.

The headmaster of a private grammar school in England, Dalgarno discussed his theories and techniques for teaching deaf students to speak in *The Deaf and Dumb Man's Tutor*, in which he explained that the senses were connected in complex ways. He believed that a person blind from birth could learn quicker than a deaf person. However, with maturity, a deaf person would surpass a blind person in learning because, Dalgarno thought, sight was more essential to education in the long run than hearing. Although he implicitly believed that a deaf person could learn to speak and speechread, he believed that writing and his manual alphabet (a variation of the ROCHESTER METHOD, which he called DACTYLOLOGY) were more practical.

Espousing a natural language approach and early language stimulation, Dalgarno believed that a deaf infant could learn as quickly as a hearing baby if given the proper stimulation.

Danish Mouth-Hand System   See MOUTH-HAND SYSTEMS.

Danish Sign Language   Considered to be the primary language of deaf people in Denmark, Danish Sign Language has about 6,000 signs and is used together with the INTERNATIONAL HAND ALPHABET introduced by the WORLD FEDERATION OF THE DEAF in 1975. This manual alphabet is now used in Norway, Denmark and Finland. In addition to fingerspelling, a MOUTH-HAND SYSTEM has become an integral part of DSL.

Deaf Danish students were first taught in 1807 using methods based on the French manual method of ABBÉ CHARLES MICHEL DE L'EPÉE. Danish students were using their own signs, but teachers supplemented these with French signs when necessary; this influence by French Sign Language is still noticeable in the Danish sign vocabulary.

Although the oral method of education was introduced in 1881, DSL was never banned from Danish schools. Today, the five deaf schools all emphasize a manual educational method.

In addition, a combination of spoken Danish and sign language is called Signed Danish. It is used, as in many other sign systems around the world, primarily when communicating between deaf and hearing people and in interpreting.

D.E.A.F., Inc. The Developmental Evaluation Adjustment Facility, Inc., is a multiservice agency serving deaf people in New England. Acting as a sister organization to GLAD in California, the agency offers independent living services, an evaluation unit, education and training and also sponsors the telephone relay (TDD) service for Massachusetts. In addition, D.E.A.F. sponsors PROJECT ALAS, a service for deaf Latinos and their families. Contact: D.E.A.F., Inc., 215 Brighton Ave., Allston, MA 02134; telephone (voice and TDD): 617–254–4041.

deaf and dumb An archaic term coined by Aristotle meaning that a person can neither hear nor speak. The term is not in favor today because of its negative implication that deaf people are also "dumb" in a literal sense.

Deaf and Hard-of-Hearing Entrepreneurs Council A group that encourages, recognizes, and promotes entrepreneurship by people who are deaf or hard-of-hearing. Contact: Deaf and Hard-of-Hearing Entrepreneurs' Council, 814 Thayer Avenue, Ste. 303 Silver Spring MD 20910; telephone (TDD) 301–650–2244; email: MACFADDEN@MACF.com

Deaf Artists of America This group was organized to bring support and recognition to deaf artists by collecting, publishing and disseminating information about deaf artists. It also provides cultural and educational opportunities and services to members and exhibits and markets deaf artists' works.

The group offers two directories—one of visual artists and one of performing artists. The directory of visual artists (such as painters, sculptors and graphic designers) includes names, addresses, telephone numbers, education, type of artist and availability, along with several photographs of artwork. The directory of performing artists lists information on individual artists and performing arts groups. It includes names, addresses and telephone numbers of actors, dancers, mimes, poets and storytellers with information on their availability, fees and willingness to travel. Contact: Deaf Artists of America, 87 N. Clinton Avenue, Suite 408, Rochester NY 14604; telephone (voice and TDD): 716–325–2400.

deaf-blindness The twin difficulties of the inability to see and hear cause special problems for the individual as well as the person's teachers and rehabilitators. The exact term used to describe people who are both deaf and blind is controversial. People who are both deaf and blind sometimes prefer their condition to be described as "deafblind" or "deaf-blind."

Some people feel that removing the hyphen to create one word separates the condition from deafness and from blindness, reflecting the unique nature of the condition. Others assert that hyphenating the words achieve this distinction. Because deaf-blindness is rare, there has been relatively little help from agencies in this country. The first federal program for deaf-blind people was legislated only in 1968.

This legislation authorized and funded the rehabilitation facility called the National Center for Deaf-Blind Youth and Adults and regional educational programs for deaf-blind students, aimed at helping states educate deaf-blind children.

Although the particular problems of deaf-blind citizens were not widely known, the 1964 rubella epidemic brought the problem to the attention of the U.S. Congress—of the 30,000 infants who suffered visual or auditory systems problems because of this epidemic, about 1,500 were born blind and deaf. In 1966, there were 564 deaf and blind students in this country, but only 177 were enrolled in school. A realization of the impending influx of deaf-blind students prompted Congress to appropriate special funds for their education in 1968.

Deaf-blind people have a loss of two senses in common, but there is wide variation among their other abilities, just as in the hearing and sighted population.

One of the problems faced by deaf-blind people is the definition of deaf-blindness: Different facilities and educational programs define it differently. Further, blindness itself is defined differently across the country. Many groups support this definition: Deaf-blindness involves visual and auditory problems so great that they prevent accommodation in programs for those who are only visually impaired or hard of hearing.

The number of deaf-blind people in the United States is hard to calculate, but a national study commissioned by the Department of Education in 1980 estimated between 42,000 and more than 700,000, depending on how deaf-blindness is defined.

Most people who are deaf-blind are over age 65 because as individuals get older, the risk of impairments increase. More women than men are deaf and blind, which may be related to a woman's longer lifespan. The study also revealed the so-called "rubella bulge" (the excess number of children born blind and deaf during the 1964–65 rubella epidemic), who were from 14 to 16 years old at the time of the study.

In the absence of epidemics, between 250 and 300 deaf-blind children can be expected to be born each year because of genetic problems, accidents and diseases.

Only 1.7% of deaf-blind people are institutionalized, which means that for every person institutionalized, more than 50 are living in the general population.

Despite this national study, many gaps in understanding this population remain. There is no available data on socioeconomic status, education, race, employment or civil status of deaf-blind people, which inhibits efforts to reach this population.

Education   Teaching a deaf-blind child is certainly difficult, but it is not impossible. According to the National Needs Assessment of Services for Deaf-Blind Persons, the major obstacle to success is the low opinion of the abilities of deaf-blind people held by parents, teachers and society.

When the Elementary and Secondary Education Act of 1968 was passed, it authorized the establishment of centers for deaf-blind children. But it was not until the passage of the Education for All Handicapped Children Act of 1975 (PL 94-142) that education for all deaf-blind children could be guaranteed, since any local agency could deny education to a student it considered too difficult (or costly) to teach. From 1968 to 1980, enrollment for deaf-blind students increased from 110 to 6,000.

According to research, even children born blind and deaf can be taught to communicate, especially if provided with early intensive intervention soon after birth. Without early efforts to stimulate deaf-blind infants, they develop stereotypical, asocial behavior in an effort to provide the stimulation they don't get from their environment. To counteract this, parents must provide continual, consistent stimulation of taste, feel, smell, movement and temperature together with enhancing whatever residual sight or hearing the child has.

Although deaf-blind children are just as intelligent as sighted and hearing children, their communication problems mean they acquire knowledge more slowly and often show self-stimulatory behavior. This behavior, which appears almost autistic, can include waving fingers, rocking and rubbing their eyes.

History   The first deaf-blind student successfully educated was LAURA DEWEY BRIDGMAN, who was taught by 19th-century educator Samuel Gridley Howe, director at the Perkins Institute for the Blind in Massachusetts. Eight-year-old Laura first learned the names of objects by feeling raised letters that spelled out their names and were pasted on the objects. She later learned the manual alphabet, although she never learned to speak.

Her educational success was followed by Helen Keller's, who was taught by another Perkins school graduate, Anne Sullivan. Keller later attended Perkins and met the elderly Laura Bridgman.

The first school with a formal program for deaf-blind students was Perkins, which established a department for the education of deaf-blind students in 1931. This was followed by seven other schools for deaf-blind students within the next 30 years. (See also KELLER, HELEN.)

Deaf Entertainment Foundation (DEF)   An organization that recognizes and encourages excellence among deaf artisans and that promotes the realistic portrayals of the deaf and hard-of-hearing world. The Deaf Entertainment Guild Directory (DEG) lists more than 150 talented people (the largest publication of its kind), including deaf, hard-of-hearing and hearing people who are fluent in American Sign Language. Contact DEF: 8306 Wilshire Blvd., Ste. 906, Beverly Hills CA 90211–2382; telephone (voice): 323–782–1344; (TDD) 323–655–1542 or 323–782–0298; website:http://www.deafentertainment.org/

Deafness and Communicative Disorders Branch   This office is part of the Rehabilitation Services Administration in the Office of Special Education and Rehabilitative Services of the federal Department of Education.

Designed to promote better rehabilitation services for deaf, hard-of-hearing, speech-impaired and language-disordered people, the office offers technical assistance to administration staff, public and private agencies and individuals and funds interpreter training programs. Contact: Rehabilitation Services Administration, Department of Education, Mary E. Switzer Building, 330 C Street SW, Room 3315, Mail Stop 2312, Washington DC 20202; telephone: 202–732–1282.

Deafness Research Foundation (DRF)   The nation's largest voluntary health organization devoted primarily to furthering research into the causes, treatment and prevention of hearing loss and other ear disorders.

Founded in 1958, this group provides grants for fellowships, symposia and research, provides information and referral services and publishes *The Receiver.*

Second only to the federal government in its research support into hearing loss and ear problems, the DRF also maintains an otologic fellowship program to aid talented third-year medical students interested in research. For example, it awarded more than $1.5 million toward research into age-related hearing loss between 1987 and 1991. Contact: Deafness Research Foundation, 575 Fifth Ave., 11th floor, New York, NY 10017; telephone (voice and TDD): 212–599–0027; website http://www.toxicnoise.com

DEAFPRIDE   A nonprofit, community-based advocacy organization that works for the human rights of all deaf people and their families. DEAFPRIDE helps groups organize and work together for change in the District of Columbia and throughout the country.

DEAFPRIDE also provides interpretative services for residents of the Washington, D.C. metropolitan area, the agencies that employ them and the programs that provide social, health, legal and educational services, including a 24-hour emergency service for medical and legal emergencies.

The organization is working for a changed society where deaf people are understood as persons with their own language and culture and who have equal access to everything society has to offer. The organization has a special focus on deaf people who have the least access to resources and education. Contact: DEAFPRIDE, Inc., 1350 Potomac Ave. SE, Washington, DC 20003; telephone (voice and TDD): 202–675–6700.

DEAFTEK.USA   The only international nonprofit organization providing computer electronic mail service for deaf and hard-of-hearing people. DEAFTEK was established in 1977 by the Deaf Communications Institute of Framingham, Massachusetts. No longer in operation, the institute was an independent organization that focused on telecommunications services and offered a range of other communications services in addition to DEAFTEK.

The computerized DEAFTEK services include electronic messages, open bulletin boards for sending news of interest to the deaf community, telex, fax, electronic mail for research projects and express mail. Either a computer with modem or a telecommunication device for the deaf (TDD) WITH ascii must be used to hook up to the service.

An electronic mail network allows a subscriber to communicate with other members of the mail network, using a computer or ASCII-equipped TDD. The system works by transferring a message from one subscriber through a central computer which then transmits the message to the receiver who subscribes to the same system. The message is delivered in seconds to the recipient's "mailbox" (user's name or number), where it remains until that person picks it up by calling the system to retrieve messages. With electronic mail, the same message can be sent to several different mailboxes, saving time and money.

To use DEAFTEK, the caller dials a local phone number to access GTE Telemail (a national electronic mail network) and then types his mailbox name and password to connect to DEAFTEK. A DEAFTEK member can send or receive messages to or from others who belong to DEAFTEK, read "bulletin boards" with news announcements about the deaf community and have access to news items, provided by *USA News Today*, which are updated hourly.

DEAFTEK is available 24 hours a day throughout the world. The service is accessible only by ASCII modems or TDDs with ASCII capability. There is a yearly fee when joining DEAFTEK on GTE Telemail and monthly user fees (like a telephone bill).

In addition, DEAFTEK offers several limited access bulletin boards, spin-off communication networks focused in one area. DEAFTEK's bulletin boards include PSYCH.NET (mental health and the deaf community), AIDS.NET (AIDS and the deaf community) and NICD.GALLAUDET, where the NATIONAL INFORMATION CENTER ON DEAFNESS posts messages. Soon to be offered will be a "federal register" for the use of the Department of Education. (See also BAUDOT CODE.) Contact: DEAFTEK.USA, c/o INTERNATIONAL DEAF/TEK, INC., P.O. Box 2431, Framingham, MA 01701; telephone: 508–620–1777 (voice/TDD).

diplacusis   A condition in which a given frequency produces a different pitch in each ear; this common problem is called binaural diplacusis. The disorder is diagnosed by having the patient adjust the frequency in one ear to equal the pitch to a reference pitch in the other ear.

Although it is normal for a person with normal hearing to have slight differences in pitch between the two ears, people with a cochlear or retrocochlear hearing problem may experience up to an octave difference in pitch.

A related condition, called monaural diplacusis, results in hearing a group of tones when only one tone is actually present.

Often, an individual is unaware of having diplacusis unless he or she is a musician.

dizziness   This sensation of unsteadiness is a mild form of VERTIGO, which is characterized by a feeling of spinning either of oneself or the surroundings.

Although most attacks of dizziness are harmless, they may occur because of a disorder of the inner ear, hearing nerve or the brain.

In labyrinthitis, a viral infection can inflame the fluid-filled canals within the inner ear, affecting balance; in severe cases, even a sudden movement of the head can cause dizziness and fainting. In the inner ear degenerative syndrome called Ménière's disease, dizziness and vertigo are common symptoms.

In more rare cases, a tumor or MENINGITIS affecting the hearing nerve can cause dizziness. Any disorder of the brain stem that connects with the hearing nerve—such as reduced blood supply or tumors—can also result in dizziness.

In cases of dizziness caused by disorders of the inner ear, some physicians may recommend antiemetic or antihistamine drugs.

Doerfler-Stewart test   An auditory test used to determine functional or psychogenic hearing loss by testing a patient's ability to respond to spondee words (two long or accented syllables) spoken in the presence of a masking noise presented through earphones. In cases of a functional hearing loss, the patient will be unable to respond consistently to words at varying intensity levels.

Dutch Sign Language   Formally known as Sign Language of the Netherlands (SLN), this sign language has five separate dialects, each related to a school for deaf students. There are about 25,000 deaf Dutch people who use sign language.

Dutch Sign Language is based on signs invented in 1827 and later formally taught in a school based on the educational principles of French deaf educator ABBÉ CHARLES MICHEL DE L'EPÉE. Developed from French Sign Language some features are similar to British and American Sign Languages. However, most other Dutch schools were oral in approach, and these students developed their own signs independent of their schools.

It is only recently that Dutch educators have begun to accept SLN based on new research findings. The language is different from Signed Dutch.

dysacusis   Meaning "faulty hearing," the term includes any hearing problem not caused primarily by a loss of auditory sensitivity.

From the word "acusis" (or "acousis"), referring to hearing, and "dys," meaning ill or painful, the word is also spelled "dysacusia" and "dysacousia." It is caused by a malfunction or injury of the central nervous system, the auditory nerve or the organ of Corti and is not helped by amplifying speech. Therefore, dysacusis is not measured in decibels.

It must be emphasized that deafness/hearing loss and dysacusis are not necessarily mutually exclusive; for example, a person may have both HEARING LOSS measured in decibels and also a dysacusis in the form of a loss of discrimination.

"Dysacusis" may also be used as a broader term meaning loss of all kinds of hearing—two or three of which may be present in the same person. On the other hand, "hard-of-hearing" implies specifically one kind of problem—loss of sensitivity.

There are several types of dysacusis, including discrimination loss for words, syllables or PHONEMES; reduced intelligibility for sentences; AUDITORY AGNOSIA; phonemic regression; and binaural DIPLACUSIS and monaural diplacusis.

dysphasia   Speech or language problem. It is thought that children with dysphasia hear sounds but can't make sense of them, or, if they can make sense, they are unable to put their responses into words. There may be problems with perception, sound discrimination, auditory memory, comprehension, word-finding, reading and writing.

Unlike adults with APHASIA (often following a stroke), there is no loss of previous function; instead, children fail to develop normal language.

Sometimes, deaf children are wrongly labeled aphasic or dysphasic, especially those who don't make progress in oral-only programs. Because there are not any clearcut tests for developmental dysphasia, careful and repeated evaluations are necessary.

E

eardrops   Eardrops are prescribed for certain conditions in the outer and middle ears but cannot affect the inner ear. Eardrops cannot restore hearing in cases of nerve damage, but they can treat itch, discomfort or ear infection in the outer or middle ears. Eardrops should only be used upon recommendation by a physician.

Ear Foundation, The   A national, nonprofit organization founded in 1971 and committed to leading the effort for better hearing through public and professional educational programs, support services and applied research. The foundation is particularly interested in problems of ear-related disorders, specifically hearing loss and balance disturbances. From its inception, the foundation has been dedicated to the continuing education of ear specialists and to the development of auditory and vestibular research.

The foundation also administers THE MÉNIÈRE'S NETWORK, a national network of patient support groups that provide people with Ménière's disease the opportunity to share experiences and coping strategies. Contact: The Ear Foundation, 1817 Patterson St., Nashville TN 37203; telephone (voice and TDD): 800-545-HEAR.

ear massage   Although it is untrue that pressing on the skull behind the ear or on the neck can improve hearing, gentle massage can restore hearing caused by a problem with the eustachian tube.

However, ear massage can also cause disarticulation of the middle ear bones and is not recommended.

When the eustachian tube doesn't equalize pressure in the MIDDLE EAR cavity (such as during an airplane flight), rubbing the ear gently, yawning, swallowing, chewing and so forth can fill the middle ear with the needed air.

ear structure   Ears collect and decipher everything from whispers to screams, and can distinguish not only one musical note from another but even the same note played on different instruments. Superbly crafted to handle our environment, ears contain a sort of gyroscope to help maintain balance, and can protect themselves against noise and selectively tune out unwanted sounds—even during sleep.

The outer and middle ears amplify some sound waves because of the way the ear canal narrows as it proceeds inward, funneling the noise. Once the sound reaches the eardrum, it is transmitted and amplified by the vibrations of the eardrum's skin. Next, the middle ear's three bones

164

(OSSICLES) receive sound through the drum and push it through the oval window into the inner ear.

Once inside the inner ear, the COCHLEA (a small-shaped system of canals located behind the oval window) takes over to interpret pitch. The cochlea contains fluid and about 20,000 tiny hair cells tuned to various pitch frequencies. When the middle ear's stirrup pushes the sound through the oval window, it makes the cochlea vibrate, and the fluid travels to the tiny hair cells where separate pitches are registered. Hair cells responsible for high notes are located near the base of the cochlea, lower-frequency cells are near the apex.

The cochlea generates tiny electrical currents, sending the sound through acoustic nerve connections to the brain, where it is decoded and presented as one of the 350,000 separate sounds a human can recognize. (See also DIAGRAM OF THE EAR; INNER EAR; MIDDLE EAR; OUTER EAR.)

ear tube   A small tube that is inserted through the EARDRUM during a surgical incision (MYRINGOTOMY) made in the eardrum to treat a chronic middle-ear effusion in children.

The tube serves to equalize the pressure on both sides of the eardrum, which allows the fluid to drain out of the ear. About six to twelve months after the operation, the tube usually falls out on its own as the eardrum heals.

Water should be kept out of the ear in children with an ear tube, and swimming is usually forbidden. (See also MYRINGOTOMY; SEROUS OTITIS MEDIA.)

earwax   A yellow or brown secretion called cerumen, earwax is produced only by glands in the outer ear canal. Any wax deeper inside the canal has been pushed there by a finger or a cotton applicator. The normal function of wax in the ear is to protect the skin of the ear canal by keeping it soft and moist.

Among people who have very narrow or hairy ear canals and among people who work in dirty or dusty environments, wax can build up until it completely blocks the ear canal. When wax is pushed into the ear canal and presses on the EARDRUM, it may sometimes cause ear noises and even dizziness, both of which disappear when the wax is removed.

Earwax is a normal part of the body's function and should not be stopped. Removing earwax with a COTTON SWAB is dangerous; probing can remove protective layers of keratin, opening the way for possible infection of skin cells. There is also a danger that the swab could be pushed through the eardrum, causing problems ranging from severe pain to total deafness. Often cotton swabs push wax farther into the ear canal, which eventually causes impacted earwax. To be kept clean, the ear only needs soap, water and a washcloth.

echolocation   The technique of locating objects by emitting bursts of sound and interpreting the echoes; used by sonar and animals such as bats.

Education and Auditory Research (EAR) Foundation   A national nonprofit association of doctors, educators and concerned citizens dedicated to providing information and resources to people who suffer from hearing problems. The EAR Foundation offers support services promoting the integration of people with hearing and balance problems into mainstream society. The foundation also provides practicing ear specialists with continuing medical education courses and related programs specifically regarding rehabilitation and hearing preservation. Finally, the group tries to educate young people and adults about hearing preservation and early detection of hearing loss, enabling them to prevent at an early age hearing and balance disorders. Contact: The EAR Foundation, 1817 Patterson St., Nashville TN 37203; telephone (voice and TDD): 800–545–HEAR; (voice and TDD): 615–329–7807; http://www.theearfound.com

Education for All Handicapped Children Act   See LEGAL RIGHTS.

education of deaf children   Deafness itself does not affect either a person's intellectual capacity or the ability to learn. Since most deaf children have hearing parents, it is important to begin exposing these children to communication as early as possible. But often, a child's hearing loss—or his parents' acceptance of it—might not come until the second year of the child's life. Even if the parents are willing to learn American Sign Language at that point, it takes time to learn before they become proficient. Crucial early interaction with some form of language has been lost.

Because deaf children of hearing parents are not exposed to a continuous language flow, they miss out on an enormous amount of language stimulation. Language delays can be offset by exposing deaf children to early, consistent visible communication methods (sign language, fingerspelling or cued speech) together with amplification and aural/oral training, if desired.

Only a small percentage of deaf children have deaf parents, but those who do have the great advantage of learning AMERICAN SIGN LANGUAGE (ASL) from the beginning. Studies show that these children progress in language development and acquisition at the same rate as hearing children learn English and outdistance their deaf peers who did not learn ASL from infancy.

Type of School   The first problem facing parents of a school-age deaf child is where to get the best education. In the past, deaf children were educated primarily in residential schools, which provided maximum exposure to the latest technology in deaf education but limited the child's family relationship.

Today, the trend is growing in favor of MAINSTREAMING the child at least part of the day at the local public school, enabling the child to live at home and remain in touch with the neighborhood. This change reflects the popularity of the mainstreaming movement and also the Education for All Handicapped Children Act of 1975, which mandates a free public education for all "handicapped" children in the least restrictive environment and sets specific guidelines to protect their rights. The act also requires each child to receive nondiscriminatory testing and an individualized educational plan that is renewed each year. (See also LEGAL RIGHTS.)

As a result, parents have many more educational options today than they did prior to the 1960s. There are four major choices: residential school, special day school, special day classes, or regular classes supplemented by special services. Each of these options is described below.

Residential schools. These schools board deaf students full time, although most programs allow the students to spend weekends at home with their families. These schools offer instructional, recreational and social programs designed for their deaf pupils. Students who live nearby may attend these residential schools as day pupils.

Day school programs. Deaf students in these programs go to a school exclusively for deaf youngsters but return home in the afternoon like other school children.

Self-contained day classes. Many neighborhood public school systems offer special classes for deaf students. Under this program, deaf students may join hearing students for physical education and art or be "mainstreamed" (put in classes with hearing students) with interpreters for some classes. Usually, these special programs provide a resource room to help deaf students get information for classes they attend with hearing students.

Regular classes. This choice, known as mainstreaming, allows deaf students to attend regular classes with hearing students for most or all of the day. Often, the deaf child may be provided interpreters, tutors and resource room teachers.

In addition, some school districts may design their own programs for deaf students, utilizing some or all of the above methods.

In high school, deaf students can choose to enter a vocational training program or take academic courses with an aim to attending college, either at a regular university or a college for deaf students, such as GALLAUDET UNIVERSITY in Washington, D.C. or the NATIONAL TECHNICAL INSTITUTE FOR THE DEAF in Rochester, New York. In addition, there are many community colleges and technical schools in the United States with special programs for deaf adults.

Manual vs. Oral Approach   In addition to the type of school, parents must make another important—and historically far more controversial—

decision. There has been no issue in deaf education more bitterly disputed over the past 200 years than the question of how students and teachers should communicate in the classroom.

The problem was made more difficult by a misunderstanding of American Sign Language by linguists in the first part of the 20th century, who insisted only spoken language was a real language. Today, linguists accept that American Sign Language is indeed a language with its own syntax and grammar and all the richness and complexity of any other language.

The manual approach was brought to this country by educator THOMAS HOPKINS GALLAUDET, who, thwarted in learning the oral English method, studied the French manual method instead. Trained at the famous Paris Institute (Institut National de Jeunes Sourds) in this method, Gallaudet introduced the manual approach to America at the first public school for deaf students in Hartford, Connecticut.

Other methods from Europe soon followed. In 1867, Bernard Engelsmann, a teacher of deaf Viennese students, introduced the German method—the oral approach—in a school for deaf children in New York City, now known as the Lexington School.

In 1878, Zenas Westervelt introduced the ROCHESTER METHOD at a school for deaf students in Rochester, New York based on a system in which deaf students are taught to speak and fingerspell English simultaneously while written English is also being emphasized.

Gradually, schools in this country began to rely on the oral approach of communication until almost all preschool and elementary classes for deaf children were oral-only and forbade the use of signs or fingerspelling. Schools emphasized oral education based on the theory that any type of manual communication would interfere with English and speech development and would keep the deaf child isolated from the larger hearing world.

But as the skills of deaf students—who have the same intelligence range as hearing children—lagged behind, educators began to question whether all-oral schools were failing large numbers of deaf people. This growing doubt was fueled by studies showing that deaf children of deaf parents out-performed deaf children of hearing parents in academic achievement, social adjustment, reading and written English skills. These studies seemed to show that not only did ASL not inhibit English fluency but apparently enhanced its acquisition. Today, few schools use an oral approach.

Manual approach supporters also argue that many children do not have the aptitude for oral instruction and that the time spent on trying to speak could better be spent developing the child's mental abilities. Further, some advocates of a manual education believe that deaf people prefer to associate with other deaf people and therefore have no need to be able to speak.

Some oral approach supporters, on the other hand, still believe that training in speech and speech reading help the child adjust to a speaking world. By learning to speak, they reason, the deaf child will not be confined to the deaf community or to those willing to use sign or a pad and pencil. They further point out that a person who can speechread and speak may find it easier to land a job. In general, oral supporters believe that orally-trained youngsters are likely to do better as more teachers are trained in this field.

All organizations of deaf educators believe that deaf children should be given the opportunity to learn to speak, but there is often heated debate as to what constitutes "fair opportunity."

Total Communication   Today, programs for deaf students are moving toward a more inclusive form of education called Total Communication, which supports a deaf child's right to be exposed to any form of communication that is effective. This includes speech, speechreading, gestures, reading, writing, FINGERSPELLING, manual codes of English, ASL and use of residual hearing.

Most programs today use a manual code of English together with spoken English.

How much the child's inability to hear will affect school performance depends on many things—the degree and type of hearing loss, the age of onset, additional handicaps, the quality of the school and support the child receives.

Typically, deaf children from ages one to three begin their education in a clinical program featuring extensive support from parents. Because 85% to 90% of deaf children are born to hearing parents, these programs often emphasize the implications of deafness and teach parents how to cope with problems. At age three, the child can attend preschool sessions with other deaf children, and by age four many deaf youngsters attend special nursery and kindergarten classes full time.

In order to learn, deaf children must devise a way to communicate. A child's hearing may be helped by hearing aids, but hearing may still be quite limited. In order to develop a consistent, two-way means of communication, many deaf children and their parents learn sign language.

electronystagmography   A test to determine the presence of damage to the body's balance system, which can help determine damage to the inner ear, by recording the electrical changes caused by eye movement. This technique has been used successfully for more than 50 years. For this test, electrodes are placed on the face above, below and beside the eyes. The patient is then placed in a variety of situations, and resulting eye movements are electrically recorded. (See also AUDIOMETRY.)

El Mudo   See NAVARRETE, JUAN FERNANDEZ DE.

employment of deaf people   Deaf people work in the same jobs as hearing people, and their deafness in itself does not prevent them from doing most jobs. In fact, according to the NATIONAL INFORMATION CENTER ON DEAFNESS at GALLAUDET UNIVERSITY, more and more deaf people have been moving into professional, administrative, managerial and technical careers. Today, they are working as physicians, dentists, lawyers, physicists, engineers and computer analysts and programmers in addition to other technical and professional positions. Prior to the 1970s, however, most deaf people were employed mainly as factory workers, craftspeople and unskilled laborers.

The movement of deaf workers into all job levels can be credited to improved educational opportunities, antidiscrimination laws, a better understanding of deafness by the general public and an increased assertiveness in the deaf community.

Unfortunately, salaries have not kept pace with the upward movement of deaf employees; the average salary of deaf workers has been somewhat less than the salary of hearing workers in similar jobs, although this gap is closing due to antidiscrimination laws.

In the 1972 National Census of the Deaf Population, employed deaf workers' median incomes ranged between 72% and 76% of that of the general population. Of these workers, 71% were in crafts, operative or clerical jobs. A 1982–83 survey of managerial, professional and technical workers with hearing problems (from mild to profound) found a median salary of $21,957—about $1,700 less than the salary of workers in similar jobs.

Many experts in the field of deafness believe deaf people still tend to be underemployed, which was certainly true prior to the 1970s. Still, the picture is changing; one study found that in 1960 profoundly deaf people were working in 28 different types of professional jobs in the hearing sector. By 1982–83, this number had almost doubled to 54.

l'Epée, Abbé Charles Michel de (1712–1789)   Born in 1712, de l'Epée was a French cleric who, upon meeting two deaf daughters of a Parisian family, saw the children's deafness in spiritual terms and wanted to teach the girls about the Catholic church in order to save their souls. Making up his methods as he went along, the cleric eventually taught the girls to read and write.

Following this experience, he opened a school in Paris in 1760 for deaf students; this became the first school that taught only deaf children and the first large community of deaf people anywhere in the world. Today it is known as the INSTITUT NATIONAL DES JEUNES SOURDS.

As he worked with his pupils, de l'Epée discovered that many of these children—especially those whose parents were deaf—communicated with each other by using systematic gestures. Suspecting that these gestures might be the "mother tongue" of deaf people, de l'Epée collected these signs and added his own "methodical" signs for gender, tense and number.

Although de l'Epée recognized the importance of speech and taught it to some of his pupils, he realized that in his classes (some as large as 60) signing was more practical. He believed that it was better to give many deaf children some idea of language—albeit a silent one—rather than teach only a small number to speak. His critics argued that SIGN LANGUAGE condemned deaf people to isolation, but de l'Epée believed it was important to allow deaf students to have their own identity. This tension between the value of sign versus the ability to speak is the core of a controversy over educational methods for deaf students that has lasted for more than 200 years. (See also SICARD, ABBÉ ROCH AMBROISE CUCURRON; SPEECHREADING.)

Episcopal Conference of the Deaf   This group, affiliated with about 50 Episcopal congregations in the United States, promotes ministry to deaf people though the Episcopal Church.

Originally called the Conference of Church Workers Among the Deaf, the group was founded in 1881 at St. Ann's Church for the Deaf in New York City to support church members working with deaf people. The organization holds annual meetings and publishes a newsletter, *The Deaf Episcopalian.*

The Episcopal Church was the first religious group in the United States to establish a congregation specifically for deaf members—St. Ann's Church for the Deaf in New York City, founded in 1852 by Thomas Gallaudet, the eldest son of THOMAS HOPKINS GALLAUDET.

Soon, a second church for the deaf was established in 1859 in Philadelphia (All Souls Church) with help from St. Stephen's Church, which had been holding special services for deaf members. All Soul's Church also became known for allowing the ordination of the first deaf Episcopal priest in 1876 in the United States. Contact: Episcopal Conference of the Deaf, 1616 Calle Santiago, Pleasanton CA 94566.

Eustachio, Bartolomeo (1510?–1571)   Roman anatomist and great pioneer of otology who described the air passage from the throat to the ear now known as the EUSTACHIAN TUBE.

Eustachio studied in Rome, becoming the personal physician to the duke of Urbino. When he returned to Rome as the personal physician to the pope, he soon became famous as an anatomist, physician, philosopher and linguist.

His discoveries span the entire field of anatomy, although his greatest contribution was the description of the shape and course of the structure that bears his name. Although the existence of the eustachian tube had been vaguely known, it was left to Eustachio to explore it fully.

Exact English   See MANUAL ENGLISH.

F

facioscapulohumeral muscular dystrophy (FSH MD)   One of the mildest forms of muscular dystrophy, some recently reported cases of FSH MD have involved SENSORINEURAL HEARING LOSS in both ears. However, not enough cases have been documented to clearly define the incidence of hearing loss associated with this condition.

This is an autosomal dominant condition, which means it can be transmitted genetically to other offspring in 50% of all cases. (See GENETICS AND HEARING LOSS.)

Falloppio, Gabriele (1523–1562)   One of the foremost Italian anatomists of his time, Falloppio of Modena was the founder of the Italian School of Anatomy and was among the first to describe the anatomy of the ear, ACOUSTIC NERVE and tympanic cavity.

fast auditory fatigue   A hearing problem that occurs in patients with a tumor on the auditory nerve in which continuous loud sounds decrease in intensity.

During a continuous sound, a normal listener hears the tone loudly at first, then less loudly because of adaptation, but the tone remains audible and at a fairly steady loudness after the first 15 or 20 seconds.

However, if the auditory nerve is partially compressed—by a tumor, for example—the loudness continues to fall until the tone is inaudible. If the intensity is increased, the tone becomes audible again but then fades out again.

fenestration   This name for an operation on the ear literally means "opening a window." Fenestration was once the treatment of choice for otosclerosis, a familial form of deafness corrected only by surgery.

In 1938, American otologist Julius Lempert discovered and first performed a fenestration, which can relieve deafness by creating a new route for sound to travel from the outer ear to the cochlea. By removing most of the bone in the middle ear, Lempert extended the outer ear canal and created a new OVAL WINDOW (or fenestra) through which sound waves could be sent to the inner ear. After a fenestration, sound by-passes the entire chain of bones (OSSICLES) in the middle ear, and although the otosclerosis is still present, the new window is located in the horizontal semicircular canal of the LABYRINTH—an area rarely affected by otosclerosis.

For 20 years, fenestration was the only surgical way to treat otosclerosis, but it was never performed casually since afterwards hearing can never again be completely normal. Although patients had a good chance for some improvement of their conductive hearing at first, most patients experienced a deterioration in hearing afterwards. Since both the eardrum and ossicles (which usually help magnify sound waves) were removed, patients experienced a hearing loss of at least 25 decibels. Many experienced unpleasant side effects, including facial paralysis, VERTIGO and suppurative (draining) ear infections. The patient must be careful of his ears for the rest of his life. Even a small amount of water in the ear can cause a serious infection; baths, showers and hair-washing can be a major problem.

Because of this, fenestration has not been the treatment of choice in otosclerosis since 1951, except for a few patients. These would include someone whose disease has progressed to the point of solidifying the entire oval window, people who have already had more than one STAPEDECTOMY (an operation to free the fixed stapes) because of closure of the oval window from otosclerosis or people born without an oval window or stapes.

For everyone else—and for those for whom fenestration did not work—stapedectomy gives more satisfactory results.

fingerspelling This system of communication involves spelling out words in an alphabetical language by using the letters of the manual alphabet—with handshapes and positions corresponding to each letter of the written alphabet.

Manual alphabets are found throughout the world, although the systems in Continental Europe and the Americas are quite different from the one used in Great Britain, where manual English uses both hands.

Manual alphabets differ from sign languages in that they are not a natural language but a method invented by educators and derived from a written language.

Fingerspelling can either be used by itself or together with sign language, when it is generally employed to spell out proper names or technical words. The alphabet can be modified for use with deaf-blind people by making handshapes and movements on the palm of the receiver of the message.

It is thought that the earliest manual alphabet was developed by PEDRO PONCE DE LEÓN in the 1500s and first published by JUAN PABLO BONET in 1620, and its roots can still be seen in many of the one-handed alphabets used today throughout the world. Even countries that do not use the Latin alphabet—such as Israel, which uses the Hebrew alphabet, or the Soviet Union, which uses the Cyrillic alphabet—still use a manual alphabet related to Bonet's.

Unrelated to Bonet's alphabet is the British two-handed system, which is used throughout the British commonwealth countries. A third type is the Swedish manual alphabet invented by Per Borg and exported to Portugal. It is the parent alphabet of the Swedish and Portuguese manual alphabets used today.

Still, other types of manual alphabets developed in countries without written alphabetic systems, such as Japan and China. Japan uses a fingerspelling system based on syllables instead of single sounds, and although a Chinese manual alphabet is being developed, most deaf Chinese draw the outline of the Chinese characters in the air or on palms.

In the American manual alphabet, conversations can be entirely fingerspelled, but among deaf individuals, fingerspelling is more often used in conjunction with AMERICAN SIGN LANGUAGE for proper names and terms for which there are no signs. Fingerspelling alone is used more often among people who are both deaf and blind, presented either at close distance or inside the hand.

It takes only a few hours to learn the individual hand shapes, but becoming fluent as a fingerspeller is quite difficult. The drawback to the method is its relative slowness; for people very experienced in its use, the average fingerspelling rate is about 60 words a minute, which is only about 40% as fast as the normal speaking rate.

Although very rarely used as the primary mode of communication in schools for deaf students today, fingerspelling combined with spoken English is known as the ROCHESTER METHOD.

Finnish Sign Language   There are two major dialects of Finnish Sign Language (FinnSL), one used by the Finnish-speaking majority and the other by the Swedish-speaking minority. (Finland has three official languages: Finnish, Swedish and Lappish). About 5,000 of the 8,000 deaf Finns use one of the two forms of FinnSL.

By far, the majority of Finns speak the Finnish dialect; 16 of the 17 schools for the deaf are Finnish. Signing is not forbidden in any of the Finnish schools for deaf students, and teachers use Signed Finnish, a pidgin type of FinnSL using the syntax of Finnish and the vocabulary of FinnSL. As is typical in many other countries, congenitally deaf Finns can use Signed Finnish, but they ordinarily do not communicate among other deaf Finns in anything other than FinnSL.

There are 37 handshapes in FinnSL: 31 are distinctive, although six of these are rarely used. Handshapes are classified into three groups: fist, one-finger and multi-finger. Further, every multi-finger handshape must include at least one finger that appears in a one-finger handshape. There are 12 locations of signs and 24 movements. In addition, the international manual alphabet has replaced the Swedish manual alphabet for spelling out place names and proper names.

Fitzgerald Key   A printed system to help deaf children learn to speak, read and write syntactically correct English sentences. The Fitzgerald Key was developed in 1929 at the Texas School for the Deaf by Edith Fitzgerald, a deaf supervising teacher.

Its set of six words and symbols help children analyze the relationships between units of connected language, enabling them to write good sentences and correct their own errors. Under the system, a child places individual words under the headings of subject, verbs and predicates, indirect and direct objects, phrases and words telling where, other word modifiers of the main verbs and "when" words and phrases.

The system is still widely used today. (See also EDUCATION OF THE DEAF.)

flat hearing loss   A hearing loss that is about the same at all important frequencies.

Flourens, Marie-Jean-Pierre (1794–1867)   This 19th-century French experimental neurologist was the first scientist to find evidence that the vestibular labyrinth is the organ of equilibrium. His experiments with pigeons showed, among other things, that hearing was not affected by destroying the nerves to the vestibular organs, but it was destroyed by cutting the cochlear nerve.

fluoride and hearing   Fluoride is chiefly used in this country to combat tooth decay, but it is believed to strengthen the bones of the body as well.

Research suggests that the COCHLEA—the strongest bone in the body—may also benefit from fluoridation of public water systems. These studies suggest that just as tooth decay decreases in areas of fluoridated water, the incidence of otosclerosis (softening and overgrowth of bone within the middle or inner ear) decreases in those same areas.

However, if otosclerosis is already present, fluoride does not appear to have any effect.

France   This country, with its long history of education for deaf students, has about 3.5 million people with hearing problems; between 50,000 and 100,000 of these use sign language as their primary means of communication. With a deafness rate at 47 out of 100,000 France has one of the lower proportions of deafness in the world.

One of the most famous schools for the deaf is the Institut National de Jeunes Sourds founded in 1790 as a school favoring the manual education philosophy. It was to this school that THOMAS HOPKINS GALLAUDET came to learn sign language and, together with French instructor LAURENT CLERC, returned to America with the manual method.

Since the early 1960s in France, physicians emphasized the early identification of hearing problems together with immediate use of hearing aids and preschool education beginning in infancy. The four largest public national institutes for the deaf are primarily residential and were founded in the 19th century or before; most private schools for the deaf are religious institutions and today make up the Federation of Institutions of the Deaf and of the Blind of France. This private group of 40 schools, mostly residential, stresses vocational training. Finally, there is a group of private nonresidential centers that teaches students from preschool age up. These centers use more innovative techniques than the older schools and take a medical approach to deaf education.

Although the history of education for deaf students stressed vocational training, there were a few students who chose instead a more academic curriculum. Today, one private institution prepares students to take the special "baccalaureate," an exam required of 18-year-olds for many jobs and for acceptance to a university. Very few deaf students pass the exam, however, and even fewer go on to university training.

MAINSTREAMING has also been introduced in France on a very limited basis; in 1980, only 346 deaf and 1,326 hard-of-hearing students attended public schools.

The oral approach in education became accepted in France following the Congress of Milan of 1880 and endured in all schools until the late 1970s.

FRENCH SIGN LANGUAGE (FSL) began making a return to popularity in the wake of the WORLD FEDERATION OF THE DEAF Congress in Washington D.C. in 1975, where French delegates were impressed at how AMERICAN SIGN LANGUAGE was accepted. As organizations have gathered to fight for the use of FSL, demand for classes and interpreter services has risen dramatically. The National Association of France of Interpreters for the Hearing Impaired was created in 1979. (See also SICARD, ABBÉ ROCH AMBROISE CUCURRON; L'EPÉE, ABBÉ CHARLES MICHEL.)

French Sign Language   The primary method of communication among deaf French people and the first sign language to earn acceptance as a separate, complete language of its own. Called LSF (Langue des Signes Française), this language was made famous by the ABBÉ CHARLES MICHEL DE L'EPÉE, leading educator of deaf students in the 19th century.

By the 18th century, LSF was a fully integrated sign language among the deaf French populace; at the beginning of the 19th century l'Epée and the ABBÉ ROCH AMBROISE CUCURRON SICARD borrowed signs from LSF, added some of their own and created their "methodical signs." This system, which included signs representing French grammatical structure, was the first attempt at applying the structures of a spoken language to a sign language.

It was during the 19th century that the great debate between oralists and manualists took place; as the debate between the French manualists and the German oralists raged, disciples of the French method were sent all around the world. As a result, traces of LSF can be found internationally, especially in the sign languages of the United States. In fact, some say more than half the signs of ASL have been borrowed from the French.

By the 1820s, French educators were arguing that deaf students should be educated in LSF, not the artificial "methodical sign" language. For the next 50 years, LSF was used in schools as a primary communication method. With the Milan Congress of 1880 came the triumph of the oral approach over sign, however, and sign language was banned in French schools by the government. But in the late 1970s, the sign language movement gathered steam again around the world.

Today in France, LSF is taught by deaf people outside the educational system, as deaf schools have not been quick to welcome back sign language. It is estimated that up to 100,000 deaf people in France use LSF.

Research suggests that LSF is grammatically similar to ASL; handshapes are quite similar between the two. Like AMERICAN SIGN LANGUAGE, there are three categories of LSF verbs: verbs that don't use personal pronouns, verbs that change direction with the use of personal pronouns ("you give me") and classifier verbs. Many similar facial expressions are also shared between the two to indicate negative sentences, questions and conditional and relative clauses. (See also FRANCE; MANUALISM; ORAL APPROACH.)

functional hearing loss (nonorganic)   Functional hearing loss exists when there is no physical reason for the patient's apparent inability to hear. It is also known as psychogenic hearing loss or hysterical hearing loss.

Instead, the person's hearing loss is primarily a result of psychological or emotional factors; the hearing mechanism itself may be completely normal. Sometimes, there is some slight damage in the ear, but the recorded hearing loss is much less than the patient reports.

Functional hearing loss is often caused by anxiety resulting from emotional conflicts and is beyond the control of the patient. In many cases, a functional hearing loss may occur at the same time as a true organic hearing problem. Called functional overlay, the problem in this case is to recognize the two different components of the hearing problem using a patient history and otologic exams.

A person with unilateral functional deafness may have a complete absence of bone conduction on the side of the bad ear and normal acuity on the side of the good ear. Such a person may even claim not to hear a shout on the bad side in spite of good hearing on the opposite side. It is these inconsistencies that help establish a functional loss.

G

Gallaudet, Edward Miner (1837–1917) This leading educator of deaf people established the first college for deaf students in the United States and fought to introduce a combined educational system integrating oral methods with the MANUAL APPROACH dominant at that time throughout the country. At a time when the rest of the world had changed to oral instruction in the wake of the Milan Congress of 1880, he clung resolutely to his belief in retaining the "natural" language of deaf people, although he did recognize the strong appeal ORAL APPROACH held for many people.

The son of a deaf mother and THOMAS HOPKINS GALLAUDET, cofounder of the first public school for deaf students in the United States, Edward Gallaudet felt a profound sensitivity toward deaf people. His understanding of their educational potential made him a leader in the field.

Although young Edward did not start out intending to focus on education of deaf children as a career, he changed his mind after his father died. He began teaching at the AMERICAN SCHOOL FOR THE DEAF in 1855 but, unhappy at the school, he left and was on the verge of heading to Chicago when he received a letter from philanthropist Amos Kendall of Washington, D.C.

Kendall, a multimillionaire, wanted Gallaudet to take over the Columbia Institution for the Deaf. Gallaudet saw this as his chance to establish his dream: a university for deaf students.

He began his job there in 1857 when he was only 20 years old, and in 1864 he asked Congress to allow the institution to grant degrees after a six-year course of study.

Gallaudet went to Europe in 1867 to study the ORAL APPROACH just being introduced in the United States, and upon his return, he submitted a plan to introduce oral instruction in combination with the MANUAL APPROACH then being taught at the school. He strongly believed in an equal emphasis on the manual approach and offered oral instruction as a separate course at the school. Other courses were taught manually, with additional classes in speechreading and speech.

In his career of educating deaf students, Gallaudet became an implacable opponent of oralist ALEXANDER GRAHAM BELL. Although the two initially disagreed politely, over time their enmity deepened. In 1895, Gallaudet accused Bell of fanaticism over the oral approach, calling him an outsider before a CONVENTION OF AMERICAN INSTRUCTORS OF THE DEAF. Bell and Gallaudet did not speak for the next five years.

Gallaudet lived to see the 100-year celebration of the American School for the Deaf, the institution founded by his father. He died in Hartford, Connecticut, in 1917.

Gallaudet, Thomas Hopkins (1787–1851)   This Connecticut theologian was a pioneer in U.S. education for deaf people and opened the American School for the Deaf, the first permanent school for deaf students in the United States at Hartford, Connecticut.

The eldest of 12 children, Thomas Gallaudet was born in Philadelphia, the son of a merchant family of deep religious convictions. A brilliant child, Thomas entered Yale at age 14 and graduated first in his class three years later; within five years, he had apprenticed with a law firm, studied literature and earned a master's degree from Yale. He graduated with a divinity degree from Andover Theological Seminary in 1814 and intended to become an itinerant preacher until a chance meeting with a young deaf girl changed his life forever.

While visiting his parents in 1814, the 27-year-old Gallaudet met ALICE COGSWELL, nine-year-old deaf daughter of Dr. MASON FITCH COGSWELL, a prominent Hartford physician. Gallaudet began trying to teach young Alice some reading and the manual alphabet and succeeded in breaking through the communication barrier by teaching her the word "hat." With the enthusiastic backing of her father, who did not want to have to send young Alice to Europe to be educated, Gallaudet was persuaded to learn the European methods of teaching deaf students so he could return and set up a school in Connecticut.

When Gallaudet's informal census of deaf children suggested there were about 80 in Connecticut, he guessed there might be at least 400 in New England and perhaps 2,000 in the entire country.

It is probable that when Gallaudet set out, he intended to study both the British method of oral instruction and the French manual style in order to develop a combined approach to education. But when Gallaudet arrived in Great Britain, the developers of the British method—the THOMAS BRAIDWOOD family—were unwilling to share their methods. Gallaudet spent some time studying educational philosophies in Scotland and then went to Paris to interview ABBE ROCH AMBROISE CUCURRON SICARD, head of the Institut Royal des Sourds-Muets, (now called the Institut National de Jeunes Sourds) who welcomed Gallaudet. At the school Sicard allowed Gallaudet to observe methods used at each level and personally taught him the manual method used at the school. Gallaudet also studied sign language with JEAN MASSIEU and LAURENT CLERC at the school.

With Sicard's permission, Gallaudet took Clerc, one of Sicard's best pupils and a master teacher himself, back to Connecticut with him in 1816 to help organize a school for deaf students. In order to garner support for the school, Gallaudet, Clerc and Mason Cogswell toured New England, presenting demonstrations at town meetings, churches and public gatherings. Clerc's presence at Gallaudet's side was proof of the possibility of educating a deaf person and their fund-raising tours were very successful.

Within six months after returning to America, Gallaudet opened the country's first permanent school for the deaf in Hartford, Connecticut. The school featured the manual (French) method of education. Soon Gallaudet's Asylum for the Education and Instruction of the Deaf and Dumb (now the AMERICAN SCHOOL FOR THE DEAF) began enrolling students from other states.

Because the school was on its way to becoming a national institution, Gallaudet was granted financial aid from the U.S. Congress to continue his programs.

By the middle of the 19th century, there were schools for the deaf in 12 states and a national college for the deaf in Washington, D.C. run by Gallaudet's son, EDWARD MINER GALLAUDET.

Most of the schools that began during the 1800s used the French method of manual instruction, a trend established with Gallaudet's American School for the Deaf in Hartford.

Gallaudet College, renamed after Thomas (formerly the Columbia Institution for the Deaf), was officially chartered by an act of Congress in 1864 and signed into law by Abraham Lincoln. It has now operated for more than 100 years as the only liberal arts college for deaf students in the world.

Gallaudet's position as leader of the movement for deaf education was helped by his talents as preacher, orator and writer, which were useful in his push for educational reform from the pulpit and the podium.

He died on September 10, 1851, in Hartford, but his interest in education for deaf students was continued by his deaf wife Sophia Fowler, a graduate of the Hartford School, and by two of their children. Their oldest child, Thomas Gallaudet, was a minister to a deaf congregation at St. Ann's Church in New York City; EDWARD MINER GALLAUDET was the first president of Gallaudet College, now GALLAUDET UNIVERSITY, in Washington, D.C.

Gallaudet Preschool Signed English system   An invented sign system based on the spoken English language and including English spelling, pronunciation and meaning. The signs used in this system feature letter initialization and compounding. (See also MANUALLY CODED ENGLISH.)

Gallaudet Research Institute   This eight-unit research group, located at GALLAUDET UNIVERSITY in Washington, D.C. is the largest institute in the world dedicated to investigating the immediate and long-range concerns of deaf people.

The institute has a multiple mission of research, teaching and service and supports broad-based research involving collaborations among scientists from many disciplines. The group brings together individuals from around the world to discuss deafness-related research and shares its information through conferences, seminars, lectures, training and consultation.

As part of its dedication to service, the institute offers a wide range of resources through its eight units, including:

- genetic counseling
- communications networks for teachers and administrators
- technological device referral
- monograph series
- demographic statistics
- projections/recommendations on needs of deaf elderly people
- "working paper" series in a wide variety of topics
- advice and consultation for researchers
- published proceedings of major deafness-related events
- technical assistance to businesses developing new devices for people with hearing losses

Firmly believing in the importance of outreach and service, institute staffers often give lectures and presentations to various groups, consult on deafness-related topics, serve on advisory boards, review and edit manuscripts and participate in peer review for funding agencies. A national advisory committee helps guide the institute's choice of research priorities, and the Office of the Dean of Graduate Studies and Research administers the institute.

The eight units in the institute are:

Center for Assessment and Demographic Studies   This unit analyzes national databases containing information on deaf and hard-of-hearing people and advises governmental agencies on national policy. Since 1968, this unit has conducted its own annual survey of hard-of-hearing children. In addition, the unit monitors hard-of-hearing students receiving special services and studies national test standardizations for hard-of-hearing students.

Center for Studies in Education and Human Development   This unit was established in 1981 to conduct research in the field of deafness. Today, ongoing research studies include how deafness affects parent-infant interaction, the earliest stages of language development and reading and writing processes. In addition, scientists are trying to develop models of the best educational environments for deaf children.

Center for Auditory and Speech Sciences   Researchers in this unit investigate ways of improving the speech perception of deaf and hard-of-hearing people through auditory, visual or tactile means. Through auditory experiments, researchers try to discover the exact types of distortions hearing problems impose on the perception of specific speech sounds. Researchers are currently developing tactile devices to aid speechreading and are investigating certain types of hearing deficits common to the elderly.

Genetic Services Center   This center was established by the institute in 1984 to explore the more than 200 known genetic forms of hearing problems as well as certain other kinds of deafness acquired through environmental means. The primary function of this center is to provide genetic evaluations and counseling sessions to help deaf people and their families understand the causes and effects of hearing loss. Staffers also consult with and train AUDIOLOGISTS, geneticists, parents, consumers and the medical community.

Technology Assessment Program   Established in 1985, this program produces information for industrial, government and consumer groups interested in improving access to technology for people with hearing problems. The unit collaborates with several technical centers to develop devices that can, for example, alert deaf drivers to approaching emergency vehicles, convert speech to text, allow deaf people to communicate in sign language or speechread over telephone lines and provide deaf-blind people with robotic fingerspelling as an alternative to braille or personal interpreters.

Culture and Communication Studies Program   This unit analyzes and compares the processes involved in acquiring language and forming cultural identities in the United States and other countries. Presently, the program's cross-cultural studies involve Spain, Italy, Mexico and some countries of Central and South America.

Mental Health Research Program   The cause and effect of mental health problems among people with hearing problems is explored by this unit, which is also working to develop better ways of testing and treating these problems. Researchers are currently studying differences in cerebral organization among hearing and deaf children, personality characteristics of deaf college students and depression among deaf adults. The program also provides information on coping strategies for people who lose their hearing in adulthood and psychologists are involved in translating standard psychological tests into AMERICAN SIGN LANGUAGE.

Scientific Communications Program   This program was created in 1987 to intensify the institute's efforts to communicate results of deafness-related research to others. In addition to its publication *Research at Gallaudet* and the institute's annual report, the group publishes research monographs, conference proceedings and working papers to help publicize results of selected studies. Contact: Gallaudet Research Institute, 800 Florida Avenue NE, Washington DC 20002; telephone: 202–651–5400 or 800–451–8834.

Gallaudet University   Located in Washington, D.C., Gallaudet University is the only liberal arts university specifically for deaf students in the world.

The school was established in 1864 on land donated by Amos Kendall, a well-known journalist, politician and philanthropist, who had become interested in the welfare and education of deaf children. Called the Columbia Institution for the Deaf and Dumb and Blind when it was incorporated by Congress in 1857, it was granted a charter in 1864 to operate a collegiate division at the request of its first superintendent, EDWARD MINER GALLAUDET. Gallaudet was the son of THOMAS HOPKINS GALLAUDET, who founded the first public residential school for deaf children in the United States.

The National Deaf Mute College opened with 13 male students, one professor and one instructor; in 1887 it admitted six women as part of a two-year experiment. Although criticized for this decision, Dr. Gallaudet allowed the women to remain, letting them live in the president's house until the experiment was considered successful and a woman's dormitory could be built.

A Normal Department was begun in 1891 to train hearing teachers of deaf students, and three years later the school's name was changed to Gallaudet College to honor Edward Miner Gallaudet's father, Thomas.

Today, Gallaudet has a student body of more than 2,200, including a limited number of hearing undergraduate students. The school includes two campuses: the original 99-acre Kendall Green campus in northeast Washington and a newer nine-acre Northwest Campus seven miles from Kendall Green. Students are accepted upon recommendation from local school districts or special schools and must have graduated from high school and have passed the Gallaudet entrance exam. Of the more than 1,400 students who take the exam, usually only half qualify for admission; of these, about 70% must take up to one year of preparatory work before they can be admitted to the first-year class.

About two-thirds of the student body have a profound hearing loss and more than one-fourth have a severe loss. Almost all students lost their hearing before school age; since 1970, most students have been congenitally deaf.

In 1988 the university elected King Jordan as its first deaf president after a one-week mass protest and demonstration initiated by the deaf community, faculty and students. The successful protest is considered by deaf people to be a historic event, and profoundly important to the deaf community.

Gallaudet continues its commitment to education, research and service and houses the world's most complete collection of materials related to hearing loss, deafness and deaf people. Its library archives contain written, visual and audio materials on deafness dating back to 1546.

Gallaudet's MODEL SECONDARY SCHOOL FOR THE DEAF opened on 17 acres on the northwest part of the Kendall Green campus in 1976, and a KENDALL DEMONSTRATION ELEMENTARY SCHOOL began in 1980 on six acres in the northeast part of campus.

Gallaudet's 288 faculty members, of whom 35% are deaf and hard-of-hearing, teach in more than 40 undergraduate and graduate programs offered through the following schools: College of Arts and Sciences, School of Communication, School of Education and Human Services, School of Management and School of Preparatory Studies. Educational programs are also offered through the College for Continuing Education.

The university grants bachelor of science or arts degrees in 26 major fields of study; its graduate school offers hearing students a two-year program leading to a master of science in audiology and both hearing and deaf students a master of arts in education, rehabilitation counseling, school counseling, educational technology and linguistics.

The Ph.D. degree in the administration of special programs is offered by the graduate school in conjunction with the Consortium of Universities in the Washington area, of which Gallaudet is a member. About one-third of these doctoral candidates have hearing problems.

Gallaudet also offers extensive noncredit courses, workshops, seminars, internships and an associate of arts degree in interpreting for hearing people who wish to become certified sign language interpreters.

The university maintains an active student government and publishes a school paper *(The Buff and Blue)*, an annual literary magazine *(Manus)* and a yearbook *(Tower Clock)*. Plays are produced twice a year and are presented in signs and voice; they are open to the public. The college has three sororities and three fraternities and a varied sports program that includes football, soccer, rugby, track, volleyball, basketball, baseball, field hockey, tennis and golf.

Gallaudet also maintains the NATIONAL CENTER FOR LAW AND THE DEAF, the International Center on Deafness, GALLAUDET RESEARCH INSTITUTE, the NATIONAL INFORMATION CENTER ON DEAFNESS and the Management Institute.

The university's Center on Deafness also features educational extension centers in cooperation with local colleges and universities. These include Ohlone College in Fremont, Calif.; Northern Essex Community College in Haverhill, Mass.; Flagler College, St. Augustine, Fla.; Kapiolani Community College, Honolulu, Hawaii; Johnson County Community College, Overland Park Kans.; Eastfield College, Dallas Tex.; Gallaudet University Regional Center, Washington, D.C.; and University of Puerto Rico; San Juan, P.R. (See also GALLAUDET UNIVERSITY ALUMNI ASSOCIATION.) Contact: Gallaudet University, 800 Florida Avenue NE, Washington DC 20002.

Gallaudet University Alumni Association   Representing more than 4,000 deaf people, the Gallaudet University Alumni Association members include about half of all alumni from the four-year college.

Founded in 1889 in Washington, D.C., the association meets twice a year and is open to graduates, past attendees of the college and people who have received an honorary degree from the school. It is an associate member of the WORLD FEDERATION OF THE DEAF and maintains more than 55 chapters throughout the United States and Canada. Local chapters raise money for student loans, scholarships and awards, athletic uniforms, and so forth and have provided money for memorials, endowment funds and travel for students participating in leadership conferences.

In addition, the association publishes the *Gallaudet Alumni Newsletter* twice a month, coordinates reunions and special events on campus and assists in recruiting, fundraising and public relations.

German Sign Language   In the former Federal Republic of Germany (West Germany), almost all prelingually deaf Germans use Deutsche Gebardensprache (DGS), a sign language with many dialects arising from various schools for deaf students.

A traditionally oral country, there has been little research into DGS, which has not generally been used in educational settings, although it is a natural communication mode among deaf people outside the classroom. When manual approaches are mentioned in schools, the reference is to Signed German.

Although similar to AMERICAN SIGN LANGUAGE in some ways, DGS—as many other European sign languages—uses more lip movements. FINGER-SPELLING, using a manual alphabet similar to the American one, is also used with DGS, although older DGS users do not know the manual alphabet. More popular is a manual system called PMS (Phonembestimmtes Manualsystem), which represents phonemes instead of letters. This system is used in schools for deaf students to teach articulation.

gestuno   The first "international" SIGN LANGUAGE, developed by members of the WORLD FEDERATION OF THE DEAF in an attempt to overcome the problem of communication at international meetings.

Gestuno is a collection of about 1,500 signs chosen for ease of use to build a basic international vocabulary. The problem of syntax was simply ignored.

The problem with this international sign language is that few people are willing to learn the new signs, the communication it allows is often too limited, and there are not enough occasions to use it to make learning gestuno worthwhile for most people.

gestural language See SIGN LANGUAGE.

ginkgo biloba A tree whose leaves have been used by Chinese herbalists for thousands of years to treat a variety of physical problems, including deafness and TINNITUS (ringing of the ears). Western herbalists today use ginkgo leaves for a variety of problems, explaining that the leaf can help expand blood vessels and improve blood flow in vessels and arteries (especially in the lower legs and feet). It also appears to boost blood flow to the brain. Herbalists believe that the leaves of the ginkgo tree may help reverse deafness caused by reduced blood flow to the nerves involved in hearing.

The leaves are available in dry bulk, in capsules or as a tincture. Standardized ginkgo biloba extract (GBE) is available in health food stores. WARNING: Ginkgo should not be used by anyone with a clotting disorder or by pregnant or nursing women. It should not be given to children without a doctor's supervision and should only be used in medicinal amounts in consultation with a health care professional. Some people are unable to tolerate ginkgo even in small doses.

GLAD An acronym for Greater Los Angeles Council on Deafness; this nonprofit group, founded in 1969, is a comprehensive service center and umbrella agency for more than 45 California groups and agencies in the field of deafness, including social, recreational and service clubs for the deaf community and educational, professional, health and religious organizations. It serves more than 1,500 hearing and deaf members.

GLAD sponsors community workshops and educational lectures and links traditional social service agencies with the deaf community. It also offers employment referral services, interpreter referrals, telephone/TDD relay services, peer counseling and advocacy. Under a grant from California's rehabilitation department, GLAD also offers the first sign language interpreter pool free of charge to deaf people. With this pool, deaf people in California have access to more than 200 qualified interpreters.

The council consults with police, hospitals, school districts and the state legislature in support of deaf services. Located as it is in the heart of the entertainment business, the council also works with producers on projects that involve deaf subjects or actors to ensure that deaf characters are honestly portrayed and that deaf actors are hired as often as possible to play deaf roles.

The council produces an extensive resource book, the *Directory of Resources Available to Deaf and Hearing Impaired Persons in the Southern California Area* and the journal *GLAD News Magazine* and maintains a bookstore carrying volumes on deafness. The council is a member of the NATIONAL ASSOCIATION OF THE DEAF. Contact: GLAD, 616 South Westmoreland Avenue,

Second Floor, Los Angeles CA 90005; telephone: 213–383–2220 (voice/TDD).

grammar   The structure of language. Grammar consists of a number of elements: *morphology* (how sounds go together to form words or (in a signed language) how the elements of position, shape and movement combine to form signs); *syntax* (how words or signs are organized in sentences); *semantics* (how to interpret the meaning of words, signs and sentences); *pragmatics* (how to participate in a conversation).

Greece   The outlook for deaf people in Greece is not encouraging since less than half the deaf citizens in the country are given any education at all. Of those who are, only 10% get more than elementary instruction.

Although it is estimated that there are at least 1,480 deaf children in the country, only 640 receive some form of special education, and there is no state provision for their education.

The National Foundation for the Protection of the Deaf and Dumb provides six educational facilities for deaf children, serving about 400 residential and day students (most in elementary schools). There are two other schools for deaf children. The schools all favor an oral approach, with an emphasis on speechreading and auditory training and no signing in class. Despite this, Greek Sign Language, with its roots in American and French sign languages, is used by more than 30,000 adult deaf Greeks.

Since there is no provision for deaf teacher training, specialists either are educated abroad or are trained simply as regular classroom instructors. There are currently no adult or higher education programs specifically for deaf people.

Although at present deaf citizens have few choices and fewer services, there is hope for the future: In 1983 a national committee began developing a comprehensive educational program for all children with hearing problems between ages 12 and 18.

H

hair cells More than 15,000 microscopic hair-like cells are located inside the inner ear in an area smaller than a fingernail. They cover the ORGAN OF CORTI—the actual part of the ear that allows a person to hear. There are about 3,400 inner hair cells in the human cochlea that extend in a row from the base to the apex of the cochlea. In much the same way, close to the lateral surface of the organ of Corti are three or four rows of about 12,000 outer hair cells. These inner and outer hair cells incline toward each other, and cilia emerge from the upper surface of the inner and outer hair cells to penetrate the tectorial membrane, which forms a roof over the organ of Corti.

When a sound wave makes the eardrum vibrate, the vibrations are carried across the middle ear by the hammer, the anvil and the stirrup, which passes the vibrations through the oval window to the fluid in the tubes of the inner ear. This makes the hairs of the organ of Corti vibrate— and the more hairs that vibrate, the louder the sound. The shorter, thinner hair cells pick up high sounds, and the longer, thicker hairs pick up low sounds. The auditory nerve picks up the messages from these hairs and sends them to the brain, where the sound is processed.

Excessive noise can overload the tiny, irreplaceable hair cells and can seriously impede the ability to hear.

hearing aid helpline This toll-free telephone number is operated by the NATIONAL HEARING AID SOCIETY for anyone who suspects a hearing loss and is uncertain what to do or who needs information about hearing loss and hearing aids. The helpline may be used by consumers to locate qualified, competent hearing aid specialists and answer questions about hearing instruments, dispensing and service.

Callers can also obtain a consumer information kit, which includes a regional edition of the membership directory of the Hearing Aid Society plus a 22-page booklet covering topics such as how hearing works, signs of hearing loss and types of hearing aids.

Information is available on ASSISTIVE LISTENING DEVICES, requirements for entering the hearing aid profession, statistics on hearing loss and hearing instruments, federal regulations pertaining to the hearing instrument industry and so forth. The helpline does not provide medical advice, recommend specific products or quote prices.

Although direct financial assistance is not available through the helpline, the helpline can provide a list of possible financial resources. All services and materials provided are free. Callers may use the helpline numbers (1–800–521–5247; in Michigan, 1–313–478–2610) Monday through Friday, 9:00 A.M. to 4:30 P.M. EST.

hearing ear dogs   Certain dogs can be trained to respond to specific sounds (a doorbell, a crying baby, a smoke alarm, an alarm clock) by making physical contact with the owner and leading him or her to the source of the sound.

The dogs, which can be any breed or size, are usually obtained at humane shelters by a nonprofit training center. At these special centers, the dogs complete a six-month program in basic obedience, specialized skills, using both voice and hand signals, and "sound keying"—zeroing in on specific noises. Most dogs are trained to alert in different ways depending on the type of sound so that the owner can distinguish a crying baby from a ringing doorbell.

After training is completed, the dog is taken to its new home, where dog and potential owner go through an intensive one-week course together. After three months of satisfactory performance by the dog, ownership is transferred and certification is granted. The dog's blaze orange collar and leash entitle dog and master to the same legal rights accorded to blind people and their dog guides.

Hearing dog programs are completely supported by donations and community service organizations; no applicant is denied a hearing dog because of inability to pay. For more information about hearing ear dogs, contact the American Humane Association, 9725 East Hamden Ave., Denver, CO 80231. (See also AMERICAN HUMANE ASSOCIATION; CENTER FOR HEARING EAR DOGS; Appendix 3.)

Hearing Education and Awareness for Rockers (H.E.A.R.)   An organization that educates the public about the real dangers of hearing loss resulting from repeated exposure to excessive noise levels. The group offers information about hearing protection, hearing aids, assistive listening devices, ear monitor systems and testing as well as other information about hearing loss and tinnitus. Further, it operates a 24-hour hotline information, referral and support network service. H.E.A.R. also conducts a hearing screening program in the San Francisco Bay area and launches public hearing awareness campaigns, programs for schools and seminars and distributes earplugs to club and concertgoers. Contact HEAR: P.O. Box 460847, San Francisco CA 94146; telephone (voice) 415–773–9590 or 415–431–3277; website: http://www.hearnet.com.

hearing-impaired   A term for hard-of-hearing or deaf persons that many in the deaf community find objectionable due to its negative connotations. The preferred term is "hard-of-hearing or "deaf.""

Hearing Industries Association (HIA)   This group is the professional association for hearing aid manufacturers and suppliers of component parts. Contact HIA: 515 King Street, Ste. 420, Alexandria VA 22314; telephone (voice): 703–684–5744; email: HIAllears@aol.com

Heinicke, Samuel (1727–1790)   This 18th-century German educator is considered to be the father of the ORAL APPROACH and founded one of the first state-supported public schools for deaf students in the world.

Although others believed that speaking was important in the education of deaf children, it was Heinicke who was convinced that speech is necessary in order to develop abstract thought. He was a contemporary of ABBÉ CHARLES MICHEL DE L'EPÉE, the founder of the MANUAL APPROACH, with whom he maintained a lifelong debate over the superiority of communication modes.

Born in Nautschutz, Germany, Heinicke joined the Saxon army after a quarrel with his father. While in the army he spent most of his time studying. Eventually, he became a tutor and in 1754 began to teach one of his pupils, a deaf boy, the manual language.

With the onslaught of the Seven Years' War in 1756, Heinicke fled the Prussian troops and eventually settled in Hamburg, where he found work as a private secretary, tutor and schoolteacher. Twenty years after teaching his first deaf student, he began to teach a second, this time abandoning the manual alphabet in favor of speech. In 1775 he published the first textbook ever written for the instruction of deaf students, and his fame as a deaf teacher grew; two years later, he was asked to establish a school for deaf students in Leipzig, Germany.

This new school, the Electoral Saxon Institute for Mutes and Other Persons Afflicted with Speech Defects, opened in 1778 as the first school for deaf students in Germany. It exists today as the Samuel Heinicke School for the Deaf.

Heinicke continued to refine his beliefs in the oral approach for deaf students during his 12 years as administrator at the school. Although he kept his methods to himself, he is known to be the world's first oralist who believed that no hearing child ever learned to speak by first learning letters. Instead, Heinicke taught deaf students the way hearing children learn to speak: first came words, which were then broken down into syllables.

Because Heinicke believed that deaf people have an inner drive to speak just the way hearing people do, he believed teaching speech was not a difficult task. Heinicke was convinced that certain tastes cause the mouth to form the correct position for certain vowels and that by substituting the sense of taste for the lost sense of hearing, Heinicke believed deaf students could be taught to articulate. In his work he used a special artificial throat and tongue designed to help students produce sounds.

Heinicke condemned the practice of operating on the tongue of a deaf child to correct speech defects since he believed that a deaf child's inability to speak was because he could not hear, not because his tongue was malformed.

Although Heinicke allowed the occasional use of signs in order to explain concepts, he required his students to speak out loud to each other in his presence.

De l'Epée and Heinicke both established schools for deaf students in their respective countries, paving the way for the idea of a free public education for deaf students and emphasizing the importance of special education for everyone who needed it. Yet although both de l'Epée and Heinicke believed in the importance of educating deaf children, they differed profoundly over how to accomplish this goal.

Heinicke maintained an ongoing debate with l'Epée over the superiority of communication methods, and was severely shaken when two universities decided that l'Epée's manual approach was superior. Heinicke was particularly distressed to learn that the University of Leipzig, with which his school was affiliated, sided with l'Epée in the controversy. Critics of his method persisted, and Heinicke continued to defend his methods. It appeared that the oral approach was waning and the manual approach was gaining momentum, but Heinicke's theories were eventually resurrected, refined and popularized many years after his unexpected death of a stroke in Leipzig, Germany on April 30, 1790.

Helen Keller National Center for Deaf-Blind Youths and Adults   The only national facility providing comprehensive services for diagnostic evaluation, rehabilitation and personal adjustment training and job preparation and placement for deaf-blind people.

The center also conducts extensive field service through regional offices, affiliated programs and national training teams, offers services to elderly deaf-blind people and maintains a national register of deaf-blind people. The organization designs and improves sensory aids and publishes *The Nat-Cat News*. Contact: Helen Keller National Center for Deaf-Blind Youths and Adults, 111 Middle Neck Road, Sands Point, NY 11050; telephone (voice): 516–944–8900; TDD (516): 944–8637; http://www.helenkeller.org

Helmholtz, Hermann Ludwig Ferdinand von (1821–1894)   A brilliant physiologist, anatomist, mathematician and physicist, von Helmholtz developed a resonance theory that each sound wave entering the ear induced vibrations in a basilar fiber that responded to the wave's frequency. It was

these vibrations, he believed, that stimulated the ORGAN OF CORTI, which transferred the vibrations to the auditory nerve. Later scientists found, however, that while the individual fibers do not resonate, the BASILAR MEMBRANE itself can create the resonance effect.

Hertz, Heinrich Rudolf (1857–1894)   This German physicist proved that light and heat are electromagnetic radiations, and he measured the length and velocity of electromagnetic waves in the laboratory. In honor of his achievements, the unit of vibration frequency, cycles per second, was named for him.

Hertz was also the first to broadcast and receive radio waves and proved that electromagnetic waves had the same properties of susceptibility to reflection and refraction as light and heat waves. (See also HERTZ; FREQUENCY.)

Holder, William   A 17th-century English rector interested in teaching deaf children to speak. His book *Elements of Speech*, detailed the position of all organs related to speech during the production of PHONEMES.

Holder advocated positive reinforcement and systematic speech development in which sounds are taught first, combined into syllables and then formed into words associated with objects.

home sign   Sometimes called homemade SIGN LANGUAGE, this refers to the gestures developed by deaf people who are isolated from the deaf community. Home sign is often the first way a deaf child communicates with hearing family members. Home signs are not the same as artificial sign languages, which are created by educators as a representation of a spoken language. (See also AMERICAN SIGN LANGUAGE; MINIMAL LANGUAGE SKILLS.)

House Ear Institute   A private, non-profit, medical research organization specializing in research into the ear—the causes of hearing loss, diagnosis and treatment—and training ear specialists and professionals from allied disciplines.

Founded in 1946 as the Los Angeles Foundation of Otology by patients of Howard P. House, M.D., the institute is supported entirely by private funds and was renamed in 1981 to honor House and his brother, William P. House, M.D., director of research.

Research at the institute includes studies of COCHLEAR IMPLANTS, HEARING AIDS, ear disease and tumors, diagnosis, hearing tests, TINNITUS, and prosthetic devices. In addition, the institute's researchers study normal and diseased tissues removed from patients during surgery. Its labs house the world's largest documented collection of temporal bones for microscopic study.

In 1981 the institute began a cochlear implant program for children, providing rehabilitative therapy and helping parents deal with issues facing deaf children. Parents' organizations sponsored by the institute include Bridging the Gap, Family Camp, Kid Safe and the Young Adult Work Program. Contact: House Ear Institute, 256 S. Lake, Los Angeles, CA 90057; telephone: (voice) 213–483–4431, (TDD) 213–484–2642.

Hubbard, Gardiner Greene (1822–1897)   This Massachusetts lawyer was passionately interested in educating deaf people, largely because his daughter Mabel (later the wife of ALEXANDER GRAHAM BELL) lost her hearing after a bout of scarlet fever at age four.

When Hubbard was told his daughter would lose her speech and could not attend school for six more years, he realized he would need to educate his daughter himself—or find a teacher who could. Aware of the success achieved by German educators of deaf students, he decided to set up a similar school in Northampton.

Hubbard was instrumental in the establishment of the Clarke Institution for Deaf Mutes, in Northampton, Massachusetts, an oral school for deaf students now called the Clarke School.

With his son-in-law Alexander Graham Bell, Hubbard founded the American Association to Promote Teaching of Speech to the Deaf, the National Geographic Society and the publication *Science,* the official magazine of the American Association for the Advancement of Science. In addition to his many entrepreneurial ventures, such as bringing gas lights and water to Cambridge, Hubbard led the presidential commission to reorganize the U.S. Postal Service and was a trustee of the Smithsonian Institution.

hysterical hearing loss   See FUNCTIONAL HEARING LOSS (NONORGANIC).

I

immune system and hearing loss   The immune system is crucial to the defense against infection of both the middle and inner ear. There is evidence that a faulty immune system can induce hearing loss and is responsible for the progression of chronic otitis media and possibly other disorders for which no cause has been found, such as Ménière's disease.

In addition, certain diseases that affect the immune system—such as AIDS—can also result in hearing loss. (See AIDS AND HEARING LOSS.)

impacted earwax   A hard plug of EARWAX firmly filling the ear canal, blocking the passage of sound to the eardrum and interfering with hearing. Symptoms are worsened if water enters the ear, causing the wax to swell.

Normally, earwax (or cerumen) is produced by glands in the skin of the outer ear canal and carried outward to the external ear. When it is produced too quickly, it builds up and forms a hard plug.

Large plugs of earwax must be removed by a physician; smaller plugs may be removed at home. A person can remove hard wax with mineral oil drops; soft wax can be removed with hydrogen peroxide drops or a commercial softener. The drops may be applied overnight and then removed by irrigating the ear with warm water from a baby ear syringe.

COTTON SWABS should not be used because of the danger of pushing wax deeper into the ear.

incus   The middle bone of the three OSSICLES of the middle ear, also known as the ANVIL.

India   It is estimated that out of India's population of more than 700 million, 800,000 are deaf; most of these live in the rural areas. Only about 5% of India's deaf children are currently in school. At a deafness rate of 66 per 100,000, India is about midway between Peru's high rate (300) and Australia's low rate (35).

Communication for India's deaf population is complicated by the fact that the country is considered trilingual, with the three languages being Hindi, English and one of the many regional languages. The education a deaf child would receive varies depending on the area in which he or she grows up.

The government is interested in helping provide services for its deaf citizens, but most resources for this purpose are limited.

India's first school for deaf students was opened in 1885; since 1900, 200 more schools have been established—none in the rural areas. Of the 200, only 14 offer secondary school education, and only a few offer vocational training. There is no school for university education for deaf students, although there are a few deaf Indian students studying at universities in the United States.

Education in India is not required, is not free and is based on an oral approach. Although most deaf Indians communicate in sign, its use in schools has been repressed.

INDIAN SIGN LANGUAGE is a highly-structured, grammatical language, and its first dictionary was just published in 1980.

Most deaf citizens are unemployed. There is no national captioning service, TELECOMMUNICATIONS FOR THE DEAF (Tdds) are not available, and there are almost no interpreters, even in large cities.

Indian Sign Language   Despite the country's official languages and more than 200 dialects, Indian Sign Language (ISL) is surprisingly universal in India; there is only one sign language, and more than one million deaf Indians communicate with it.

In general, the signs of the Indian system do not relate to any of the European sign languages, although there are a few signs similar to BRITISH SIGN LANGUAGE and its FINGERSPELLING system.

Because ISL is not used in schools, most deaf speakers use the pure, natural sign language. Initial research in ISL suggests its grammar is complex and is not similar to any of languages of India.

Ingrassia, Giovanni (1510–1580)   Born in Recalbuto, Sicily, Ingrassia was one of the most well-known Renaissance anatomists, and a contemporary of EUSTACHIO and FALLOPPIO. A professor in Padua, Naples and Palermo, and adviser to the king, he was among the first to describe the tympanic cavity and the OSSICLES and was credited with discovering the STAPES in 1546.

inner ear   An extremely intricate portion of the ear deep within the skull that contains the AUDITORY NERVE and the balance mechanism of the body in a winding maze of passages called the LABYRINTH.

The front of the inner ear, which resembles a snail shell and is concerned with hearing, is called the COCHLEA. The rear part, concerned with balance, is a series of three SEMICIRCULAR CANALS at right angles to each other and connected to a cavity called the VESTIBULE.

These canals contain hair cells continually bathed in fluid, some of which are sensitive to gravity and acceleration and others to position and movements of the head. This sensory information is registered by the cells and conveyed by nerve fibers to the brain.

Institut National des Jeunes Sourds   Also called the Paris Institute, this institution was founded by ABBÉ CHARLES MICHEL DE L'EPÉE in the 1700s and is today the oldest permanent school for deaf students in the world.

Begun with a grant from King Louis XVI, the school managed to stay open during the French Revolution. L'Epée began the school by teaching two sisters in his home and by the late 1760s had six students; 10 years later there were 30 students, and at the time of l'Epée's death in 1789, there were more than 60.

After the death of l'Epée, the school was run by ABBÉ ROCH AMBROISE CUCURRON SICARD, who convinced the French National Assembly that aid for handicapped students was a natural duty. In response, the assembly nationalized the school in 1791, naming it the National Institution for the Congenitally Deaf (Institut National des Sourds-Muets de Naissance).

The years of the French Revolution were difficult, and Sicard, the school's director, was imprisoned at least twice as a suspected Royalist. He was saved at last by a petition from his deaf students. Sicard directed the spartan program for 32 years until his death in 1822 at the age of 80. At that time, the school had 150 students, all whom used SIGN LANGUAGE (Old French Sign Language).

After the Catholic church was reestablished in France following the Revolution (in 1801), the school began to emphasize religion for its deaf student. Contact: Institut National des Jeunes Sourds, 254 rue Saint Jacques, 75005, Paris, France; telephone: 33-1-435-48280

intensity   The strength of a sound the brain perceives as loudness; usually measured by the amplitude of its wave. It is also measured in decibels.

International Catholic Deaf Association   A group promoting ministry to Catholic deaf people and responding to spiritually-related requests worldwide.

In general, Catholics have not had separate congregations for deaf members, although they do provide worship services in which an interpreter or priest signs the spoken portion of the mass. However, there are a few deaf Catholic churches in the United States, including St. Mary Magdalene Church for the Deaf (Denver, Colorado), Mother of Perpetual Help Church for the Deaf (Omaha, Nebraska), St. Francis of Assisi Catholic Church and Center for the Deaf (Landover Hills, Maryland), St. John's Deaf Center (Warren, Michigan) and the Catholic Deaf Center (New Orleans, Louisiana). (See also NATIONAL CATHOLIC OFFICE OF

THE DEAF.) Contact: International Catholic Deaf Association, 8002 S. Sawyer Road, Darien IL 60567; telephone (TDD): 630–887–9472; email: KgKush@aol.com

International Congress on the Education of the Deaf

For the past century, international meetings have been held to discuss education for deaf students, although early meetings rarely involved deaf educators or deaf persons at all.

For the first 100 years, no group administered these international meetings; a meeting could be called simply whenever a group within a country invited representatives from other countries to meet. But in 1975 in Tokyo, an International Congress Committee made up of the chairs of the three preceding congresses was finally established.

Many different topics were discussed at these meetings, but the prime controversy for almost 100 years was the debate between the ORAL APPROACH and the MANUAL APPROACH. The oral approach was the early favorite, and the second international Congress of Milan 1880 had an enormous effect on the education of deaf students around the world when convention participants decided that speech was "incontestably superior" to sign.

Further, Milan congressional delegates decided they preferred the oral approach over the simultaneous use of signs and speech as well. Milan resolutions cited the long-term benefits of oral education and devised procedures to introduce the oral approach into the schools.

The only votes against these pro-oral approach resolutions were an English delegate and the American delegates led by EDWARD MINER GALLAUDET. The oral-manual controversy continued to rage in nearly all of the congresses up until 1980, when delegates at the Hamburg congress decided the controversy was pointless and that both the oral and manual approaches could be helpful to deaf persons.

International Games for the Deaf

See WORLD GAMES FOR THE DEAF.

international hand alphabet

See INTERNATIONAL MANUAL ALPHABET.

International Hearing Society (IHS)

A professional association that represents hearing instrument specialists who test hearing and select, fit and dispense hearing instruments. It is a leading consumer advocate and conducts programs on competency qualification, education and training and promotes specialty-level accreditation for its members.

Founded in 1951 by a group of hearing instrument specialists, the society is active in promoting the highest possible standards for its members. Its directory lists members of the hearing health profession approved by the qualifications board of the society. The group also publishes a journal, *Audecibel* and provides consumer information through a toll-free helpline. Contact: International Hearing Society, 20361 Middlebelt, Livonia MI 48152; telephone (helpline): 800-521-5247.

International Lutheran Deaf Association   Nonprofit organization that promotes Lutheran ministry for deaf people throughout the Lutheran Church-Missouri Synod. The group, which publishes *The Deaf Lutheran,* holds an annual convention. Contact: International Lutheran Deaf Association, 1333 S. Kirkwood Road, St. Louis MO 63122; telephone (voice): 314–965–9917, ext. 1315; (TDD): 314–965–9000; V/T: 800–433–3954.

international manual alphabet   A manual alphabet devised by the WORLD FEDERATION OF THE DEAF and used primarily in Scandinavian countries.

International Organization for the Education of the Hearing Impaired   See ALEXANDER GRAHAM BELL ASSOCIATION FOR THE DEAF.

International Phonetic Association alphabet (IPA)   The most widely used phonetic alphabet, which is used to describe the segmental sound of speech. Most of the symbols in this alphabet are variations of Roman letters and can be used to describe speech in any language or dialect.

A sentence transcribed into a phonetic alphabet would allow a person to correctly speak the transcription, even if in a language that has never been heard.

A phonetic symbol represents a letter as a type of shorthand to describe how that sound is produced. For sounds that also have small differences in how they are pronounced, the alphabet uses basic and secondary symbols called diacritics, which are placed above or below (or before or after) the primary symbols. These diacritical marks indicate differences in sound.

The phonetic symbols used in dictionaries are not generally the IPA but the dictionary's own phonetic symbols, which are defined for readers using key words.

interpreters   See ORAL INTERPRETERS; SIGN LANGUAGE INTERPRETERS.

interpreters and the law   Since the 1960s, federal and state governments have enacted several laws requiring that a certified interpreter be provided for hard-of-hearing people during various court proceedings.

Unfortunately, although each state has some type of law guaranteeing an interpreter for a deaf person, many of the laws are vague, simple or unclear. Some laws state that courts and judges may appoint an interpreter when "necessary," but it is unclear who pays for these services, what the qualifications of the interpreter must be or what "necessary" means. Some states have comprehensive laws stating that interpreters should be appointed at the time of arrest in all civil and criminal cases, for the preparation of depositions, during commitment hearings, before grand juries, for a state exam needed for employment with the state and in juvenile proceedings.

Under state law, it is generally up to the judge to decide the qualifications for interpreters; some states do require consultation with the local or national REGISTRY OF INTERPRETERS FOR THE DEAF.

In criminal proceedings, most states will pay for an interpreter, and some states will pay for these services during civil proceedings as well.

Hard-of-hearing and deaf persons have the right under federal and state law to use the services of interpreters upon their request. When a hard-of-hearing or deaf person states a preference for an oral interpreter, the court must do its best to find one.

The situation is a little more clear in federal courts. When the federal government brings a criminal or civil action against a deaf individual, the law requires that the court appoint a qualified interpreter; in other situations, the federal court can appoint an interpreter if it so chooses. (See also COURT INTERPRETER'S ACT.)

interpreter services   See ORAL INTERPRETERS; SIGN LANGUAGE INTERPRETERS.

intra-aural muscles   The two muscles contained in the middle ear, known separately as the TENSOR TYMPANI and the STAPEDIAL MUSCLE. Their action is reflexive and bilateral and may be initiated either by intense acoustic stimulation or by irritation of the tissues of the external or middle ears.

A number of functions for these muscles have been suggested, but only two are generally accepted: The muscles assist in maintaining the OSSICULAR CHAIN in its proper position, and they act to protect the internal ear from too much stimulation by inhibiting ossicular movement.

Some research data suggest that the intra-aural muscles under moderate levels of tension and at certain frequencies slightly enhance the transmission of sound by the middle ear.

Irish Sign Language   There are three sign systems used in the Republic of Ireland—two based on manual English systems and one indigenous, informal method.

The newest system, called Irish Sign Language, is a manual code for English with one vocabulary for both men and women, unlike the older system with separate styles for men and women. It was introduced in the late 1970s by the Unified Sign Language Committee.

Most signs in the new system are based on the first letter of the word in English and are grouped so that many words of similar meaning will use the same basic sign but with different handshapes. This new sign language is used in some sign language classes taught outside traditional deaf schools and in the manual classes in the oral deaf schools. However, many people in the Irish deaf community prefer the old sign language system.

This older system is also a manual code for English and uses gender-specific vocabularies. Brought over from France in the 1800s, the French signs were modified to express English grammar and also split into "feminine" styles for use with the deaf girls' schools and more "masculine" for the deaf boys' schools. Today, the two vocabularies differ as much as 30%, although boys and girls can still understand each other.

Finally, the "informal" sign language, known as Deaf Sign Language, is used by deaf people in informal settings and is less accepted than the first two. It is believed this informal method is derived from the old sign language used in the Irish schools, but it does not parallel English grammar. Like all natural sign languages, however, it does appear to have its own grammatical system.

To a degree, portions of Irish sign systems have been exported to both South Africa and Australia.

Israel   Although there have been no definitive studies of the deaf population in Israel, estimates suggest that the incidence of deafness in Asiatic-African Jewish children and Israel's minority (predominantly Arab) group is about double that of European-American children. This unexpected incidence of hearing problems is probably due to the incidence of intermarriage within these cultures.

By age one, most of the country's deaf children are referred to one of the nationwide nonprofit institutions designed for deaf infants. Two of these centers use Total Communication; three use the oral approach. At these centers, parents are offered a range of services, including sign language classes, special discussions groups and home training. By the age of five or six, most deaf Jewish children are mainstreamed into state-supported kindergartens; about 10% attend special kindergartens designed for deaf pupils only. Once a child reaches elementary age, there are several options: a special school for deaf children, integrated classes, mainstreaming or a special school for multidisabled children.

Until 1976, all school programs used the oral approach; today educators use a combined approach (speech and ISRAELI SIGN LANGUAGE). At high school age, a student can choose to attend a vocational high school, integrated classes or mainstreaming.

In addition, the government offers its deaf citizen job placement and training services and private tutoring for deaf children in regular classes.

Israeli Sign Language was developed in the early 1900s and was eventually unified during the late 1950s with the establishment of the Association of the Deaf. In 1977, a signed Hebrew alphabet was created.

In general, Israel's heritage and comparatively concentrated number of deaf citizens has led to a wide network of services and programs for the deaf community.

Israeli Sign Language   About 5,000 deaf Israelis use Israeli Sign Language (ISL), a relatively new language continually infused with new signs from other countries as immigrants come to Israel. In addition, a FINGER-SPELLING system for Hebrew was adapted from the American MANUAL ALPHA-BET and includes 16 handshapes for Hebrew.

Still considered a very new language, ISL appears to be very flexible regarding sign order. The modifying sign follows the sign for the thing it modifies (for example, cat fat) and quantifiers precede the sign for the thing quantified (four horses) or bracket the thing quantified (four horses four). Israeli sign language also has major structural characteristics as in other sign language, such as the simultaneity of signs.

Although deaf schools in Israel have been completely oral since the first school was founded in 1934, teachers today use some ISL signs in their oral classes.

Italian Sign Language   Still widely considered to be simple gestures in Italy, research has found the sign language of deaf Italians is indeed a complete language with a complex structure and grammar.

The structural features of LIS (Lingua Italiana dei Segni) are different from other languages, and the Italian spoken language influences LIS in the use of speechreading and articulation. FINGERSPELLING is rarely used, although there is an old and a new manual alphabet. The older method, used primarily by older deaf Italians, is a two-handed system employing hands and the face. The new version, used by younger deaf Italians, is a one-handed system using only handshapes.

There is no census information available on the number of people who use ISL, and it is not used in the all-oral school systems.

Italy   The exact number of deaf citizens is not known, but a 1980 survey suggests that there may be at least 70,000 profoundly deaf people in Italy, with the rate of deafness higher in the southern regions of the country. In general, hearing loss occurs in about 8-10% of the general population.

Although there is a significant lack of good services and programs for them, deaf Italians do have a strong community among themselves, including a national organization for the deaf, and promote Italian Sign Language LIS (Lingua Italiana dei Segni).

The government provides special services only for preschool through age 14, either in special, mostly residential schools or mainstreamed with hearing children. The ORAL APPROACH is generally the preferred educational mode of communication, and sign language is generally prohibited in class, although it is tolerated elsewhere. In actuality, most deaf students and adults communicate in sign.

J

Japan   About 320,000 adult Japanese have hearing problems, and the programs and services for this population have improved since World War II. The presence of deafness in Japan appears to be growing, according to demographic reports. Census data from 1947 found 118 out of 100,000 to be prelingually deaf; figures rose to 225 per 100,000 in 1970.

Education is compulsory between ages 9 and 15, and in Japan deaf and hard-of-hearing children are treated separately: Deaf children are educated in special schools, and hard-of-hearing children attend special classes or are mainstreamed. Special school populations, however, are decreasing as more and more deaf students are attending regular classes and going to a university.

Most schools in Japan use the ORAL APPROACH, although more and more schools are introducing CUED SPEECH; students use sign language among themselves. Although JAPANESE SIGN LANGUAGE is not yet considered a language, since it does not match the expressive forms of the Japanese oral language, efforts are being made to make it more systematic.

The Japanese Association of the Deaf and Dumb, with 20,000 members, serves as an advocate for improved services for deaf Japanese. The association offers an annual convention and an annual sports meeting and has local branches in many areas throughout Japan. In addition, the Japanese Society for the Study of Education for the Deaf is a national network of 5,000 teachers in deaf schools. Deaf adults can expect a lower standard of living than hearing Japanese, and less than 32% of all Japanese deaf people are employed at all. Still, the outlook has improved since new laws require public agencies and private businesses to hire a certain number of physically disabled people.

Japanese Sign Language   More than 95% of the 320,000 deaf Japanese are assumed to be able to understand Japanese Sign Language (JSL), called "Shuwa" (hand talk).

Since all deaf schools are officially oral except for a few that use the simultaneous method (communication combining speech, sign and fingerspelling), JSL does not play a large part in the educational system. In the classes that use the simultaneous method, teachers use Signed Japanese or manually coded Japanese. Their sign language, called simultaneous methodic signs, uses FINGERSPELLING to represent suffixes and postpositions. In general, this language is not accepted by people in the deaf community, who use Pidgin Sign Japanese in communicating with deaf and hearing Japanese. Pidgin Sign Language is also used on TV programs, lectures and so forth.

Still in the early stages of research, JSL is not yet well understood by linguists.

Jena method   Developed by Karl Brauckmann in Jena, Germany, the Jena method is a system of teaching SPEECHREADING that focuses attention on the syllable and rhythm patterns in speech.

Jewish Deaf Congress   This organization (formerly known as the National Congress of Jewish Deaf) has served as an advocate for religious and cultural ideals and fellowship for Jewish deaf people since it was established in 1956. It serves as a clearinghouse for information about religious, educational and cultural programs for deaf Jews and represents them in projects involving nursing homes, interpreters, legal rights, demographic studies, education, sports and so forth. Publications include *The J.D. Quarterly.* The congress maintains a Hall of Fame honoring well-known deaf Jews and has been active in the campaign against offensive signs and terms for the words *Jews* and *Jewish.* The group also participated in founding the World Organization of Jewish Deaf People in Israel in 1977 to serve deaf Jews in Israel and Europe. In the 1960s, the group established an endowment fund to provide for the education of deaf rabbis. The congress holds biennial conventions in major cities. Contact: Jewish Deaf Congress, 9420 Reseda Boulevard Ste. 422, Northridge CA 91324; telephone (TDD): 818–993–2517.

The Job Accommodation Network (JAN)   This international toll-free consulting service is not a job-placement service, but an information source about job accommodations and the employability of people with hearing problems. JAN also provides information regarding the Americans with Disabilities Act (ADA). It is located at West Virginia University in Morgantown WV. Contact JAN by telephone (voice and TDD): 800–526–7234; website: http://janweb.icdi.wvu/edu/

Junior National Association of the Deaf   This group, affiliated with the NATIONAL ASSOCIATION OF THE DEAF, tries to develop leadership, scholarship and service among deaf high school students. The organization carries out its mandate by creating opportunities for hands-on experience through participation in various extracurricular activities and a youth leadership camp.

The first Junior NAD national convention was held in 1968 at Gallaudet University, with 120 student delegates from 36 chapters in schools for deaf students. The association also publishes the *Junior NAD Newsletter.*

Justinian Code   During the reign of Justinian I from A.D. 527–565, all of Roman law was codified, including the legal rights of deaf citizens (which were basically non-existent).

Deaf Romans could not marry, and legal guardians were appointed to handle their affairs. The code was more lenient for the adventitious deaf person, allowing those with acquired deafness to handle their own affairs if they could write.

K

Keller, Helen Adams (1880–1968)   This world-famous Alabama woman, blind and deaf from early childhood, became one of the best-known advocates of the education for blind and deaf students and was hailed for her achievement as a writer and lecturer.

She was born June 27, 1880, the daughter of a former officer in the Confederate army. A severe illness at 19 months destroyed both her sight and hearing, and she quickly deteriorated from an energetic, bright child into a spoiled, rebellious youngster who was almost impossible to handle.

Aware that the Perkins Institute for the Blind in Massachusetts had successfully educated a deaf-blind girl 50 years earlier, Helen's parents—on the advice of ALEXANDER GRAHAM BELL—sought help from the institute in educating Helen.

The institute recommended a former graduate, Anne Mansfield Sullivan, then 20 and partially blind herself. Sullivan arrived March 3, 1887, and began trying to teach young Helen names of objects by pressing the manual alphabet into her hand. Eventually, Sullivan managed to break through Helen's dark and silent world when Helen finally connected the feel of the water running over her hand to its manual sign.

A remarkably bright child, Helen's vocabulary increased rapidly, and she went on to be educated at the Horace Mann School for the Deaf in Boston and the Wright-Humason Oral School in New York City, where she learned to read and write in braille. She graduated cum laude in 1904 from Radcliffe, where Sullivan spelled lectures into her hand.

Keller—a close friend of the oralist Bell—was likewise a confirmed oralist who had learned to speak by feeling vibrations in Sullivan's larynx. Although far from perfect, her voice was understood by those who knew her well. Still, aware of the controversy between oral and manual methods of communication, she tried to find a common ground, admitting that no method was perfect and that deaf people need every advantage they can get.

Although her voice required interpretation in public, she became a noted lecturer for 12 years. Eventually, she became affiliated with the American Foundation for the Blind and spent many years traveling and speaking all over the world for this group.

In addition to lectures, Keller was a prolific writer; she wrote speeches, letters, magazine articles and books, including: *The Story of My Life* (1903), *The World I Live In* (1908), *Out of the Dark* (1913), *Midstream*

(1929), *Helen Keller in Scotland* (1933), *Helen Keller's Journal* (1938) and *Teacher: Anne Sullivan Macy: A Tribute by the Foster-Child of Her Mind* (1955). Although known all over the world, Keller lived within a small, protected circle: the ever-present, possessive teacher (Sullivan), Sullivan's husband John Macy and, later, an assistant. In her middle years she intended to marry but decided against it in the face of her mother's reluctance to "lose" her daughter.

A relentlessly kind woman, Keller was a suffragist strongly opposed to racism and war; she joined the Socialist party and ardently supported the Bolshevik Revolution.

Of her blindness and deafness, Keller considered deafness to be the greater loss, and her efforts to help those who were both blind and deaf led to the establishment of the HELEN KELLER NATIONAL CENTER FOR DEAF-BLIND YOUTHS AND ADULTS in Sands Point, New York.

Kendall Demonstration Elementary School   Originating as a school for deaf pupils in the Washington, D.C. area in 1857, the Kendall school became a national demonstration elementary school in 1970 when Congress mandated it provide not only an education to local students but also conduct research into a deaf education for dissemination across the country.

Public Law 91-587 set up the school as a demonstration center and emphasized that it must stress innovative auditory and visual devices, excellent architecture and works of art. Legislation also set up a new high school in 1966 for deaf secondary students located at GALLAUDET UNIVERSITY campus.

Students at Kendall range from young infants to 15-years-olds who must live in the national capital region (the District of Columbia, northern Virginia and nearby Maryland counties) and have a hearing problem severe enough to warrant placement in a special class. Among its 200 commuter students, 90% have a severe to profound hearing loss and the other 10% have a severe to moderate loss. About 30% have a disability in addition to hearing problems. The school includes a parent-infant program and a pre-school, primary, intermediate and middle school. Because it was designed as a demonstration school, Kendall often serves as a product testing ground and also supports applied and basic research. (See also MODEL SECONDARY SCHOOL FOR THE DEAF.)

L

labyrinth, inner ear   This section of the INNER EAR contains the nerve endings of the vestibular nerve (the nerve of equilibrium) and the AUDITORY NERVE (nerve of hearing).

Diseases of the labyrinth may affect both nerves or only the auditory nerve, causing hearing loss, or only the vestibular nerve, disrupting balance and causing VERTIGO. Common inner ear diseases include congenital nerve deafness (a defect of the hearing nerve in the COCHLEA), viral nerve deafness (a hearing impairment caused by a virus, such as mumps, measles or flu), deafness from ototoxic drugs, skull fracture, noise exposure, labyrinthitis, acoustic neuroma, Ménière's disease or presbycusis.

language   Symbols, words or signs that are composed by strict rules and arranged into sentences also governed by strict rules. All languages have symbols, and all languages have rules about how those symbols are grouped together to form sentences. In spoken languages, symbols are made up of sounds in particular ways; in sign languages, symbols are made up of body movements and positions.

The study of language, called LINGUISTICS, is still a relatively new science and is often controversial, but its basic tenets are universal. All spoken languages have rules about which sounds can be put together in certain ways to form words and sentences; similarly, natural sign languages have rules as well. But in sign language, grammatical rules govern body positions, facial expressions and movements.

Languages can differ at even the smallest levels, in the way in which sounds combine to form words and in the word order used to form sentences.

In English, word order usually follows the subject-verb-direct object format ("I love you"). In other languages, this word order is different; for example, in French, word order is subject-object-verb ("I you love"). Some languages, such as Latin, have no required word order at all but discriminate subjects from objects by word endings.

Because linguistic research into sign languages is still in its infancy, studies are only beginning to provide information on its syntactic rules. The key to understanding the grammatical structure of sign languages is to study the way signers use space.

People, places or objects not in the immediate area will be assigned a spatial location (to the left or right, for example). The signer can indicate the subject and object by moving the verb from one location to another.

For example, by first assigning the right location to "Sam" and the left location to "cat," the signer moving the sign "see" from right to left means "Sam sees the cat."

Contrary to the widespread assumption that infant babbling requires normal hearing and an ability to speak aloud, recent research suggests that the brain seems to possess some type of unified capacity for learning both signed and spoken language. Psychologists at McGill University in Montreal studied five infants, two of whom were deaf and whose deaf parents' first language was sign. The three hearing babies had hearing parents who did not use sign language. When researchers videotaped babies at ages 10, 12 and 14 months alone and with their parents, they found that both deaf and hearing babies engaged in their own brand of babbling. Hearing infants initially produced strings of sounds and syllables, emitting their first words by age 1. The two deaf babies babbled with their hands, starting out with basic hand shapes for letters and numbers that they saw their parents use. Hand movements and shapes gradually grew more complex until the first linguistic signs emerged also by age 1.

lateralization   Sound vibrations presented to one side of the head will move through the bones of the skull toward the opposite COCHLEA. Whether the sound reaches the cochlea depends on the decibel level of the sound. All sounds will lateralize, but not all will be heard by the opposite cochlea.

law   See COURT INTERPRETER'S ACT; LEGAL RIGHTS.

legal rights   A number of laws have been enacted since the 1970s guaranteeing legal rights for deaf people. They include:

Rehabilitation Act of 1973   Called the "Bill of Rights" for disabled people, this act was designed to make sure that programs receiving federal funds can be used by all disabled people. The four major sections of the act prohibit discrimination and require accessibility in employment, education, health, welfare and social services.

Section 501:   This section, which applies to federal government hiring practices, requires each executive department and agency to have an affirmative action plan for the hiring, placement and advancement of qualified handicapped people.

Section 502:   This section creates the ARCHITECTURAL AND TRANSPORTATION BARRIERS COMPLIANCE BOARD, which ensures compliance with a 1968 federal law regarding architectural barriers in federally-funded buildings and public transportation systems.

Section 503:   This requires affirmative action for qualified handicapped persons by people who have contracts or subcontracts with the federal government worth more than $2,500 a year or who employ more than 50 people.

Section 504:   This prohibits any form of discrimination against individuals with disabilities in any federally-supported program or activity, including most public and some private schools, nursing homes, museums and airports.

Public Law 94-142   Now known as the Individuals With Disabilities Act, this federal law guarantees public education to handicapped students in the least restrictive environment. It was signed into law on November 29, 1975, by President Gerald Ford.

The law provides states with funds for special education and imposes specific requirements on how such education should be provided— emphasizing special education and related services, protecting the rights of handicapped children and their parents and providing for the assessment of the effectiveness of programs.

The definition of handicapped children includes hard-of-hearing and deaf children, with "deaf" defined as: "a hearing impairment which is so severe that the child is impaired in processing linguistic information through hearing, with or without amplification, which adversely affects education performance." The law defined "hard-of-hearing" as an impairment—either fluctuating or permanent—that affects a child's educational performance.

The act defines "deaf-blind" as a "concomitant hearing and visual impairment" that causes such severe communication and other problems that these children cannot be accommodated in special education programs designed just for deaf or for blind children alone.

The act further provides that each child must have an individualized education program (IEP), a signed, written agreement renewed yearly, that includes a statement about the child's current abilities, annual goals and short-term educational objectives, specific services and the extent of participation in regular educational programs. The IEP is prepared with input from parents, teachers and school administrators.

According to information from the Department of Education, the number of hard-of-hearing students served by this law has steadily decreased over the past 10 years, due to the aging of children deafened in the RUBELLA epidemic of 1963 to 1965. Since the implementation of public laws aimed at assisting handicapped children, the number of hard-of-hearing and deaf students below 21 years of age decreased 19% between 1977–78 and 1985–86.

Public Law 97-410   The Telecommunications for the Disabled Act of 1982 addresses the issue of compatibility between hearing aids and telephones.

The law provides that all coin-operated telephones must be hearing-aid compatible; credit card phones must also be compatible unless there is a compatible coin phone nearby. Further, emergency phones (elevator phones, police and fire call boxes) and new public phones in businesses and public buildings must be compatible and an employer must supply a compatible phone on request by a deaf employee.

Hotels and motels must also specify compatibility when installing new phones until 10% of the rooms have compatible phones. Further, new phones installed after 1985 in hospitals, convalescent homes, homes for the aged, prisons and other confined areas must be compatible.

Public Law 88-565   Also known as the Vocational Rehabilitation Act, this law provides a number of direct services for deaf people and other disabled Americans. It includes funding and services for continuing education in a university or technical school and funds research and demonstration grants influencing deaf education.

The law led the way for expanded services and organizations for deaf people, including the REGISTRY OF INTERPRETERS FOR THE DEAF, the Professional Rehabilitation Workers with the Adult Deaf (now known as ADARA, the AMERICAN DEAFNESS AND REHABILITATION ASSOCIATION) and the Council of Organizations Serving the Deaf.

Amendments enacted in 1965 (PL 89-333) extended federal support even further to include education as well as rehabilitation and provided for interpreter services in a wide variety of settings.

Public Law 85-905   This important legislation for the deaf community created the Media Services and Captioned Films Branch in the Bureau of Education for the Handicapped, granting deaf people accessibility to entertainment and educational films. Additional laws (PL 87-715 and 91-230) set up a national advisory committee on deaf education, enlarged the focus of Media Service and Captioned Films and funded a National Center on Educational Media and Materials for the Handicapped to be located at Ohio State University at Columbus.

Public Law 100-533   The National Deafness and Other Communication Disorders Act of 1988 established the NATIONAL INSTITUTE ON DEAFNESS AND OTHER COMMUNICATION DISORDERS within the National Institutes of Health. The law addresses not only hearing disorders but also balance, voice, speech, language, taste and smell.

This law requires the program include investigation into the etiology, pathology, detection, treatment and prevention of all forms of disorders of hearing and other communication processes. It also requires research into diagnostic, treatment, rehabilitation and prevention techniques; prevention and early detection of these disorders; and the environmental agents that influence hearing disorders. Finally, the law establishes a data system to collect, analyze and distribute information from patients, a national information clearinghouse and multipurpose research centers.

Public Law 87-276   In response to a shortage of teachers for deaf students, this law was signed on September 22, 1961, by President John F.

Kennedy to provide stipends for undergraduate and graduate study. As a result, the number of approved university teaching training centers doubled.

Public Law 88-136   This legislation set up an advisory committee on deaf education, which began in March 1964 under the leadership of Homer Babbidge. The subsequent "Babbidge Report," which highlighted and analyzed problems in deaf education, was partly responsible for the subsequent creation of the MODEL SECONDARY SCHOOL FOR THE DEAF located on the GALLAUDET UNIVERSITY campus in Washington, D.C.

Vocational Education Act of 1963   This law allowed residential schools for deaf children to qualify for supplementary funding for their vocational departments; amendments in 1968 to this law required that at least 10% of the federal funds allocated for vocational education be set aside for handicapped students.

Public Law 89-36   This law, signed on June 8, 1965, by President Lyndon Johnson, established the NATIONAL TECHNICAL INSTITUTE FOR THE DEAF and an advisory committee to administer it. Of 28 competing colleges and universities, the Rochester Institute of Technology in New York was awarded the job.

linguist   A person who uses highly-specialized skills to analyze language and associated cultural patterns in research or applied LINGUISTICS. Current research in the field of deafness includes studies of the history and development of AMERICAN SIGN LANGUAGE, comparative sign languages and language development of deaf children. Applied linguistics is especially useful in schools, where a professional can analyze language patterns of individual students and help the teacher devise strategies to develop new language skills. (See also SIGN LANGUAGE.)

linguistics   The study of language as a system, involving an investigation into its nature, structure, units and modification. Theoretical linguistics tries to establish a theory of the underlying structure of language, isolating the structure of language from actual language production. It does not take into account language acquisition or usage. Applied linguistics tries to use the findings and techniques of the scientific study of language for a range of practical tasks, especially to help improve the teaching of language.

Linguistics of Visual English (L.O.V.E.)   One of the five main manually coded English systems, this one was developed by Dennis Wampler. In this system, stress was placed on signing by morpheme (a word that conveys meaning and cannot be broken down into a smaller word). This system, similar to SEE-2 and SIGNED ENGLISH, features the use of symbols adapted from William Stokoe's symbols in the *Dictionary of American Sign Language* to show how signs were made, rather than depending on words or pictures to depict signs. This system is not widely used. Because it's considered to be a signing system rather than a language, some people claim that exposure to L.O.V.E. doesn't give children the complete linguistic access needed to internalize whole language.

lipreading   See SPEECHREADING.

Little Theatre of the Deaf   Working under its parent company, the NATIONAL THEATRE OF THE DEAF, the Little Theatre has presented stories, fables and poetry to young audiences for more than 20 years.

The theater uses body movement, sign language and hearing interpreters to bring both classic literature and original works to life. Programs are presented in schools, parks, museums, theaters and libraries throughout the United States and in other places, such as India, the Far East and Scandinavia.

Now composed of two companies of five actors each, the theater offers one-hour performances that include short stories, fables and often an introduction to sign language. The actors form living sculptures during "Your Game," a program using suggestions from the audience to illustrate ensemble performances, such as a washing machine or a videocassette player in fast forward.

The 31-year old theater, where deaf and hearing actors team to present performances in sign language and spoken words, is the country's oldest, continually producing touring theater. The theater set a global record February 1998 in Antarctica when it became the world's first theater to reach all seven continents. Contact: THE NATIONAL THEATRE OF THE DEAF, 5 West Main St., PO Box 659, Chester CT 06412; telephone (voice): 860–526–4971, (TDD): 860–526–4974.

Lombard test   A special test for functional hearing loss in which masking sounds are introduced into the ears while the subject talks. The test is positive if the subject raises the intensity level of his voice in order to hear himself above the masking sound and negative if his voice remains at a fixed level. (See also AUDIOMETRY; FUNCTIONAL HEARING LOSS [NONORGANIC].)

M

mainstreaming   The process in which a student with hearing problems attends some—or all—classes in a regular school for hearing students. (See also EDUCATION OF DEAF CHILDREN.)

manual alphabet   See FINGERSPELLING.

manual approach   Method of communication among deaf people using sign language and fingerspelling. Those who believe in the importance of manual communication consider it is a natural mode of communication for deaf people, that deaf people should be encouraged to use signs and they should be allowed to sign in school. Opponents of the manual approach generally reject sign language, at least for the purpose of education.

There are intermediate positions between the two ends of the manual-oral spectrum. Some supporters of oral communication agree with the use of FINGERSPELLING in many settings but not in schools; others approve of mouth-hand systems of communication, such as CUED SPEECH.

Many schools in the United States today have tried to reach a compromise between the manual and oral methods by combining the two approaches.

The manual approach was referred to as the "French method" during the 19th century and was the preferred educational method of ABBÉ CHARLES MICHEL DE L'EPÉE of Paris. At the same time, German deaf educator SAMUEL HEINICKE of Leipzig was promoting the oral approach.

L'Epée, as director of the French Royal Institute for the Deaf and Dumb in Paris (now the Institut National des Jeunes Sourds), promoted the use of what he called "methodical signs" for the education of deaf students, becoming the first proponent of sign language usage in schools. Because l'Epée did not believe there was any logical connection between sounds and ideas, it did not matter to him whether a person spoke or signed thoughts—each would be equally useful. All education was taught through his methodical signs, except for proper names for which he used fingerspelling. Still, l'Epée did teach speech and SPEECHREADING as well.

It was at the Paris Institute that THOMAS HOPKINS GALLAUDET learned how to educate deaf children, and it was therefore the French manual method he took back home to the United States. From the beginning of the first permanent school for deaf students in 1817, which Gallaudet founded, until the late 1860s, all instruction in the United States (some 26 separate schools) was based on the manual method.

But in the 1840s, educators began to tour Europe and bring back reports of the oral progress in English and German schools. Eventually, when parents of some deaf children did not want their children to learn signs, they formed a school in 1867 with the assistance of John Clarke, who donated $300,000 to start the first purely oral school in America, the Clarke School of Northampton, Massachusetts.

A more recent refinement of the manual approach is called Total Communication, which implies acceptance, understanding and use of all methods of communication. Proponents of this theory believe people with hearing loss should be exposed to all methods, emphasizing whatever enables them to learn and communicate effectively. (See also SIMULTANEOUS COMMUNICATION.)

manually coded English   All artificially developed codes that try to represent the English language in sign form are known as manually coded English (MCE). Typically, these systems have been developed primarily for the educational system to help build English language skills by manually incorporating many English language features.

In the past 20 years, a number of these codes have been developed, including SEEING ESSENTIAL ENGLISH (SEE 1), SIGNING EXACT ENGLISH (SEE 2) and SIGNED ENGLISH. All were designed to improve deaf students' English scores.

These codes, also known as manual English, are just that—codes, not languages—that reflect the structure and vocabulary of English. Generally, these systems use AMERICAN SIGN LANGUAGE signs in English word order, along with new signs that have been created to represent English parts of speech normally omitted from ASL. These manually coded systems therefore parallel the word and sentence structure of English.

However, manually coded English can be confusing to those used to American Sign Language. Whereas in English (and MCE) one word can have many meanings, ASL would assign a different sign to each separate meaning of the word. For example, the ASL sign for "run" (meaning a gait) is different from the run in a stocking or running for office.

Preliminary studies suggest these systems may improve students' grammar, but they are cumbersome to use, taking as much as twice as long to sign a word as it would to say it. Because of this, many students and teachers began to drop required signs. In response, Harry Bornstein, the author of Signed English, in 1982 came up with a pared-down version, although he continues to advocate that teachers and parents of young children slow down and sign accurately.

Use of these manual systems outside the classroom is not popular with the majority of deaf people, who view the system as an attempt to interfere with or eliminate ASL. (See also SIGN CODES.)

Martineau, Harriet (1802–1876)   This strong and independent journalist was remarkable for her outspokenness during the Victorian era; she became one of the most famous writers of her time.

Born June 12, 1802, in Norwich, England, to a radical Unitarian family, her severe, painful hearing problem began at the age of 12. Within six years she was severely deafened but was reluctant to use an ear trumpet.

Extremely well-educated for her time, Martineau wrote about economics, education, sociology and philosophy for the leading periodicals of her day, making enemies for her unorthodox views along the way. A believer in mesmerism (hypnotism), her subsequent views on religion (she espoused a form of atheism) brought her even more criticism.

On a visit to the United States, she was appalled at the treatment of women and Indians, and her strong antislavery views made her a controversial speaker.

Despite this, her home in the Lake District was a beacon to other well-known philosophers and writers, including William Wordsworth, Matthew Arnold, Charlotte Brontë, Ralph Waldo Emerson and Nathaniel Hawthorne.

She also wrote widely about deafness and the problems deaf people encountered, ridiculing hearing people for meddling in the affairs of the deaf community and blaming parents and teachers for inadequate education of deaf children.

maskers   See TINNITUS MASKER.

Massieu, Jean (1772–1846)   This brilliant, outgoing educator, together with the ABBÉ ROCH AMBROISE CUCURRON SICARD, helped develop the manual method of education taught at the famed Paris Institute.

Born in 1772 near Cadillac, France, Massieu was one of six children, all deaf, who communicated among themselves in the family's own system of manual signs. Sent to a school for deaf children in Bordeaux, Massieu met Abbe Sicard, who taught him how to read and write. When Sicard was named head of the Paris Institute, both men moved to Paris in 1790.

As the French revolution exploded around them, Massieu and Sicard worked to establish education for deaf people. Massieu worked as instructor at the school, together with LAURENT CLERC, and helped teach THOMAS HOPKINS GALLAUDET their manual method of education. Upon Sicard's death in 1822, Massieu was fired for sexual indiscretions and moved to Aveyron, where he became headmaster of a local school for deaf students, retiring in 1839.

mastoidectomy   A surgical procedure to remove the mastoid portion of the temporal bone, thereby removing the infected air cells within the bone caused by mastoiditis, otitis media or cholesteatoma. It may also be used in the repair of a paralyzed facial nerve. It is performed less frequently today because of the widespread use of antibiotics in the treatment of acute OTI-TIS MEDIA and acute mastoiditis. Most mastoidectomies are performed behind the ear under general anesthesia.

There are several types of mastoidectomy, including antrotomy, cortical, modified radical, radical and a combined approach.

Antrotomy   Now almost obsolete, this operation involves the clearing and draining of the infected bone.

Cortical   Also called a simple or Swartze mastoidectomy, this procedure is used in acute and masked mastoiditis, a severely draining ear and recurrent otitis media. It involves removal of all cells of the mastoid bone.

Modified Radical   This procedure is used for cholesteatoma not involving the MIDDLE EAR but confined to the attic and mastoid, in which part of the bony wall is removed. It is also called a Bondy operation.

Radical   This operation for otitis media and, rarely, cholesteatoma involves removal of the tympanic membrane (EARDRUM), the OSSICLES, the posterior wall of the external canal, the diseased tissue and the mastoid. This converts the mastoid and middle ear into a single, healthy cavity. Unfortunately, a conductive hearing loss of up to 50 dB is usually expected because the middle ear ossicles are removed, although a TYMPANOPLASTY may offset some of the loss. There may also be a partial or complete sensorineural hearing loss if the footplate of the STAPES is dislodged.

Combined   This treatment for cholesteatoma, also called an intact canal wall mastoidectomy, avoids leaving a mastoid cavity by clearing the mastoid cavity and the middle ear of cholesteatoma while preserving the posterior canal wall. Unfortunately, some of the disease may be overlooked and left behind, which is why some otologic surgeons perform routine follow-up surgeries in several years.

Ménière's Network, The   A national network of patient support groups administered by the EAR FOUNDATION to provide people with the opportunity to share experiences and coping strategies. Contact: The Ear Foundation, 2000 Church Street, Box 111, Nashville, TN 37326; telephone (voice and TDD): 800-545-4327. http://www.theearfound.com

mental health services   Finding adequate mental health services has become easier in recent years.

Accurate and appropriate diagnosis and treatment requires a working knowledge of the educational, psychological, social, cultural, linguistic, communication and emotional aspects of deafness—and fluency in sign language in particular.

Significantly, it has been demonstrated in the past 10 years that deaf people do respond to and benefit from the various methods of therapy used with hearing clients, as long as treatment is carried out using the preferred communication mode and style of the deaf individual.

There are a number of ways to locate sources of mental health services for deaf and hard-of-hearing people. State and community agencies serving people who are deaf and hard-of-hearing, in addition to community referral centers, often maintain files on service providers working with specific populations in a state. These include:

- State offices/commissions for deaf and hard-of-hearing people
- Community service agencies for deaf and hard of hearing people
- Hearing and speech agencies
- State school(s) for deaf children
- State departments of mental health

Other resources include:

- *Mental Health Services for Deaf People (1992)* A 210-page directory that identifies more than 350 U.S. mental health programs and services for deaf people, including information on services, accreditation, fees, special programs, and accessibility. Copies are available for $4 plus $2.25 shipping/handling from Gallaudet Research Institute, The Center for Assessment and Demographic Studies, Gallaudet University, 800 Florida Avenue, NE, Washington DC 20002–3965.
- *National Directory of Alcohol and Other Drugs Prevention and Treatment Programs Accessible to the Deaf (1995).* This directory, identifies programs reporting that they are culturally and linguistically accessible to deaf consumers. Copies are available for $35 plus $5 shipping/handling from Rochester Institute of Technology, Campus Connections Bookstore, 48 Lomb Memorial Drive, Rochester NY 14623–5604.
- *Standards of Care for the Delivery of Mental Health Services to Deaf and Hard-of-Hearing Persons.* The seven chapters of this document present an up-to-date description of the mental health resources and standards of care for deaf and hard-of-hearing persons. Included in the binder are descriptions of the population, referral into the mental health system, methods of access, specialized services, specialized resources and skills. The appendices include a list of state coordinators of mental health services for deaf and hard-of-hearing persons, residential facilities for deaf adults, and residential programs for deaf children and adolescents with emotional/behavioral disturbances. Copies are available for $64.95 plus $4.75 shipping/handling from: National Association of the Deaf Bookstore, 814 Thayer Avenue, Silver Spring MD 20910.

mental illness Research has shown that the rates of psychological disorders and mental illness are about the same for both the deaf and hearing populations. However, the lack of access to quality mental health services for deaf patients often precludes preventive mental health care.

In addition, hearing mental health professionals tend to diagnose psychological disorders and mental illness in deaf patients where none exist because they are unfamiliar with the educational, psychological, social, cultural, linguistic and communication aspects of deafness and are unable to use sign language to communicate.

To the inexperienced mental health professional, deaf people may appear to be psychologically disturbed or mentally ill when in fact they are not, according to Barbara A. Brauer, Ph.D., psychologist and research scientist at the Mental Health Research Program at GALLAUDET RESEARCH INSTITUTE. Because AMERICAN SIGN LANGUAGE and English have very different structures, styles and syntax, the English comprehension and writing levels of deaf people may appear pathological when in fact they are normal. Standardized tests are also culturally biased, as the tests are given in the context of the hearing experience, which may in many respects be different from the deaf experience. Consequently, the results often yield erroneous information about psychologically healthy deaf individuals.

For this reason, a number of psychological and personality tests have been translated by Dr. Brauer into American Sign Language on videotape as part of Gallaudet University's Mental Health Research Program. According to Dr. Brauer, preliminary findings suggest normal profiles for most deaf individuals tested.

Mercer, William (1765–1839)   Little is known about the early life of this deaf American painter, other than that he was born deaf in Fredericksburg, Virginia in 1765, the first of five children. At the age of 18, he was sent to be apprenticed to Charles Willson Peale, a well-known Philadelphia artist. For three years, Mercer boarded with the Peale family and studied painting under the master artist.

Mercer's artworks include *The Battle of Princeton,* and a half portrait of his grandmother, Mrs. John Gordeon (both of which are owned by the Historical Society of Pennsylvania), and an oval miniature of a Virginian official (owned by the Virginia Historical Society of Richmond).

Although Mercer returned to Fredericksburg in 1786, where he continued to work as a painter, no other pictures by him are known to have survived.

methods of instruction   There are currently four primary methods of instruction for deaf students used in the United States—the oral, auditory, Rochester, and simultaneous methods—as well as a more recent method—total communication.

Oral Approach   Also called the oral-aural method, children learning under this system are taught through SPEECHREADING (lipreading) and amplification of sound; they express themselves by speaking. Gestures and signs are prohibited.

Auditory Method   This system concentrates on helping children develop listening skills by relying primarily on hearing. Early reading, writing, and speechreading (lipreading) are discouraged. This system is generally used for people with moderate hearing loss, but it is sometimes used with profoundly deaf students as well.

Rochester Method   Rarely used in this country today, this system combines the oral approach with FINGERSPELLING. Children receive input through speechreading, amplification and fingerspelling, with great emphasis placed on reading and writing.

Simultaneous Method   This features a combination of the oral approach plus signs and fingerspelling. Children are taught through speechreading, amplification, signs and fingerspelling.

Total Communication   In addition to the above four methods, Total Communication has received widespread attention in the past several years. According to the Conference of Executives of American Schools for the Deaf, Total Communication is a philosophy incorporating aural, manual and oral modes of communication to ensure effective communication with and among deaf people.

Mexican Sign Language   Known as LSM (Lenguaje de Señas Mexicanas), this sign language is used throughout Mexico by many of its more than 1.3 million deaf citizens.

As is typical for sign language, LSM does not parallel Spanish grammar. Sign meaning can be altered by varying speed, size and duration of the sign, and placement of signs depends on context. As in written Spanish, a sign for "question" appears at the beginning of the sentence.

There are no manual codes that follow Spanish language structure, such as the manual codes for English in the United States.

Education is still widely oral in Mexico, although deaf educators are working to include LSM in the schools.

Mexico   With more than 1.3 million deaf and hard-of-hearing citizens there has been growth in the number of services provided for deaf people in Mexico, although there is still much more to be done in the field of education for deaf students and in the training of deaf teachers. According to a 1940 census, the prevalence rate of deafness in Mexico was 39 per 100,000; the count rose to 46 per 100,000 in the 1974 census. Still, this represents a fairly low rate compared to those of other developed nations that report data on deafness, which range from 35 per 100,000 to 300 per 100,000.

Mexico does not have any national organizations or regional groups for deaf people, although there are two deaf sports associations. Although education for deaf Mexicans began in the late 1860s, few new schools were established until the middle of the 20th century as the educational philosophy changed from the MANUAL to ORAL approach. In 1951 the first institute for deaf people in Latin America was established, called the Mexican Institute of Speech and Hearing (IMAL). The institute, primarily oral, offers courses for teachers, audiologists, speech pathologists, technicians and deaf people, conducts research and provides social services.

minimal language skills   A controversial term meaning a diminished communication repertoire of some individuals with hearing loss. This term replaced the negative "low verbal" description used before the 1970s, which was incorrectly used to label people who were proficient in AMERICAN SIGN LANGUAGE but not in spoken English.

Minimal language skills does *not* mean a person has problems with spoken language (especially English), has problems speech-reading or is illiterate. A person who is not competent in sign language *or* in spoken language may be said incorrectly to have minimal language skills.

Miss Deaf America   A national competition designed for young deaf women between the ages of 18 and 28 who have already won their state competitions, it takes place during the biennial convention of the NATIONAL ASSOCIATION OF THE DEAF. Miss Deaf America serves as a role model for young deaf people and increases awareness of deafness among the general public through her appearances around the country. The pageant's goal is to encourage and foster future leaders and is one of several youth programs of the National Association of the Deaf.

The MDAP began as a vision of the late Douglas J. Burke, who in 1966 established a National Cultural Program within the NAD for the purpose of finding the hidden talents of deaf people in the visual arts. As a way of discovering deaf actresses at an early age, Burke created the Miss Deaf America Talent Pageant as a part of the National Cultural Program.

The first pageant took place in Miami Beach during the 1972 NAD Convention, with just five contestants; in 1976, the word *talent* was removed, and it simply became known as the Miss Deaf America Pageant, following closely the structure of the Miss America Pageant. Women are judged across a broad spectrum of categories including community service, academics, current events and deaf culture.

Model Secondary School for the Deaf (MSSD)   Established by an act of Congress on October 15, 1966, the MSSD was designed to provide an outstanding example of a secondary school program for students with hearing problems and to stimulate the development of similar programs around the country.

Congress stipulated that the school should serve as a regional high school to prepare deaf students for college or a vocational career and should upgrade education for deaf students, using the newest research in testing, methodology and curriculum development.

In the beginning, admission requirements mandated that students be at least 14 years of age and have a third-grade reading level, a hearing loss of 70 decibels or more in the better ear and no other major problems. (These criteria were loosened following the passage of PL 94-142, the Education for All Handicapped Children Act.)

Students attending MSSD come primarily from Maryland, Delaware, Pennsylvania, Virginia, West Virginia and Washington, D.C., although students from other states are admitted if there is space. In that case, preference is given to students who have no access to a full-service high school.

Today, the school—located on 17 acres in the northwest corner of GAL-LAUDET UNIVERSITY—includes residence halls, health facilities, dining rooms, an infirmary and playing fields and serves about 400 deaf students a year. If offers students a continually-updated curriculum of more than 180 courses, including foreign language, art and theater arts. About 75% of the students live on campus; the rest commute from nearby Washington. Approximately 70% of MSSD students continue their education after graduation.

The school also offers a wide variety of interest clubs, a yearbook and service organizations, such as the Junior National Association of the Deaf.

The school provides curriculum development, workshops, seminars and internships for professionals and graduate students. School staff publish *Perspectives,* a professional journal for teachers, and *The World Around You,* a national high school student publication.

Input is received from the Parent Advisory Council and a National Advisory Council, which helps maintain goals and direction. (See also KENDALL DEMONSTRATION SCHOOL.)

mouth-hand systems   Mouth-hand systems are not a language but an aid to the visual transmission of spoken languages using handshapes close to the mouth to differentiate PHONEMES that look the same when spoken. (Phonemes are a family of closely related speech sounds regarded as a single sound; for example, the "r" in "bring," "red" and "car.") Used as aids for speechreading and speech training, there are two major forms of mouth-hand systems: CUED SPEECH and Danish.

Cued Speech   Cued speech was developed in 1966 as a speechreading support system which (in English) uses eight hand configurations and four hand placements near the mouth to supplement visible speech. Each "cue" (hand placement or configuration) identifies a special group of two to four speech sounds. The combination of cues and mouth movements makes all the essential speech sounds appear different from each other so that the spoken message is clarified.

The hand configurations and locations are called "cues," not cued speech, which is the combination of the cues with speech (the cues are not readable alone).

Each hand configuration identifies a group of consonants; each hand location identifies a group of vowels. Further, cued speech can be used to indicate approximate voice pitch for each syllable uttered, which is important in tonal languages (such as Thai, Cantonese, Mandarin and Igbo).

For example, in Cantonese, the syllable "ma" can mean "mother," "scold," "horse," or "right?" depending on the pitch. Tone cueing is also helpful in speech theraphy. In order to cue a tone, a person changes the inclination of the cueing hand to indicate changes in pitch.

Cued speech has been adapted to many languages, and audiocassette lessons designed for self-instruction by hearing persons are available. The system is generally the same in all languages.

Proponents believe cued speech makes spoken language visually clear and solves the communication problem at home and that it helps children learn a spoken language more easily. It is also an easily-learned system, taking only about 12 to 20 hours to master.

Initial research does suggest that cued speech helps make the spoken language clear, but the long-term effectiveness of the language is not known. Cued speech is not widely used by adults in the deaf community.

Danish   The mouth-hand system was invented in 1900 in Denmark by Georg Forchhammer, head of a deaf oral school, who believed that visual communication was necessary. Married to a deaf woman, he realized it would be helpful to improve SPEECHREADING capability by making similar-sounding words clear.

In the Danish system, there are 14 different hand positions, each making clear a sound that is hard to speechread. Hand positions are designed to symbolize the sound, and the most-often used sounds are the easiest to make.

Easy to use, the system is the most common visual aid in Denmark by hard-of-hearing people who don't know sign language. On the other hand, this system tends to slow down communication and is tiring to read or produce over a period of time.

Among the Danish deaf population, the mouth-hand system is used as a way to improve speech training and has also become a part of SIGN LANGUAGE in much the same way that the MANUAL ALPHABET is used in conjunction with other sign languages. In Denmark, the system is used to spell out names and words with no equivalent in Danish sign language.

This system can be used with any language, with additional shapes used for sounds that are not made in Danish. These hand positions have been developed for use in English, French, German, Swedish and Norwegian.

multisensory teaching approach   This method, one of two philosophies used in teaching speech to deaf and hard-of-hearing children, calls for the use of all sensory channels—hearing, sight, feel—as opposed to the AUDITORY-ORAL METHOD, which teaches the child to rely solely on the auditory system, however flawed.

The proponents of the multisensory method believe that the hard-of-hearing or deaf child has an auditory system that is inadequate for the development of good speech and that this calls for the use of other senses, including sight and touch. (See also SPEECH TRAINING.)

myringoplasty   See TYMPANOPLASTY.

myringotomy   A surgical procedure used to open the eardrum to drain the middle ear cavity. It is usually performed in children to treat persistent middle ear effusion (a sticky secretion in the middle ear cavity causing hearing loss). This hearing loss may become permanent if the condition isn't treated. Before antibiotics, a myringotomy was used to treat acute otitis media by releasing the pus, relieving pressure on the eardrum.

While the patient is under general anesthesia, the otolaryngologist makes a small incision in the eardrum, removing most of the fluid by suction. At the same time, a small tube may be inserted in the hole to allow any remaining fluid to drain into the outer ear. The patient can leave the hospital the next day, and the tube usually falls out several months later as the hole in the eardrum closes. A second operation may be needed to insert another tube if the condition does not clear up.

Some experts advocate the use of allergic management or decongestive therapy, which eventually allows the effusion to clear. Unfortunately, the hearing loss that occurs while the effusion exists may cause developmental problems in children. Some research suggests that long-term treatment with antibiotics may help clear some cases of effusion.

N

NAD Legal Defense Fund   Established in 1976 to handle lawsuits aimed at protecting the rights of deaf Americans, the Legal Defense Fund is totally funded by the NATIONAL ASSOCIATION OF THE DEAF. The fund strives to provide protection in the areas of employment, education, physical and mental health care, welfare and social services, judicial and law enforcement and insurance. (See also NATIONAL CENTER FOR LAW AND DEAFNESS.) Contact: NAD Legal Defense Fund, National Association of the Deaf, 814 Thayer Avenue, Silver Spring, MD 20910; telephone: 301-587-7730.

name sign   A sign used in the deaf community that serves as the first, middle and last name of a person.

Since most deaf children do not have deaf parents, most deaf offspring of hearing parents receive a name sign from their deaf peers or teachers once they begin school. Name signs can change in different groups of people or when a person's status changes, such as after marriage.

Name signs may be descriptive, in which they describe a person's physical characteristics; research has discovered that many of these emphasize negative physical characteristics, such as being overweight or having a scar. Arbitrary name signs (usually given by deaf parents) all have alphabetically-based handshapes affiliated with the first, middle or last name.

FINGERSPELLING is also sometimes used to spell out an abbreviated form of the name.

narcotics and deafness   Deafness from overuse of narcotics has been rarely reported. However, recent studies show that overuse of a combination of the narcotic pain reliever hydocodone and acetaminophen (a product called Vicodin) can lead to total deafness. Typically, hydrocodone and acetaminophen in combination are often used to alleviate pain. This rapid and progressive hearing loss has been treated successfully with cochlear implant.

National Association for Hearing and Speech Action   This organization was founded in 1910 in New York City to advocate and provide information for deaf and hard-of-hearing people and is the consumer affiliate of the AMERICAN SPEECH-LANGUAGE-HEARING ASSOCIATION.

The group operates a toll-free speech and hearing helpline (800-638-TALK) and has produced brochures and television public service announcements promoting healthy hearing.

The association was first called the American Association for the Hard of Hearing and was designed for people interested in teaching SPEECHREAD-ING to hard-of-hearing people. During the 1920s, the association moved to Washington, D.C., and led an aggressive campaign to prevent hearing problems and establish screening programs in schools.

In 1966 the association was renamed the National Association of Hearing and Speech Agencies and emphasized community organization and professional service, education, diagnosis and research.

Its final name change occurred in 1972. Today, its members are involved in promoting the interests of people with speech and hearing problems and emphasizing consumer advocacy, prevention and social action.

Contact: 10801 Rockville Pike, Rockville MD 20852.

National Association of the Deaf (NAD)   NAD is a consumer advocate organization concerned about and involved with everything affecting opportunities for the more than 22 million deaf and hard-of-hearing people in the United States.

With 50 affiliated state associations and more than 22,000 members, NAD changed its orientation in 1960 from a group of individuals to a federation of state associations. The first association founded by deaf people, it was founded in 1880 by a group of deaf leaders concerned that deaf people were not included in the decision-making processes affecting their own lives.

In 1964, the group abandoned its policy of allowing only deaf people to become members, but today less than 100 of its more than 22,000 members can hear. Most of these 100 are professionals who work with deaf clients.

Today, NAD serves as a clearinghouse of information on deafness and is an advocate for the employment of deaf people. The organization promotes the use of AMERICAN SIGN LANGUAGE and supports the philosophy of TOTAL COMMUNICATION—the right of all deaf people to select and use any form of communication, including SIGN LANGUAGE, gestures, writing, reading, FINGERSPELLING, SPEECHREADING and listening with amplification.

Over the years, NAD has received a number of federal grants to conduct the first national census of deaf Americans, to set up a communication skills program and to establish the REGISTRY OF INTERPRETERS FOR THE DEAF, among others.

NAD—together with its affiliate state association in Massachusetts—operates D.E.A.F., INC., a rehabilitation facility serving the deaf population in New England, and administers a survey research organization, the Deaf Community Analysts. The organization also subsidizes the NAD LEGAL DEFENSE FUND, the International Association of Parents of the Deaf and the JUNIOR NATIONAL ASSOCIATION OF THE DEAF and holds an annual leadership camp for deaf youth.

Finally, the NAD publishes a national monthly tabloid, *The Broadcaster,* featuring columns, articles, a special sports section and advertisements of special interest to the deaf community. Its quarterly magazine, *The Deaf American,* carries full-length feature articles on topics of interest to the deaf community. NAD also publishes and sells books on deafness and sells assistive devices for deaf people.

Its home office, Halex House, is located in Silver Spring, MD, where it offers for sale more than 200 books on various aspects of deafness. The NAD is a member of the WORLD FEDERATION OF THE DEAF. (See also MISS DEAF AMERICA.) Contact: National Association of the Deaf, 814 Thayer Ave., Silver Spring, MD 20910; telephone (voice and TDD): 301-587-1788.

National Black Association for Speech-Language and Hearing   A nonprofit organization dedicated to sharing information about communication impairments and differences among black people; professional development of SPEECH-LANGUAGE PATHOLOGISTS, AUDIOLOGISTS and students; and advocacy of quality service delivery to the black community.

National Black Deaf Advocates, Inc.   This organization promotes leadership, deaf awareness and active participation in the political, educational, religious and economic processes that affect the lives of deaf black citizens. Contact: National Black Advocates, Inc., P.O. Box 5465, Laurel MD 20726; telephone (voice): 410–418–8676; (TDD): (301)–206–2802; e-mail: couthen61@aol.com.

National Board for Certification in Hearing Instrument Sciences   Founded in 1981, the NBC-HIS is a voluntary non-profit organization devoted to the recognition of people who are qualified to provide competent hearing instrument services to hard-of-hearing patients.

Board certification is conferred upon hearing instrument specialists who meet specified criteria and demonstrate professional competence.

National Catholic Office for the Deaf   This group organizes workshops and provides information and teaching materials for the religious education of hard-of-hearing people. It also coordinates preparation programs for pastoral workers. (See also INTERNATIONAL CATHOLIC DEAF ASSOCIATION.) Contact: National Catholic Office for the Deaf, 7202 Buchanon Street, Landover Hills MD 20784; telephone: (voice) 301–577–1684 (TDD) 301–577–4184.

National Center for Law and Deafness   The first national center designed to meet the legal needs of the deaf population, which had been located at GALLAUDET UNIVERSITY in Washington, D.C. The center, which was abolished by Gallaudet in 1997, had been designed to provide a variety of legal services and programs for the deaf community.

The center provided free assistance to Gallaudet University students and low-income hard-of-hearing people in the Washington, D.C., area. The clinic primarily handled common legal problems (wills, immigration, consumer issues, landlord-tenant disagreements and so forth).

During the school year, law student interns—supervised by staff attorneys—worked at the center, gaining valuable experience in meeting the legal and communication needs of deaf people. The law schools at both George Washington University and Catholic University offered courses in conjunction with the law center.

The center's attorneys tried to eliminate discrimination caused by the communication barriers between deaf and hearing people in education, employment, health care, legal services and governmental programs. Efforts included technical assistance with federal and state statutes and regulations dealing with interpreter services, civil rights of deaf people and the right to good mental and physical health care. Center attorneys also provided information to a variety of groups, including other lawyers, employers, schools and the federal government, on issues that affect deaf people.

Importantly, the center concentrated on the areas of television and telephone access for deaf people and was instrumental in petitioning the FCC to require all TV stations to present emergency information in visual form; it also helped the Public Broadcasting Service reserve LINE 21 to be used for closed captioning.

Interpreters were available for interviews at the center, and all staffers were trained in sign language.

Many of the center's tasks have been taken over by the NAD LEGAL DEFENSE FUND, which maintains an office at the National Association of the Deaf in Silver Spring, Maryland. The defense fund represents deaf and hard-of-hearing people with discrimination problems and helps provide education and legal aid. Contact: NAD Legal Defense Fund, 814 Thayer Avenue, Silver Spring, MD 20910 (301) 587-7730.

National Congress of Jewish Deaf (NCJD)   See JEWISH DEAF CONGRESS.

National Cued Speech Association   The membership organization which provides advocacy, information and support on the use of CUED SPEECH. Members include both families and professionals in the field of deafness. The association's board of directors are geographically diverse and each regional director provides services for people in his or her area. Publications of the association include the *Cued Speech Journal* and newsletters *On Cue* and *On Cue News Flash*. Contact: National Cued Speech Association, 23970 Hermitage Rd., Cleveland, OH 44122; telephone (voice and TDD): 800–459–3529; website: http://www.web7.mit.edu/cuedspeech/

National Foundation for Children's Hearing Education and Research (CHEAR) This nonprofit organization's main objective is to further the growth of medical deafness research. Founded in 1969, CHEAR raises money for research for a cure or alleviation of nerve deafness. The group also helps parents and the public understand deafness and works to improve education and educational facilities for deaf and hard-of-hearing students. For the past 20 years, CHEAR has made medical research grants and has awarded incentive scholarship prizes to hearing-impaired students. Contact: National Foundation for Children's Hearing Education and Research, 928 McLean Ave., Yonkers NY 10704; telephone: 914–237–2676.

National Fraternal Society of the Deaf This group was founded in 1901 by a group of young deaf adults interested in forming a fraternal society solely for deaf people and in providing low-cost insurance protection denied to deaf individuals at that time. (Insurance was denied because at the beginning of the 20th century, insurers thought that deaf people didn't live very long and were prone to accidents.)

The society was incorporated as a mutual benefit organization by the state of Illinois in 1901, and by 1984 there were 106 divisions with assets totalling $9 million. Although it began strictly as a men's fraternal organization, by 1937 it was able to form social auxiliaries; in 1951 women were granted regular insurance membership.

Today, the society provides low-cost insurance to deaf and hard-of-hearing people, granting membership with the purchase of a life insurance policy. The society also insures deaf children, hearing children and grandchildren of deaf members and hearing adults involved in the field of deafness. The society holds conventions every four years and publishes a bimonthly newsletter, *The Frat.*

In addition to providing insurance, the society each year awards more than 50 savings bonds to outstanding deaf or hard-of-hearing graduates of deaf schools and 10 university scholarships to deaf students. The NFS gives annual All-American awards to outstanding deaf football and basketball players and an annual Athlete of the Year award to a deserving deaf athlete. The society also maintains a library of books and videos on deafness. Contact: National Fraternal Society of the Deaf, 1118 S. 6th St., Springfield, IL 62703; telephone: (voice) 217–789–7429; (TDD) 217–789–7438.

National Index on Deafness, Speech and Hearing See DEAFNESS SPEECH AND HEARING PUBLICATIONS, INC.

National Information Center for Children and Youth with Handicaps This group collects and shares information helpful to handicapped youths, sponsors workshops and publishes newsletters. Contact: National Information Center for Children and Youth with Handicaps, P.O. Box 1492, Washington, D.C. 20013; telephone (voice and TDD): 703–893–6061.

National Information Center on Deafness   Located on the campus of GALLAUDET UNIVERSITY, this unit provides information on several aspects of deafness and on the university itself. Information on careers in the field of deafness, assistive devices, hearing loss and aging, education, resource listings, reading lists and so forth is available to the public. The center maintains contact with a multitude of resources and experts at Gallaudet and around the country and shares information through ELECTRONIC MAIL networks. Contact: National Information Center on Deafness, Gallaudet University, 800 Florida Avenue NE, Washington DC 20002; telephone: (voice) 202–651–5051, (TDD) 202–651–5052; website: http://www.gallaudet.edu/~nicd/

National Institute for Hearing Instruments Studies (NIHIS)   The educational division of the NATIONAL HEARING AID SOCIETY, NIHIS accredits educational programs in the hearing instrument sciences as offered by approved providers or the institute.

National Institute on Deafness and Other Communication Disorders   This institute is one of the National Institutes of Health and was established in 1988 to conduct and support research and training on disorders of hearing and other communication processes. These disorders include diseases affecting hearing, balance, voice, speech, language, taste and smell.

The institute, which was established by the National Deafness and Other Communication Disorders Act of 1988 (Public Law 100–533), requires a wide range of research and development programs, including investigations in the etiology, pathology, detection, treatment and prevention of all forms of hearing disorders and evaluations of diagnosis, treatment, rehabilitation and prevention techniques. Emphasis is also placed in early detection of disorders in infants and the elderly and on exploring environmental causes of deafness. Contact: National Institute on Deafness and Other Communication Disorders, National Institutes of Health, 31 Center Dr., MSC 2320, Bethesda, MD 20892; telephone: (voice) 800–241–1044; (TDD) 800–201–1045; website: http://nih.gov/nidcd

National Rehabilitation Information Center   A rehabilitation information service and research library that provides reference, research and referral services, conducts custom database searches, publishes a quarterly newsletter *NARIC Quarterly,* and disseminates rehabilitation-related information. The center offers a database called REHABDATA, a computerized listing of rehabilitation literature. Contact: National Rehabilitation Information Center, 8455 Colesville Road, Suite 935, Silver Spring, MD 20910; telephone (voice) 800–346–2742; (TDD) 301–495–5626; website: http://www.naric.com

National Research Register for Heredity Hearing Loss   A clearinghouse for people interested in research on hereditary hearing loss. The register informs participating families of new research projects applicable to them and updates all families on the progress of ongoing research through its newsletter. Contact: National Research Register for Heredity Hearing Loss, Boys Town National Research Hospital, 555 30th Street, Omaha NE 68154; telephone (voice and TDD): 402–498–6631.

National Technical Institute for the Deaf (NTID)   This school is the world's largest technological college for deaf students and was established in 1965 in Rochester, New York. It is a federally-funded institution located on the campus of the Rochester Institute of Technology (RIT).

The institute's 2,100 deaf students may select from courses in 34 programs in business, computer science, engineering technology, photography and printing. The institute is one of nine colleges of RIT, sharing campus facilities, library, bookstore and athletic areas. Students may also pursue a bachelor's or master's degree in other colleges at RIT, including the Colleges of Applied Science and Technology, Business, Engineering, Fine and Applied Arts, Graphic Arts and Photography and Liberal Arts. Nearly 20% of RIT's deaf students are enrolled in another college of RIT.

Instructors at NTID use SIGN LANGUAGE, speech and FINGERSPELLING, and students may use whatever communication mode they prefer. Although instructors in other RIT courses don't use sign language, professional interpreters and trained notetakers are available. Deaf students may also obtain interpreters for student activities, counseling, theater, sports, religious services and cultural events.

The school was established with the National Technical Institute for the Deaf Act (PL 89–36), which created the school and provided that the institute must be established within a school that already existed. The law defined NTID as a postsecondary educational and residential institution with a range of basic responsibilities. The Rochester Institute of Technology was selected as the host school by a national advisory board from among 20 applicants.

Applicants to NTID must be U.S. citizens with an overall achievement level of eighth grade with good grades and have a hearing loss of 70 dB or greater without a hearing aid in the better ear.

In addition to educating deaf students, NTID cooperates with other institutions in deafness research and offers a range of programs to improve the quality of deaf education in the United States. In addition, RIT and the

University of Rochester cosponsor a graduate program that qualifies secondary school educators to work with deaf people.

A placement program is offered for NTID graduates, 95% of whom find jobs upon graduation. NTID also staffs the National Center on Employment of the Deaf, which assists both employers and deaf people seeking jobs. Contact: National Technical Institute for the Deaf, Rochester Institute of Technology, 52 Lomb Memorial Dr., LBJ Building, Rochester, NY 14623; telephone: (voice and TDD) 716–475–6906; website: http://www.rit.edu/~418www/index.html

national temporal bone banks   This program, administered by the Deafness Research Foundation, maintains four regional centers serving more than 100 hospitals in seeking the bequest of internal auditory structures from individuals with ear disorders for research and specialist training. Contact: Deafness Research Foundation, 9 E. 38th St., New York, NY 10016; telephone: 800–535–DEAF.

National Theatre of the Deaf (NTD)   A professional ensemble of deaf and hearing actors, this theater company uses mime, body language and SIGN LANGUAGE augmented by reverse interpretation of the signs for hearing audiences. Founded in 1970, the company has given more than 5,000 performances of classical repertory as well as original works in 24 countries.

The company's 14 professional actors put on a new play each fall and go on tour for 27 weeks to the major theaters of the world; it is the only theatrical company to have performed in all 50 states. The NTD has appeared on many TV specials and on *Sesame Street* and received a Tony Award in 1977 for theatrical excellence. In 1984, the group represented the United States at the Los Angeles Olympics Arts Festival, and in 1986 it became the first Western theater company to tour the People's Republic of China.

Most of the actors are deaf, and the cast takes English scripts and translates them into a theatrical form of sign language, which may also include new signs created to express a dramatic point. Two hearing actors also translate orally for the primarily-hearing audiences who come to the shows.

In addition to formal performances, the company supports the LITTLE THEATRE OF THE DEAF for young audiences and presents numerous workshops and lecture-demonstrations. The company also supports a professional theater school during the summer to teach deaf individuals basic and advanced theater skills at the company's headquarters in Chester, Connecticut.

The National Theatre of the Deaf is located at the Hazel E. Stark Center, a converted mill and residence housing offices, rehearsal space, classrooms and theater shops. Funding for the theater comes from grants, gifts, performances and the Media Services and Captioned Films section of the Bureau of Education. (See also PROFESSIONAL SCHOOL FOR DEAF THEATRE PERSONNEL.) Contact: The National Theatre of the Deaf, 5 West Main St., P.O. Box 659, Chester, CT 06412; telephone: (voice) 860–526–4971, (TDD) 860–526–4974; website: http://www.NTD.org

Navarrete, Juan Fernandez de (1526–1579) Also known as "El Mudo" (the mute), Juan Fernandez de Navarrete was born in Spain and became deaf at age three from unknown causes. As a child, he began to draw as a way of communicating and received his first art lessons in his hometown of Logrono. Eventually he was sent to study art in Italy upon his teacher's recommendation.

He toured the primary cities of Italy, studying art as he went, until King Philip II of Spain summoned him to Madrid, where he became the most important of the group of Spanish and Italian painters commissioned to work in the famed monastery and royal palace of the Escorial.

A member of the Madrid school, El Mudo painted during a time of transition in the Spanish art world. He was the first to abandon the mannerist movement, which had begun in the 16th century, and was the bridge to the naturalists of the 17th century. Almost all of his paintings are religious in nature; those that remain at the cloister of the Escorial hang in the gallery of the upper cloister.

El Mudo died on March 28, 1579, in Toledo, Spain before completing his commission to paint the pictures for 30 altars in the Basilica of the Escorial.

Netherlands About 3.4% of this population of 14.4 million is hard-of-hearing, and about 28,000 of these are deaf, representing a fairly low rate of deafness.

There are five state educational centers for deaf students, including preschool, elementary and vocational training, with varied programs offering day and residential, oral and TOTAL COMMUNICATION approaches. Few students are mainstreamed or are educated beyond high school.

The oral approach has been the basis of social interchange in the Netherlands from preschool to adult aftercare programs, but more and more experts are beginning to acknowledge the value of the manual.

Adult deaf people communicate with a blended form of Signed Dutch, DUTCH SIGN LANGUAGE and lip movements.

neurogenic communication disorder The inability to exchange information with others because of hearing, speech, and/or language problems caused by impairment of the nervous system (brain or nerves).

New Zealand   This tiny country of only three million people includes a scattered deaf population of 1,690 deaf and hard-of-hearing students in various types of classes, programs and schools.

The first state oral school for deaf students in the world was opened in 1880 by Gerrit Van Asch, whose work was praised by ALEXANDER GRAHAM BELL. Beginning in the 1940s, a host of changes were introduced: free hearing aids, formal teacher training, nursery school and guidance programs for parents and students.

Since 1960, educators for deaf students in New Zealand have tried to develop new, expanded services, serving classes for deaf children in ordinary elementary and high schools with special teachers and for students mainstreamed in regular classes. They have also developed two state residential schools. Further, the schools for deaf students are affiliated with polytechnic colleges and community colleges; they also send deaf students to regular universities.

As in many European countries, New Zealand for many years favored the oral approach; today, it has modified this approach to include TOTAL COMMUNICATION with a standardized SIGN LANGUAGE system (the Australian or Victorian) and two-handed FINGERSPELLING.

Because of the country's small size, no one school limits itself to one communication mode but consults with parents in deciding which method to use with each individual child.

Although many deaf people in New Zealand are not hired in positions that fully utilize their abilities, the increased availability of further education has raised the standard of living for deaf people.

Because the school system relied on oral instruction for many years, no formal sign language system was developed. Most deaf New Zealanders do communicate with signs they originated, but no fingerspelling is used. With the introduction of Total Communication, two-handed fingerspelling and a wide range of signs has been introduced.

Nigeria   The exact number of deaf people in Nigeria is difficult to ascertain since there has been no census of this population, but it is estimated that there are about 70,000 deaf citizens out of a population of 80 million. About 7,000 of these are believed to be between six and 18 years of age.

Too often in this country, deafness in children is unnoticed or ignored by illiterate parents; many infants are born at home, and physicians may rarely see these children. In addition, the society looks negatively at deaf children and their parents, and therefore many are hidden away. Because most cases of deafness occur after birth and during adolescence or adulthood, many deaf Nigerians can learn to speak fairly well.

Today, there are 20 schools for deaf students in addition to special classes in regular schools, and about 50 deaf Nigerian students study in the

United States each year. Most schools use the American MANUAL ALPHABET and SIGN LANGUAGE.

noise blocker   Also called an automatic signal processor, these are innovative devices operating on the theory that most noise occurs at low pitch; consequently, they are designed to pick up the low pitch sounds and automatically reduce their noise level.

However, if the wearer's speech discrimination is poor, the noise blockers may not help, particularly if the noise is coming from large groups of people talking.

nonhuman signing   Manual communication taught to nonhumans (typically apes) in an attempt to teach these animals language.

The earliest attempts to teach apes to communicate focused on speech rather than SIGN LANGUAGE. Although years of research occasionally produced an ape that could utter one or two words, forcing the apes to produce vocal human speech was doomed from the start because of the different vocal apparatus between the species.

The first successful attempt at teaching apes communication came in 1966, when two researchers, R. Allen and B.T. Gardner, taught their 10-month old chimpanzee, Washoe, AMERICAN SIGN LANGUAGE (ASL). They began Washoe's training by raising her in the social environment of their own family, living with humans by day and in a separate house trailer at night. In addition, Washoe could play in the back yard with a sandbox, gym and a large tree.

Since chimps lack the ability to produce speech and because in the wild they use gestures to communicate, the Gardners chose to teach Washoe ASL because it was a gestural and human language.

In Washoe's first four years, she acquired more than 130 signs, using them spontaneously and in correct context. She carried on everyday conversations, initiated conversation and commented to and questioned her human companions. She could ask about friends who were not there and generalized her signs to a variety of uses. For example, she would sign "dog" not just for a real dog but for photos of dogs and sounds of barking dogs.

Further study with Washoe looked at the capacity of chimps to use cross-modal transfer between auditory words and visual signs. Researchers also compared individual differences between chimps, generic and specific use of signs, comprehension, use of prepositional phrases and the conceptual use of signs.

Still, the Gardners' research with Washoe was criticized in the late 1970s by people who argued that the conclusions of the Gardners and others were false because the evidence was ambiguous, suggesting that the Gardners wanted to believe Washoe could sign and were therefore biased, and that scientists inadvertently cued the chimp. Critics also charged that the form and structure of the ape's signs showed no resemblance to ASL.

In 1978, researchers tried to design a study to answer critics, stopping all signs around the chimp except for seven signs: who, what, want, which, where, sign and name. Researchers believed if Washoe's infants acquired sign language, it was because they had learned it from her.

After Washoe's first infant died, a 10-month-old male was given to her to adopt. Eight days later, little Loulis used his first sign: "person." At 15 months, he started using two-sign combinations, and five years later, he used 54 different signs—all learned from Washoe and signing chimp friends. Loulis was therefore the first chimp to acquire human language from another chimp.

In 1980, three new chimps were raised in their early years at the Gardners' house, intended for testing in cross-chimp communication. To control the use of human signing, the chimps were videotaped and observed on monitors from a separate room in 20-minute segments three times a day for 15 days, thereby restricting access to their human caretakers.

In the 15 hours taped, 617 chimp conversations were recorded. Together with research from another study examining many more conversations, scientists found that almost 90% of these chimp "conversations" centered around play, reassurance and social interactions. Only 5% had to do with food.

nonmanual behaviors   The features of AMERICAN SIGN LANGUAGE that are not portrayed with the hands. These include facial expression, head and body movement and posture.

nonverbal communication   Nonverbal communication includes tone of voice and noises, shrugs, body position, facial expressions and gestures to enrich and modify speech. Hearing people generally assume this nonverbal communication is inferior to speech, because it is less variable and not a systematic form of language.

SIGN LANGUAGE, however, is *not* a form of nonverbal communication. Deaf people use nonverbal communication in much the same way hearing people do. The reason why sign languages have often been misclassified as nonverbal systems of communication is probably because their form is visual-gestural, which is also the most common form of nonverbal communication among hearing people.

Northhampton vowel and consonant charts   A printed system to help deaf children learn to speak, read and write syntactically correct sentences.

Devised in 1884, the system uses alphabet symbols to describe English pronunciation and was first used for teaching how sounds and words were related in reading. It is now more commonly used to help develop speech.

Norwegian Sign Language   There are three major sign dialects of Norwegian Sign Language (NSL), spoken by about 4,000 deaf Norwegians, which originate with the three schools for the deaf.

In these schools, teachers use a manual code for Norwegian called Signed Norwegian, together with speech in addition to signs. As is typical around the world, Norwegian students use SIGN LANGUAGE when speaking among themselves outside of school.

In addition to NSL, the INTERNATIONAL MANUAL ALPHABET developed by the WORLD CONGRESS OF THE DEAF and considered to be the best system for deaf-blind people, has been used since 1970.

Since the 1970s, there has been a growing demand for the use of NSL in education by the deaf community.

Unlike AMERICAN SIGN LANGUAGE, NSL vocabulary uses almost no fingerspelled signs. It does, however, emphasize the use of lip movements of spoken words.

O

open-set speech recognition Understanding speech without visual clues (speech reading).

oral approach A communication method that stresses the use of speech among deaf and hard-of-hearing people together with SPEECHREAD-ING and auditory training as a way of merging with the hearing world.

The roots of the oral approach may be traced to the 1500s, when a Spanish monk named PEDRO PONCE DE LEON taught the deaf children of nobility at his monastery. Using his own methods, he taught the children to use language, speech and speech-reading. His methods were handed on to other Spanish teachers of deaf children at the end of the 16th century, including Manuel Ramirez de Carrion. At about the same time, JUAN PABLO BONET published what was the first book describing oral teaching methods for deaf students.

Gradually, the oral method movement spread throughout Europe and found a special home in Germany in the 18th century, where SAMUEL HEINICKE became its leading proponent. Heinicke, a devout oral proponent, opened the first German school for deaf students in 1778. At the same time in England, the Braidwood family headed by THOMAS BRAIDWOOD was opening oralist schools for deaf children using its own secret methods of instruction.

In 1819 American educator THOMAS HOPKINS GALLAUDET came to the Braidwoods to learn the oralist tradition. When the Braidwoods refused to reveal their methods to Gallaudet, he went on to France to learn the manual method, which he subsequently brought back to the United States.

The MANUAL APPROACH was the sole method of instruction for deaf students up until the mid-1800s, when the Clarke School opened in Northampton, Massachusetts. From then on, aided by the European success of oralist education, the tide began to change in the United States, and from 1880 to 1930 oralism replaced the manual approach as the primary method of instruction. After World War I, about 75% of American deaf pupils were taught almost entirely by the oral method.

As time went on, however, schools began combining their methods; elementary students were taught orally, with signs used in some classes in high school. But studies in the 1960s and 1970s found that the educational achievement of deaf children educated orally fell short of their hearing peers and that students taught in sign from the beginning generally functioned at a higher level.

The 200-year debate over the oral and manual methods centers on the place in society in which a deaf person should fit. Those who supported the oral approach in this country were generally opposed to the segregation of deaf people and did not approve of special camps, churches or social organizations. Critics of the oral approach, on the other hand, believed in maintaining deaf culture and in making accommodations in communication and social organizations.

Oral supporters (whose chief champion was ALEXANDER GRAHAM BELL) promote the use of hearing aids, speechreading and speech as the right of all deaf children and do not favor the use of sign language in schools. In fact, for many years, sign language was forbidden in oral schools. This objection to sign is primarily because proponents of the oral method believe it is too difficult to learn two languages at once (speech and sign). However, not all object to sign language as a means of communication *outside* the school.

There are also differences of opinions among oral method supporters over auditory, multisensory or CUED SPEECH teaching methods. The first method uses auditory training and specialized training that does not emphasize speechreading.

The multisensory teaching method is more traditional, encouraging students to use speechreading, body language or tactile methods to communicate. Some multi-sensory programs also permit the use of FINGERSPELLING.

Cued Speech supporters believe in the cued speech system, which supplements what a person hears with a hearing aid, a combined form of speechreading and hand cues. (See also TOTAL COMMUNICATION; SIMULTANEOUS COMMUNICATION.)

Oral Deaf Adults Section (ODAS)   A service organization, this group was formed in 1964 as part of the ALEXANDER GRAHAM BELL ASSOCIATION FOR THE DEAF. Its members choose to communicate through spoken language and SPEECHREADING and have joined together to encourage the oral-aural approach in educating deaf children. Supporters of the oral approach believe students can learn to communicate effectively using speech, speechreading and auditory training.

The section was founded by H. LATHAM BREUNIG and ROBERT H. WEITBRECHT, the developer of teletypewriters (TTYs) for deaf people. It publishes a membership directory and a newsletter for members, offers educational scholarships and plans outings for families with deaf children.

The group maintains its own member speakers' bureau in order to portray these deaf adults as role models for younger deaf people.

oral interpreters   Persons skilled in the specialized interpreting ability of translating the meaning of spoken words by silently mouthing a speaker's words for a deaf person who prefers the oral approach. Oral interpreters use no sign language and are skilled in substituting words for those that are difficult to speechread. However, oral interpreters are used by only a very few deaf people.

Oral interpreters are also available to repeat to a hearing audience a spoken message from a deaf person whose speech may not be clear. They use a variety of skills and techniques to convey the message and emotions of the speaker; these are most helpful when the person with a hearing loss does not use sign language.

An oral interpreter may not be the best interpreter for a person who uses listening skills and SPEECHREADING since it is difficult to watch an oral interpreter while listening to the speaker. Because of the delay between the sound of the speaker's voice and lip movements of the oral interpreter, the oral interpreter is always several words behind the speaker.

Oral interpreters are certified by the REGISTRY OF INTERPRETERS FOR THE DEAF, the only national professional organization in the United States that certifies both oral and SIGN LANGUAGE interpreters. The registry lists interpreters in various specialties, including legal, medical and educational interpreting. In 1979, the registry established a separate certification process for oral interpreters similar to the one for sign language interpreters. Three oral interpreting certifications are awarded by the registry: Two for different levels of accuracy by hearing candidates and one for candidates with hearing problems.

Oral interpreters are listed with local and state chapters of the Registry of Interpreters for the Deaf, local speech and hearing centers, the Office of Vocational Rehabilitation, the ALEXANDER GRAHAM BELL ASSOCIATION FOR THE DEAF, a school or college with support services for hard-of-hearing students and programs and agencies serving hard-of-hearing people.

A hard-of-hearing person does not have to pay for oral interpreters under several conditions. For example, Section 504 of the Rehabilitation Act of 1973 requires that interpreting services for hard-of-hearing people must be provided free for all meetings, classes and other group activities sponsored by an agency that receives federal funds and has 15 or more employees. In an educational setting, the Education for All Handicapped Children Act of 1975 (PL 94–142) requires that the services of an interpreter must be written into a student's individual educational plan. Such an interpreter service would then be paid for by the child's school. At the same time, hard-of-hearing or deaf parents must also be given an interpreter for parent/teacher conferences and meetings. In addition, federal law requires the federal court to appoint a qualified interpreter in criminal or civil actions against a hard-of-hearing person, and the court must provide an oral interpreter if so requested. Most states also pay for an interpreter in criminal proceedings; several pay for an interpreter in civil cases as well. (See also INTERPRETERS AND THE LAW.)

organ of Corti   The organ of Corti is contained in the COCHLEA and is the most important part of the hearing process.

The organ is covered with many fine hairs arranged like the strings of a harp, with the shorter, thinner hairs picking up high sounds and the longer, thicker hairs picking up low sounds. When a sound wave makes the eardrum vibrate, the vibrations are carried across the middle ear by the hammer, the anvil and the stirrup, which pass the vibrations through the oval window to the fluid in the tubes of the inner ear.

This makes the hairs of the organ of Corti vibrate; the more hairs that vibrate, the louder the sound. The AUDITORY NERVE picks up the message from these hairs and sends it to the brain, where the sound is processed.

ossicular chain   Attached to the eardrum is a chain of three small bones called the ossicular chain. Located in the pea-sized middle ear cavity, the ossicles are the smallest bones in the human body and are full size when a child is born.

The individual bones are smaller than a grain of rice: the bone attached to the eardrum is the malleus (hammer); the second bone is the incus (anvil); and the third is the stapes (stirrup). As sound waves move the eardrum, it moves the ossicles. The three bones actually serve as a type of level that transfers the energy of the sound waves from the outer ear through the MIDDLE EAR into the INNER EAR.

ossicular interruption   A separation of the three tiny ossicles that carry sound vibrations from the eardrum membrane to the fluid inside the inner ear. It is caused by an infection or by a blow to the head.

The separation usually occurs at the weakest point of the OSSICULAR CHAIN, where the anvil (incus) joins the stirrup (stapes). A partial separation causes mild hearing impairment; a more complete separation results in a severe hearing loss.

Ossicular interruption can be diagnosed by hearing tests that indicate the hearing nerve in the inner ear is normal but sound is not being conducted from the eardrum to the inner ear.

Treatment of ossicular interruption is one of the most successful operations to restore hearing—performed by an otolaryngologist, it involves repositioning the ossicles so they can again conduct sound. (See also OSSICULOPLASTY.)

ossiculoplasty   Surgical repair of the middle-ear OSSICLES to treat hearing loss, usually caused by chronic ear infection or cholesteatoma or a temporal bone fracture. Ossiculoplasty may be combined with MYRINGOPLASTY or MASTOIDECTOMY. (See also OSSICULAR INTERRUPTION; TYMPANOPLASTY.)

osteoma   An osteoma of the ear canal is a bony knob close to the eardrum, occurring particularly in people who swim frequently in cold water. Unless the growth blocks the ear canal and therefore interferes with hearing, it does not need to be removed.

otolaryngology   A specialty medical field concerned with treatment and surgery of the ear, nose, and throat and related structures of the head and neck.

It includes cosmetic facial reconstruction, surgery of benign and malignant tumors of the head and neck, management of patients with loss of hearing and balance, endoscopic examination of air and food passages and treatment of allergic, sinus, laryngeal, thyroid and esophageal disorders. (See OTOLARYNGOLOGIST.)

otology   The branch of medicine concerned with the ear. As in many other fields of medicine, the roots of the practice of otology began well before recorded history, although actual surgery on the ear did not begin before the 18th century.

Some of the first descriptions of early otology are found in the *Ebers Papyrus*, written about 1600 B.C., in which Egyptian priests specialized in ear treatments. These treatments might include injections into the ear of olive oil, red lead, bat's wings, ant eggs or goat's urine. By the fifth century, Pythagoras was exploring the physics of sound; he constructed a musical scale by listening to different pitches that occurred when a blacksmith struck his anvil with different hammers.

It was in the 19th century that modern otology began, with the surgical advances of Sir Astley Cooper in London who cut into the eardrum to ease certain cases of deafness. Parisian surgeon Gaspard Itard explored the diseases of the ear while Marie-Jean-Pierre Flourens discussed the action of the SEMICIRCULAR CANALS and realized that the acoustic nerve has branches for hearing and for balance. By 1860, Prosper Ménière reported the case of a girl with VERTIGO, nausea and TINNITUS during a fatal illness, and in 1851 ALFONSO CORTI, an Italian anatomist, published his studies about the organ that now bears his name.

otorhinolaryngology   The full name of the surgical specialty focusing on diseases of the ear, nose and throat. (See also OTOLARYNGOLOGY.)

otoscope   An instrument used for examining the ear that includes magnifying lenses, a light and a funnel-shaped tip that is inserted into the ear canal. The instrument can be used to inspect the outer ear canal and the eardrum, and to detect certain diseases of the MIDDLE EAR.

P

Paget-Gorman sign system (PGSS)   A sign language system designed by Sir Richard Paget and further developed by Lady Grace Paget and Dr. Pierre Gorman of Great Britain.

It developed in almost total isolation from the language of the deaf community; the sign vocabulary of PGSS is not related to BRITISH SIGN LANGUAGE and is not intelligible to British deaf people. Children learning PGSS have nothing linguistically in common with deaf adults.

paracusia willisiana   The ability to hear speech better in a noisy environment. Named for Dr. Thomas Willis, the English physician who described it in 1672, paracusia willisiana occurs in people with all forms of CONDUCTIVE HEARING LOSS.

Normally, a person in a noisy environment will raise his voice about 40 decibels louder in order to be heard above the background sounds. The person with a conductive hearing loss at frequencies that match the background noise won't be able to hear it but will be able to hear the speaker's voice well at an intensity level 40 decibels higher. With a pure conductive disorder, the sense organ is normal, and the speech at this louder decibel level will be completely understandable. On the other hand, a person with normal hearing hears not only the speaker's louder voice, but the entire range of background noise as well. Finally, a person with sensorineural hearing loss has more trouble hearing in noise because of the masking effect.

Pereira, Jacobo Rodriguez (1715–1780)   This 18th-century Portuguese teacher is known as the first teacher of deaf students in France. Born in Berlanga, Portugal, Pereira moved to Bordeaux, where he demonstrated his techniques before the Parisian Academy of Science.

Advocating a low student-teacher ratio, Pereira accepted payment for his work depending on how quickly his pupils progressed. He used a one-handed manual alphabet that represented phonic qualities, not letters—the position of the fingers indicated the position of the speech organ used in making that sound. Similar to CUED SPEECH, this alphabet was used as a pronunciation aid.

perichondritis   An unusual infection of the cartilage of the outer ear, this disorder is caused by an organism and can be contracted while swimming in polluted water or by an injury.

This microorganism, *Pseudomonas aeruginosa*, creates a greenish brown musty discharge from the outer ear canal. Perichondritis can be suspected when the outer ear is tender, red and thicker than normal. Prompt treatment will prevent a permanent deformity of the outer ear.

peripheral auditory system   All of the anatomic structures from the pinna or auricle (actual ear visible on the outside of the head) to the end of the auditory nerve in the brain. Generally, the system is divided into three parts: the outer, middle and inner ear structures.

Any problem with the conduction of sound in the OUTER EAR (such as excess wax) or the MIDDLE EAR (such as fluid) that blocks the transmission of sound to the INNER EAR can result in a conductive hearing loss.

If there is a problem with the sensory cells in the COCHLEA located in the inner ear, however, both the ability to hear and understand the sound will be affected; this is called a sensory hearing loss.

If a hearing problem is caused by a condition affecting the hearing nerve to the brain (also called the auditory nerve), the resulting hearing problems is called a neural loss. Since it is common for both a sensory and a neural loss to occur at the same time—or it may be impossible to tell the difference between them—such a loss is often called a sensorineural loss. A mixed hearing loss results from conditions affecting both the conductive and sensorineural structures.

Philippines   About 300,000 people of this republic have hearing problems.

For many years, there was only one school for deaf students—the Philippine School for the Deaf, but by 1982 there were more than 2,000 deaf students enrolled in state-run educational programs. In addition, there are a number of private schools for deaf students throughout the country, serving a total of less than 400 pupils.

Communication modes vary from school to school and often change as administrators come and go. Deaf students may continue their education past high school, either with short-term vocational courses or college.

The schools may vary in their communication styles, but many graduates of deaf schools communicate as adults in sign language; those who have not gone to school use natural signs.

phonemes   The essential and smallest elements of a finite number of speech sounds. They are the code signals that give meaning to speech. Phonemes are really abstractions, a bit like an averaging of the types of sounds that actually occur in speech.

For example, the phoneme "t" in the words "cat" and "tea" sounds very much the same yet is produced very differently. In "cat," the "t" sound is really just a stop made with only a very slight explosion of breath.

The same "t" sound in the word "tea" is exploded with an audible breath. There are many different variations of pronouncing the phoneme "t," which are called its ALLOPHONES.

phonetics   The study of the smallest units of language. (See also LINGUISTICS.)

phonology   The study of how the smallest units of language (PHONEMES) can be combined to form words or signs. (See also LINGUISTICS.)

phonophobia   An extreme sense of discomfort caused by sounds above the threshold of hearing.

Pidgin Sign English (PSE)   A sign language system most often used by hearing people learning to communicate with deaf people. Also called Sign English, it combines the English word order and simplified grammatical structure with the vocabulary and nonmanual features of AMERICAN SIGN LANGUAGE. Signs for definite and indefinite articles are omitted, and only one sign is used for the verb "to be," unlike the MANUALLY CODED ENGLISH systems.

Another name for PSE is "Siglish." (See also SIGN LANGUAGE; SIGN LANGUAGE CONTINUUM; SIMULTANEOUS COMMUNICATION.)

pitch   The perception of sound frequency, measured in terms of the number of cycles per second at which a sound wave vibrates. Pitch can vary with the intensity, duration or complexity of the sound vibration.

In music, "perfect" pitch (also called absolute pitch) is the very rare ability to identify the position of a tone within an octave (in other words, the ability to identify a note, A through G, without using a reference pitch). Perfect relative pitch is the ability to identify a note with the aid of a reference pitch. Perfect relative pitch is more common and is a skill that can be learned.

Plater, Felix (1536–1614)   A 17th-century Swiss physician who published a detailed study of the bones of the ear, including the way in which sound is transmitted through the bones of the head.

In his book, Plater described both sensorineural and conductive deafness. He understood that the root of deafness was found sometimes in the brain and sometimes in the cavity of the ears. He found that if the cause of deafness is found in the brain, there is no cure. Plater is also known for his descriptions of the presence of TINNITUS in many of his deaf patients.

polymography   The process of taking X rays of the inner ear.

Ponce de León, Pedro (?–1584)   This 16th-century Benedictine monk is considered to be the father of education for deaf people and is thought to have been the first person to invent a method to teach deaf students.

Ponce de León was born in the province of León in northern Spain and entered a local monastery in 1526. Taking as his first pupil a man who had been denied admittance to the Benedictine order because he could neither hear nor speak, Ponce de León taught him to speak so he could make his confession. This student, Gaspard Burgos, went on to write several books of his own.

When transferred to a monastery in the mountains of north-central Spain, he met the two deaf sons of the wealthy marquis of Berlanga, Juan Fernandez de Velasco. The marquis' family was known for hereditary deafness, probably caused by intermarriage. Becoming close to Francisco and Pedro Velasco, aged 9 and 12 respectively, Ponce de León taught them both to speak. Pedro also learned how to write, speak and read books in Latin, Italian and Spanish before his death at age 30. Ponce de León also taught about 12 other deaf people to speak, including the marquis' deaf daughters Bernardina and Catalina.

He next established a school at the Ona monastery for teaching wealthy deaf students to talk, beginning his teaching with writing and progressing to speech. Historians believe he taught speech to his students by tracing letters and indicating pronunciation with his lips. Historians also suspect that the manual alphabet he used was probably the same one published by the Franciscan monk Melchor Yebra in 1593. This alphabet is almost identical to the one used by 16th-century deaf teachers JUAN PABLO BONET and Manuel Ramirez de Carrion, who also taught deaf members of the Velasco family.

Ponce de León is also assumed to have used signs in the education of his deaf pupils, since the Benedictines took strict vows of silence and had developed their own signs as a result.

In addition, he is said to have written a book, *Instruction for the Mute Deaf,* which was probably lost during the social upheavals common in Spanish monasteries at that time. Although books and documents from the monastery of Ona were sent to the National Archives in Spain, Ponce de León's book has never been found.

postlingual deafness   Deafness occurring after language has been acquired. (See also ADVENTITIOUS DEAFNESS.)

prelingual deafness   Deafness occurring before language skills have been acquired.

Professional Rehabilitation Workers with the Adult Deaf   Known today as the AMERICAN DEAFNESS AND REHABILITATION ASSOCIATION, ADARA was formed in 1964 under the above name as a way to separate people who worked with deaf people from the organization for rehabilitators who worked with all disabilities.

Professional School for Deaf Theater Personnel   America's only professional theater school for deaf students has offered deaf actors a concentrated four-week session in basic and advanced theater since 1967.

The faculty includes professional stage actors, academic instructors and company members of the NATIONAL THEATRE OF THE DEAF. Courses include acting, directing, playwriting, dance, costume design, fencing, storytelling, set design and Japanese dance and theater. Deaf and hearing teachers instruct both deaf students and hearing students involved in deaf culture who are proficient in sign.

The program is accredited by Connecticut College and is supported by the U.S. Department of Education's special education program. Full scholarships for 20 deaf Americans are granted each year. The application process each year ends April 15 for the session beginning in June. Contact: National Theatre of the Deaf, Hazel E. Stark Center, Chester, CT 06412; telephone: 203–526–4971 (voice), 203–526–4974 (TDD).

Project ALAS   A nonprofit service organization affiliated with D.E.A.F., INC. Project ALAS (Spanish for "wings") offers services for deaf Latinos and their families on the East Coast. Contact: Project ALAS, c/o D.E.A.F., Inc., 215 Brighton Avenue, Allston MA 02134; telephone (voice and TDD): 617–254–4041; email: imvelez@aol.com

PSYCH.NET   A computer-accessed bulletin board on an ELECTRONIC MAIL system that allows professionals in the fields of mental health and deafness to communicate. This type of electronic mail service provides cheap and instantaneous access to other subscribers.

PSYCH.NET is a limited access bulletin board, part of a larger system called DEAFTEK.USA. People wishing to become a user must first join DEAFTEK.USA, which requires an annual fee and monthly charges depending on usage. There is no charge to join PSYCH.NET, although an application is required. (See also ASCII; BAUDOT CODE.)

psychogenic hearing loss   See FUNCTIONAL LOSS (NONORGANIC).

Public Law 94–142   See LEGAL RIGHTS.

Public Law 97–410   See LEGAL RIGHTS.

Public Law 100–533   See LEGAL RIGHTS.

Puerto Rican Sign Language   There are at least four varieties of Puerto Rican Sign Language (PRSL) used today on the small Caribbean commonwealth island. It is similar to AMERICAN SIGN LANGUAGE and is believed to have developed from the introduction of ASL in the early 1900s. American Sign Language was brought to Puerto Rico in 1907 by nuns who founded a deaf school; in the 1950s a Spanish teaching order of nuns introduced the oral approach and forbade SIGN LANGUAGE.

Puerto Rican Sign Language is different from ASL in that it does not use FINGERSPELLING and has many signs that are different or do not appear in ASL. Its structural characteristics, as in other sign languages, include the use of space to show relationship between objects or ideas, classifiers and size- and shape-specifiers and the use of compound signs to describe new ideas.

In addition, Signed Spanish, which uses signs in Spanish word order, is used by deaf persons in communicating with Spanish-speaking hearing people. Signed English is used by deaf Puerto Ricans who were educated in mainland United States. Of the two, Signed Spanish is more commonly used in Puerto Rico to communicate with hearing people, especially for interpreting and watching television.

Q

Quota International, Inc. A service group whose major project, Shatter Silence, helps individuals with hearing and speech handicaps. The group publishes *The Quotarian,* offers fellowships and conducts an annual Outstanding Deaf Woman of the Year program. Contact: Quota International, Inc., 1420 21st Street NW, Washington DC 20044; telephone (voice and TDD): 202–331–9694.

R

radio for the deaf   The Pennsylvania School for the Deaf in Philadelphia established the first and largest radio network for deaf people who have specially tuned home radio receivers connected to a telecommunication device for the deaf for printout.

At the station, words are coded on a teleprinter, punched on paper tape and then converted into audible tones sent via telephone to Temple University's FM station. There, the tones are broadcast within a 30- to 50-mile radius as a type of "captioned radio."

Rainbow Alliance of the Deaf   A national organization serving the deaf gay and lesbian community, this group has 24 chapters throughout the United States and two in Canada. Contact: Rainbow Alliance of the Deaf, 10902 Bucknell Dr. 1312, Wheaton, MD 20902; telephone: (TDD) 702–804–6476; website: http://www.rad.org

receptive aphasia   See AUDITORY AGNOSIA.

receptive skill   The ability to understand what is being communicated in both FINGERSPELLING and SIGN LANGUAGE.

Registry of Interpreters for the Deaf (RID)   The largest national organization of interpreters in the United States. The registry maintains a national list of people skilled in the use of AMERICAN SIGN LANGUAGE and other sign systems.

The RID provides information on interpreting and evaluation and certification of interpreters for deaf people. When it was first established in Muncie, Indiana in 1964, the organization was designed simply as a way to register certified interpreters. But in the early 1970s, the registry began to expand its interests: It set up both the first national certification system and the first performance evaluation for interpreters in the world. At the same time, interpreter associations were founded at the local and state level to advocate legislative reform in the area of interpreter laws.

Today, RID consists of more than 3,000 members—most certified interpreters—who work to further the profession of interpretation of American Sign Language and English. Its national office produces the bimonthly newsletter *Views* and serves as a clearinghouse of information about interpretation. (See also COURT INTERPRETERS ACT; INTERPRETERS AND THE LAW; ORAL INTERPRETERS; SIGN LANGUAGE INTERPRETERS.) Contact: Registry of Interpreters for the Deaf, Inc., 511 Monroe St., Suite 1107, Rockville MD 20850; telephone (voice and TDD): 301–779–0555.

Rehabilitation Act of 1973   See LEGAL RIGHTS.

Rehabilitation Reengineering Research Center on Hearing Enhancement and Assistive Devices (RERC)   The RERC promotes and develops technological solutions to problems confronting individuals with hearing loss. Current projects include assistive devices for deaf and hard-of-hearing people, detection of hearing loss in infants using OTOACOUSTIC EMISSIONS TESTS, development of ASCII standards for TTY modems, and evaluation of the use of assistive technologies in the community and workplace. The Center provides information and referral for consumer questions on assistive technology and research. Contact: RERC, Lexington School for the Deaf/Center for the Deaf, 30th Avenue and 75th Street, Jackson Heights NY 11370; telephone: (voice and TDD) 718–899–8000. ext. 212; internet website: http:///idt.net/~reslex.

residential schools   See EDUCATION OF DEAF CHILDREN.

retracted eardrum   When the pressure inside the middle ear is lower than the pressure on the outside in the external canal, the eardrum is gradually pushed inward by the extra pressure from the outside. Sometimes the eardrum can be pressed so far into the middle ear that it touches the cochlea itself, almost completely obliterating the middle ear.

This retraction occurs during a head cold, an allergy attack or an infection in the back of the nose and throat, any of which force the eustachian tube closed so that no air can get into the middle ear. In such a situation, the air normally present in the middle ear becomes locked in, and some of it is absorbed by the lining of the middle ear, reducing the pressure in the middle ear.

This can reduce the efficiency of both the eardrum and the OSSICULAR CHAIN in transmitting sound to the inner ear, although the amount of retraction is no indication of the amount of hearing loss. The amount of hearing loss is determined instead by the site and type of damage in the ossicular chain, and this cannot be determined by appearance alone.

reverse interpreting   See SIGN-TO-VOICE INTERPRETING.

Rochester Method   See FINGERSPELLING.

Ronsard, Pierre de (1524–1585)   This "Prince of Poets" was one of the outstanding writers during the French Renaissance and was responsible for a renewed interest in poetry. He was deafened at age 15, a loss that diverted his interests from a diplomatic career toward literary pursuits. Today he is considered to be one of the leading poets in the history of French literature.

He was born on September 11, 1524, in Possoniere castle, the son of a noble family, and embarked at a young age on a career as a diplomat in the royal household. Unfortunately, in 1540 an ear infection and high fever resulted in a severe hearing loss that eliminated further advancement as a diplomat.

Much to his father's displeasure, Ronsard turned to a career in literature. Although he took preliminary steps toward the priesthood, his heart was never in it. After the death of his father, life as a literary figure became easier, and he began to study poetry and literature more seriously.

In 1547, Ronsard joined with Joachim du Bellay, who was also deaf, in forming a group of aspiring poets. He was also frequently at the royal court, eventually earning a job administering kneeling cushions and holy water for the king.

Ronsard published his first collection of poems in 1560 and was at this time an important spokesman at court and defender of the Catholic faith. Still, he was best known for his love poetry, although it is not known to what extent he pursued these relationships in actuality.

S

saccule   One of the structures of the INNER EAR, this is a small sac located in the VESTIBULE, which encapsulates a single sensory patch called a MACULA. The macula, which resembles the letter *j*, lies against the inner wall of the vestibule directly over the bone.

The UTRICLE and the saccule together with their maculae are also called otolith organs and gravity receptors (since they respond to gravitational forces). These receptors—particularly the utricle—are important in the righting reflexes and in maintaining the contractions of the muscles that keep the body standing upright.

The role the saccule plays is less well understood, although it is believed it may respond to vibration and backwards-forwards positions of the head.

Of the two, the utricle seems to be the dominant receptor.

SAI   See SOCIAL ADEQUACY INDEX.

SAL   See SENSORINEURAL ACUITY LEVEL.

Schenck, Johannes   A 16th-century physician who explored the etiology of deafness.

Schenck was able to describe the idea of hereditary deafness by exploring the case of a family with several children with congenital deafness. He also discussed how a person might lose the ability to hear following an injury.

Scotland   There are an estimated 4,000 deaf adults in Scotland, with another 2,000 students receiving help for some form of hearing loss.

The history of deaf education in Scotland is long, beginning in 1769 with the establishment of a school operated by THOMAS BRAIDWOOD in Edinburgh. As in the United States, deaf education in Scotland has gone through constant evolution, beginning with an emphasis on residential schools and now centering on MAINSTREAMING. Similarly, philosophies of communication have included the ORAL and MANUAL approaches and TOTAL COMMUNICATION.

Today, most deaf children attend regular schools, and about 25% go to special units or schools. The scattered deaf population in the country, together with its isolated location, has made services sometimes difficult to provide for this population.

Since the 1970s, pressure has grown to provide more schools closer to home, with a resulting growth in local clinics and programs for deaf people. But the quality and type of programs still varies considerably from town to town.

SEE 1   See SEEING ESSENTIAL ENGLISH.

SEE 2   See SIGNING EXACT ENGLISH.

S.E.E. Center for the Advancement of Deaf Children

The S.E.E. (SIGNING EXACT ENGLISH) Center is a nonprofit organization dedicated to improving the communication and English literacy skills of hard-of-hearing children and hearing language-delayed students.

Signing Exact English (SEE 2) is a manual communication system first published in 1972; the center was established in 1984 in response to requests for workshops, materials and information for implementing S.E.E. 2 in homes and schools across the country.

The center provides information, materials and referral services for new parents emphasizing the importance of early communication stimulation for preschool children utilizing the S.E.E. 2 approach. It also provides information for training and evaluating sign language instructors and educational interpreters in the use of S.E.E. 2.

Further, the group offers videotapes and helps educators, audiologists, psychologists and speech therapists implementing S.E.E. 2 as part of a total communication program and provides support for research assessing the impact of S.E.E. 2. Contact: The S.E.E. Center for the Advancement of Deaf Children, P.O. Box 1181, Los Alamitos, CA 90720; telephone: 562–430–1467.

Seeing Essential English (SEE 1)

One of at least five separate codes for English, SEE 1 takes much of its sign vocabulary from AMERICAN SIGN LANGUAGE.

SEE 1, published in 1971, was the first MANUAL CODE FOR ENGLISH system. David Anthony, the congenitally deaf son of deaf parents born in England, originally began SEE 1 as a graduate degree project in 1962 at GALLAUDET UNIVERSITY.

The system features the sound-spelling-meaning principle: That is, each criterion is used to determine a sign for a particular word. A single sign is used when two of these three are the same. Therefore, "I have a right to vote," "It's on the right" and "you're right" would be signed the same ("right" in this case sounds and is written the same way but has different meanings), but the word "write" would use a different sign since it sounds the same but has a different spelling and meaning.

Seeing Essential English has specific signs for morphemes, suffixes and prefixes.

Self Help for Hard of Hearing People, Inc. (SHHH)   A volunteer educational organization devoted to the interests of people who cannot hear. The group's activities include social activities, education, advocacy and consumer activism.

The group publishes *Shhh*, the only bimonthly journal in the United States written specifically for hard-of-hearing people and offering information on hearing loss, assistive technology, coping techniques and personal experiences for more than 200,000 readers.

The organization also offers referral and advisory services and operates an information and resource center. Contact: Self Help for Hard of Hearing People, Inc., 7910 Woodmont Ave. Ste. 1200, Bethesda, MD 20814; telephone: (voice) 301–657–2248, (TDD) 301–657–2249. website: http://www.shhh.org

semantics   The interpretation of the meaning of words, signs and sentences. (See also LANGUAGE.)

semicircular canals   Also called the LABYRINTH, this very important organ inside the inner ear is connected to the cochlea but does not contribute to the sense of hearing.

The semicircular canals are three small fluid-filled loops that help maintain balance by sending information about the position of the head through the vestibular branch of the AUDITORY NERVE to the brain. Infections or other problems in the middle or inner ear may directly or indirectly affect these canals, causing DIZZINESS or VERTIGO. Thus, some deaf children have difficulty with balance and may learn to walk later than a hearing child.

sensory aphasia   See AUDITORY AGNOSIA.

sensory cells   Located on the surface of the basilar membrane are sensory cells, which together with supporting cells form the ORGAN OF CORTI. Decades ago, it was shown that the production of sensory cells in the ears of mammals stops before birth and that these cells are produced only during embryonic development. This meant that damage to sensory cells later in life was irreparable; it became the basis for considering nerve deafness a permanent condition.

However, recent basic research with animals has shown that under certain conditions sensory cell production can be reactivated in mature damaged ears and that these regenerated cells contribute to recovery of hearing.

Scientists of the NATIONAL INSTITUTE OF HEARING AND OTHER COMMUNICATION DISORDERS believe it is reasonable to expect that within 10 to 20 years progenitors of regenerated sensory cells will be cloned from animals and will aid in the development of ways to recover hearing in humans.

Sicard, Abbé Roch Ambroise Cucurron (1742–1822)   This pioneer of education for deaf students led the Institut National des Jeunes Sourds established by ABBÉ CHARLES MICHEL DE L'EPÉE in 1760.

Born near Toulose on September 28, 1742, little is known of his early life; he was sent to Paris to be trained by l'Epée because of his educational gifts. After l'Epée's death, Sicard succeeded him and ran the school with an iron hand for 32 years.

Sicard's early success in educating his prize pupil JEAN MASSIEU assured him fame and the position of headmaster at the Paris institute.

Sicard's educational method was based on a combination of writing and a system of "methodical signs" developed by l'Epée. This system borrowed some signs from French sign language and invented some others to represent the grammatical structure of French, which represented the first effort at linking a sign and spoken language. Sicard also emphasized extensive grammar drills for his students. In fact, Sicard was widely recognized in France for his excellence as a grammarian, winning him faculty appointments, book contracts and a role as leader of a committee to revise the *Dictionary of the French Language*.

Often dictatorial and unyielding, Sicard's strength and popularity helped him lead his institution through the stormy years of the French Revolution, a time when many clerics were imprisoned as potentially monarchistic.

side-tone   Auditory signal that gives a speaker information about his own speech.

Siglish   Another name for PIDGIN SIGN ENGLISH, Siglish is a form of signing using the vocabulary of AMERICAN SIGN LANGUAGE in English word order along with some FINGERSPELLING and the use of ASL features such as directionality.

sign codes   At least four codes for English have been invented, although they all adapt much of their sign vocabulary from AMERICAN SIGN LANGUAGE. Each of these codes tries to duplicate the structure of English in different ways.

Unlike PIDGIN SIGN ENGLISH, these coded English systems use invented signs that correspond directly to English grammar and vocabulary. By matching a sign to a part of English, these systems become codes for English instead of a separate language.

These sign codes were developed in the United States as a way of providing a visual representation of English to improve school performance.

Codes include SEEING ESSENTIAL ENGLISH (SEE 1), SIGNING EXACT ENGLISH (SEE 2) and SIGNED ENGLISH.

Developed in the early 1970s, some of these code systems are still used in schools today, although they remain controversial among some deaf people. The invented codes have aroused hostility in the deaf population who believe their native sign languages have not been given dignity and who feel these sign codes create linguistic distortions.

The sign codes now in use are a result of the increasing acceptance of nonoral communication and the wish to teach deaf children the majority oral language by manual means. These codes have been developed as a system, very different from the native and pidgin sign languages that evolved naturally.

Sign codes were developed because it was assumed that oral language can be learned more easily this way rather than by using a native or pidgin sign language. They seem to be easier for parents to learn, since they involve only switching a mode of communication, not learning an entire new language. (See also MANUALLY CODED ENGLISH.)

Signed English   This is a manually coded English system used to represent spoken English. Developed in 1973 by Gallaudet University educators Harry Bornstein, Karen Saulnier, Lillian Hamilton and Ralph R. Miller Sr., it is considered to be the least complicated of the manual systems. Signed English includes manual gestures signed in the same word order as English, used with speech, to provide a clear language environment for a hard-of-hearing child. It is similar to SEE-1 and SEE-2.

Signed English features two kinds of gestures: sign markers and sign words. A person using Signed English can match each spoken English word with a sign word or with a sign word and a sign marker. Each of the 3,500 sign words matches the meaning of a separate word in English, with all its various meanings. Sign words do not represent any sounds or spelling. The 14 sign markers represent the most frequent grammatical changes (such as singular, plural, possessive). With a vocabulary limited to 3,500 sign words and 14 affixes, it is not possible to represent the whole English language. But by choosing the most-commonly used English words to transcribe into sign words and affixes, the system is complete enough for most general needs. The manual alphabet can be used to supplement vocabulary.

Learning Signed English is facilitated by an extensive series of texts and posters, which include its main reference text, *The Comprehensive Signed English Dictionary*, three other texts, 50 children's books and three posters. The problem with this system and also with SEE-1 and SEE-2 is that they are slow. Although they are easier for hearing people to learn than American Sign Language, they slower to use because, signs usually take twice as long as words to produce. This means that the average idea takes twice as long to express.

Research suggests that most parents and many teachers who are trying to use this system end up leaving out many of the grammatical markers and that many children who are exposed to them end up modifying them to more ASL-like forms. (See also MANUALLY CODED ENGLISH.

Sign English   See PIDGIN SIGN ENGLISH.

Signing Exact English (SEE 2)   This manual communication system is one of the most commonly used manually coded English systems in schools. It was developed in 1972 by Gerilee Gustason, a deaf teacher who lost her hearing at age five; Donna Pfetzing, mother of a deaf child; and Esther Zawolkow, daughter of deaf parents.

SEE 2 uses only one sign to represent an English word that may be expressed by several signs in AMERICAN SIGN LANGUAGE, depending on the meaning of the word in context. Hand signs for words, prefixes and endings are used to give a clear manual representation of English.

In much the same way as Seeing Essential English (See 1), Signing Exact English utilizes the sound-spelling-meaning principle. Although both systems define words either as basic, compound or complex, their definitions of these categories are very different. In Signing Exact English, basic words are words that can have no more taken away and still form a complete word, such as "run" or "trot." Compound words are two or more basic words put together, if the meaning of the words separately is consistent with the meaning of the words together.

Complex words are basic words with an added ending, such as dogs and running. Signing Exact English has signs for about 70 different endings.

According to a 1978–79 survey, the SEE 2 system is the most widely used sign method used in schools and classes for hard-of-hearing students in the United States. Programs have used this system to support spoken English emphasized in a TOTAL COMMUNICATION approach.

Sign Instructors Guidance Network (SIGN)   The original name for the AMERICAN SIGN LANGUAGE TEACHERS ASSOCIATION.

sign language   Sign languages are widely used by deaf people all over the world. Although each country has its own national sign language with its own visual-gestural signs, the sign language does not conform to the grammatical rules and structure of the native language. Within each country there are also different sign language dialects that reflect racial, ethnic or geographical differences. These dialects differ mostly in idiomatic expressions rather than grammar or syntax.

sign language continuum   The range in manual communication, from the completely English representation used in schools to the non-English pattern with its own grammar and syntax used by the deaf community.

sign language interpreter   A person skilled in the ability to translate the meaning of spoken words into sign language as the words are spoken and to translate sign language into English as signs are formed.

Technically, sign language interpretation is only used when describing the communication process between a hearing person and a person using a true sign language, such as AMERICAN SIGN LANGUAGE. A person interpreting to or from a manually coded form of a spoken language (such as SIGNED ENGLISH) is actually "transliterating," not "interpreting."

Sign language interpreters today are trained to practice their skill in a variety of settings: the legal, educational, medical, diplomatic and business areas. They are also trained to translate from either signed to spoken language or from spoken language to sign (also called sign-to-voice or voice-to-sign). Most importantly, they try to accomplish their communication task without becoming personally involved in the activity and without adding or subtracting any information in either direction.

In addition to standard sign language interpreters, specialized interpreters may at times be necessary. A person who is deaf and blind, for example, may need a specially-trained deaf-blind interpreter. This person can spell words in the deaf person's hand rather than perform traditional sign language. Oral interpreters silently mouth the speaker's words for the deaf person without signing and are skilled in substituting words for words that are difficult to speech-read.

In addition, special settings may require special knowledge or responsibilities on the part of the sign language interpreter. One of the most common places to find an interpreter is in school—from elementary to university. An interpreter is most often needed when the deaf student is mainstreamed and must communicate with many hearing students and teachers.

Interpreters in a medical setting will encounter technical terms and may find medical personnel unfamiliar with the role of an interpreter. Mental health interpreting requires sensitivity in other ways since the importance of accurately communicating in both directions can be of critical importance to treatment success. Legal interpreting also involves extensive technical language in very formal settings.

Due to a range of new legislation and educational opportunities affecting deaf people in the mid-1960s, the demand for qualified sign language interpreters suddenly exceeded the limited supply. At about this time, California State University/Northridge, the NATIONAL TECHNICAL INSTITUTE FOR THE DEAF and three regional technical vocational programs opened their doors to deaf students. In response to a much greater need, these schools also set up programs to train interpreters. At the same time, the NATIONAL REGISTRY OF INTERPRETERS FOR THE DEAF was established.

Up to that time, it was assumed that if a person could sign, he could interpret; no research had been done into exactly how interpreting was done or the best way to train an interpreter. Because of this, the first interpreter classes focused simply on teaching American Sign Language, which ended up producing a people who could converse primarily in PIDGIN SIGN ENGLISH. But in 1973, a federal grant established the Interpreter Training Consortium composed of six colleges charged with developing a curriculum for sign language interpreters.

Eventually, experts realized sign language interpreters must be both bilingual and bicultural; therefore, interpreting training courses must include comparative English/ASL linguistic and cultural analyses; text analysis; consecutive and simultaneous interpreting skills; and an overview of the profession (ethics and business practices). From a six-week course, the education of an interpreter has gradually developed into a formal four-year bachelor degree program of study, which may well progress to a graduate-level program.

All types of interpreters are listed with local and state chapters of the Registry of Interpreters for the Deaf, the only national organization that certifies both oral and sign language interpreters. (See also COURT INTERPRETER'S ACT; ORAL INTERPRETERS.)

sign-to-voice interpreting   Previously called reverse interpreting, sign-to-voice interpretation is now the preferred term for translating from a signed language to speech. Reverse interpreting is no longer used because it is now recognized that one direction of interpretation is not more important than another. (See also COURT INTERPRETER'S ACT; ORAL INTERPRETERS; REGISTRY OF INTERPRETERS FOR THE DEAF; SIGN LANGUAGE INTERPRETERS.)

sign writing   A method of writing down the symbols used in SIGN LANGUAGE. Many ways of sign language writing have been invented by many different researchers for many different reasons.

One of the main problems with sign writing is that the words do not convey the whole message of the sign language sentence. As a way to improve this problem, sign writers write various marks above and below the written word to stand for facial action or body position. But the fact that there is no standard system for these additional descriptors makes sign writing sometimes difficult for everyone to understand.

sim-com   See SIMULTANEOUS COMMUNICATION.

simultaneous communication   This communication mode combines the use of speech, signs and FINGERSPELLING and is said to offer the benefit of seeing two forms of a message at the same time. The deaf person speechreads what is being spoken and simultaneously reads the signs and finger-spelling of the speaker. In this country, users of simultaneous communication (or sim-com) at times put AMERICAN SIGN LANGUAGE signs in English word order while speaking.

Simultaneous communication is often confused with TOTAL COMMUNICATION since many people use the latter term when they mean speaking and signing at the same time. In the strictest sense, total communication actually refers to a philosophical attitude toward education using all forms of communication; simultaneous communication is one of those forms.

The communication method appeared in early 20th-century American following the oral approach as encouraged by ALEXANDER GRAHAM BELL. As educators began to argue over the importance of oral education, more and more classrooms switched from all-manual communication to a combined method using speech, signs and fingerspelling. The combined method meant that part of a student's day might be taught in sign and part in speech and SPEECHREADING. Students might also be divided according to percent of hearing loss; some might be taught orally, others manually.

Eventually, the conviction of the importance of speaking and speechreading grew to the point where most teachers decided they should speak all the time, and by 1950 most elementary school programs were completely oral. Some teachers still believed in the importance of sign, however, and therefore these instructors paired speech with signing.

But by the late 1960s, educators were disappointed with the poor results of oral-only programs and encouraged by the superior performance of offspring of deaf parents who used sign language from birth. Thus the use of simultaneous communication began an upsurge. By the late 1970s, hundreds of programs for deaf students had abandoned the oral-only approach and started to use sim-com, calling it total communication.

Today, sim-com is the most frequently-used method of communication in deaf schools across the country. It is also the standard method of communication at Gallaudet University.

Sim-com is also frequently used by a deaf and a hearing person in communication, particularly if the hearing person is not fluent in sign, or in a group of people that includes a person who cannot sign. Deaf people, however, almost never use sim-com among themselves; for many, speech had been forced on them for many years and represents a denial of their own language and culture.

Generally, it is not possible to speak English and sign in American Sign Language, since the word order and structure of ASL is fundamentally different from English. Instead, educators and proponents of sim-com have adapted ASL in order to speak English and sign at the same time. The adaptations include using a form of signing called PIDGIN SIGN ENGLISH, a manual code for English, or an older form of signing modeled after English.

Pidgin Sign English uses signs while relying on English to provide a simplified grammatical structure. The manual codes for English include a range of systems developed in the early 1970s that also use signs and English grammatical structure, together with new signs created to represent English articles, pronouns, and affixes (such as -ing, -ed, -s).

These codes include SIGNED ENGLISH, SEEING ESSENTIAL ENGLISH (SEE 1), SIGNING EXACT ENGLISH (SEE 2). Finally, older signers sometimes use modeling English in which the meaning of ASL signs are not changed and English articles or affixes are simply dropped. However, these adaptations are not strictly separated and are often used in combination, because the differences are not well understood by people not fluent in sign.

Simultaneous communication has been controversial because it satisfies neither the proponents of the oral or manual approach. Oralists, who would like to eliminate all signs, believe sim-com doesn't teach good speech skills; those who favor the manual approach counter that the English-linked manual codes usually used in sim-com are pidgin languages.

There are problems with sim-com as well. It is very difficult to speak and sign at the same time and requires such a great deal of concentration that it can inhibit communication. Further, hearing people often do not sign everything they say, which makes it hard for deaf people to follow what they are trying to communicate.

Studies of simultaneous communication have revealed that a person's oral English often deteriorates when speaking and signing; at the same time, the meaning of signs often does not match the meaning of the English words. Further, when speaking and signing together, communication tends to bog down and go much slower than when signing or speaking alone.

Studies of whether simultaneous communication actually helps deaf students learn English have reached conflicting conclusions; it is apparent that these students improve in using a manual code for English but not necessarily in English skills. Studies also do not agree on whether or not deaf students understand and learn better from teachers who use simultaneous communication.

simultaneous interpreting   This form of communicating requires the interpreter to mouth and sign everything that the speaker is saying, as opposed to manual interpreting, in which not everything is mouthed. (See also SIGN LANGUAGE INTERPRETERS.)

Smith, Erastus (1787–1837)   This Texas folk hero was the chief scout and spy for General Sam Houston, commander in chief of the Texas army.

Erastus "Deaf" Smith was born to a large family near Poughkeepsie, New York. A sickly, solitary child, Smith lost his hearing during early infancy and received little education thereafter.

Nineteen years later he visited what is now Texas, moving there permanently in 1821, where he was known as "el Sordo" (the Deaf One). After marrying a Spanish woman, he was granted Mexican citizenship and became fluent in Spanish despite his severe hearing problem. The two lived in San Antonio, which at the time was part of Mexico.

A loyal Mexican citizen, he never suspected Texas would one day petition to join the United States. But with the beginning of the Texas Revolution in 1835, Smith's neutrality was soon over; upon returning to his home in San Antonio one day, he found the town occupied by Mexicans and under siege by Texans. When the Mexicans fired on him and refused to let him return to his home, Smith joined General Stephen F. Austin and the Texas forces.

Because he was so familiar with the area, Smith was invaluable to the Texan army, becoming scout to Sam Houston en route to the Alamo. It was Smith who brought back the only two survivors of the massacre there, Mrs. Almeron Dickerson and her baby daughter. It was also Smith's advice to Houston that assured the Texan's victory at San Jacinto, where Santa Anna was captured and Texas gained its independence from Mexico.

Smith died from a lung problem in Richmond on November 30, 1837. Deaf Smith County in Texas is named in his honor.

social adequacy index (SAI)   A measure of the degree to which a patient has problems in hearing and understanding speech. The SAI is computed from the results of speech reception thresholds and speech discrimination tests.

Social Security and hearing loss   The Social Security Administration has two benefit programs for people with a hearing loss who meet their state's requirements for "disability": Supplemental Security Income (SSI) and Social Security Disability Insurance (SSDI). Both benefits are awarded to children or adults who meet the criteria for being disabled and—in the case of SSI—for financial need. To be eligible for SSDI, a working adult must have paid Social Security at least five of the last 10 years.

Society of Hearing-Impaired Physicians (SHIP)   This organization assists physicians, other health professionals, medical students and prospective medical students whose hearing impairment may necessitate different tools and/or approaches to medical practice and training.

sound conduction Sound waves move outward in all directions by back and forth movements of molecules through solids, liquids or gases.

Each complete back-and-forth movement (oscillation) is called a cycle, and the number of cycles generated by a sound source every second is known as the frequency. The term "hertz" (abbreviated Hz) represents cycles per second and is named after HEINRICH HERTZ, a famous scientist who studied sound.

Human ears can detect sounds within a frequency range of 20 Hz to 20,000 Hz; the range of speech lies mostly between 100 and 8,000 Hz. The higher the frequency, the higher the pitch or tone; almost all of the sounds we hear are combinations of many frequencies. Sounds used in hearing tests that are only one frequency are called pure tones.

A sound wave's pressure on the surface it contacts is a measure of the sound's intensity, or power. The greater the intensity of the sound waves on a person's eardrum, the louder the sound that is heard. A sound that is just barely able to be heard is the threshold intensity.

In order to test hearing, it is important to be able to measure the intensity of sounds heard; therefore, an internationally-accepted sound pressure level has been set to correspond approximately to that of a threshold intensity for a sound with a frequency of 1,000 Hz. Other sound pressures are compared to this reference pressure on a scale measured in decibels (dB), a name taken from the inventor of the telephone, ALEXANDER GRAHAM BELL. Sound intensities on this scale increase tenfold for every 20-dB difference in sound pressure.

There are two ways for sound to be conducted through our ears—air and bone conduction. Air conduction occurs when sound moves from the external ear (pinna) to the middle and inner ears. Bone conduction occurs when sound vibrations are transmitted through the skull bones directly to the cochlea.

A blockage in the external or middle ears means an overall reduction in all sound intensities but not a total hearing loss, since sound is also routed through bone.

sound spectrograph A device that records the continually changing intensity levels of frequency components in a complex sound wave via a filter analyzer.

sound wave A pressure area produced by vibration moving through air or water, causing reactions in the ear that the brain interprets as sound. (See also SOUND CONDUCTION.)

Spain This country, which has a deaf population of 20,000, has a deeply-rooted tradition of educating deaf students.

More than 400 years ago, a Spanish monk named PEDRO PONCE DE LEÓN first taught deaf people to speak. Today there is a range of special elementary and secondary schools specializing in deaf education that use a wide variety of approaches. Although some schools favor MAINSTREAMING, this method is opposed by schools who favor the oral approach.

Most deaf children begin school at age four and continue to 18; there are vocational courses open to them but no special university for deaf students. If a deaf student wishes to earn a degree at a regular university, he or she must do so without the use of an interpreter. For this reason, there are not many deaf graduates of Spanish universities.

Deaf Spaniards have a strong community, and communicate in SPANISH SIGN LANGUAGE, although dialects vary from province to province. There are special telephone devices available, but few deaf Spaniards have them in their homes. Television captioning has not yet become available.

Spanish Sign Language   The origins of Spanish Sign Language are unknown, but today sign language is used by virtually all Spaniards. It has few dialects, although its grammar is complex and poorly understood by modern linguists.

There seems to be no well-defined subject-verb-object word order in SSL. Verbs are made using one gesture, adding prefixes or suffixes as needed. FINGERSPELLING is rarely used and then only for proper names for when there is no gestural sign.

At present, the teaching of sign language in Spanish schools is under debate; some schools allow SSL and others do not. (See also SPAIN.)

speech frequencies   In audiometric testing, these are the pure-tone frequencies that can best predict the level at which speech can be understood (500, 1,000 and 2,000 Hz).

speech-language pathologist   A specialist in human communication, its development and its disorders. Also known as a speech pathologist or speech therapist, the speech-language pathologist evaluates and treats persons with communication problems resulting from total or partial hearing loss, brain injury, cleft palate, voice pathology, emotional problems, foreign dialect, development delays, stroke, learning disabilities and so forth. They also provide clinical therapy to help those with speech and language disorders, and help them and their families understand the disorder and develop better communication skills.

In most settings, speech-language pathologists perform screening tests of auditory acuity and tympanometry (a measure of middle ear function). Only a speech-language pathologist is certified to make recommendations for the type of speech language treatment required. Treatment could include a specific program of exercises to improve language ability or speech together with support from the client's family and friends.

To practice speech-language pathology, states require a master's degree in speech-language pathology, more than 300 hours of supervised clinical experience and successful completion of a certifying exam.

speechreading   The preferred term for lip-reading, a way of recognizing spoken words by watching the speaker's lips, jaw and tongue movements. Speechreading is the least consistently visible of the communication choices available to deaf people; only about 30% of English sounds are visible on the lips, and half are homophonous (that is, they look like other words). For example, the words "kite," "height" and "night" look almost identical.

The ability to speechread is often contingent on the visibility, shape and configuration of the speaker's mouth. For example, it may be difficult to speechread someone who mumbles, who has a beard or who has no teeth.

Some deaf people become skilled speech-readers, especially if they can supplement what they see with some hearing. Many don't develop much skill at speechreading, but most do speechread to some extent. Because speechreading requires considerable guesswork, very few deaf people rely on speechreading alone when exchanging important information.

One system that has been designed to be used with speechreading is CUED SPEECH, developed by Dr. Orin Cornett of Gallaudet University. Cued speech is a method in which hand movements and location are used to make all of the sounds produced on the lips clear to the speechreader. (See also VISEME.)

speech therapist   See SPEECH-LANGUAGE PATHOLOGIST.

speech training   Teaching speech to profoundly deaf individuals has been the center of a number of controversies in deaf education for hundreds of years. Today, controversy centers on how well deaf people can be taught to speak and the best methods to achieve that goal. Some still question the need to teach speech to deaf students at all.

The wide range of teaching methods vary according to the size of the speech unit taught and the number of senses the student uses in order to learn speech. Those methods that emphasize small units of speech (syllables and speech sounds) are called analytic; methods that teach units of speech no smaller than syllables and stress the importance of connected speech fall into the synthetic category.

speech training aids   Devices that display speech electronically to teach those who cannot hear how to use their voice. One of the newest is the

Matsushita speech system being evaluated jointly at the Lexington School for the Deaf in New York and the City University of New York. With this speech system, which was developed in Japan, a speech therapist and client wear special sensors inside the mouth and on the nose that are linked to a computer. When the therapist pronounces a sound or a word, the computer generates an image on a video screen that illustrates the position of the tongue within the mouth, the vibration of the nose and the intensity of the voice. The student learns to pronounce the sound or word by trying to produce the same pattern on the screen.

According to Esther Lustig of the Lexington School, the device is still in the early stages of research but shows "great promise." Originally used in Japan, the school is testing it for use with American English-speaking students and are helping develop English language software for deaf individuals in the United States.

"It's a long-range project because you have to make sure the improvement you see is a result of the machine and not other factors," Lustig explained. "You need a sampling over a period of time." The school has been testing the system since February 1989. Although Lustig emphasized that the system is still in the experimental stages, she reports anecdotal improvement among students who use it.

Other devices have been developed including a computer-based system for children with displays that resemble video games and a laryngograph, which monitors the action of the larynx from two plates held against the throat, displaying voice pitch coordination with other movements and voice quality.

stapedectomy   The removal of the STAPES and its replacement with a prosthesis. The purpose of this operation is to treat hearing loss caused by OTOSCLEROSIS, a familial form of deafness that is curable only by surgery. Otosclerosis causes the base of the stapes (stirrup), the innermost of the three bones in the middle ear, to become fixed to the opening of the inner ear by an overgrowth of spongy bone. This interferes with the stapes' ability to transmit sound to the inner ear.

While the patient is under a local or general anesthetic, a surgeon using laser and microscopic techniques opens the ear canal and folds the eardrum forward. All (or most) of the stapes is removed, and a plastic or metal prosthesis is inserted into the entrance to the inner ear; the other end is attached to the incus. The eardrum is then repaired.

Sound now travels from the eardrum to the two normal ear bones, then through the prosthesis and a vein graft to the hearing nerve.

Antibiotics are usually used up to five days after surgery to prevent infection; packing and sutures are removed about a week after surgery. Hearing shows improvement within two weeks and continues to get better over the next three months.

Good candidates for a stapedectomy are patients who have fixed stapes from otosclerosis and a CONDUCTIVE HEARING LOSS of at least 20 dB with a speech discrimination score of at least 60%. Patients with a severe hearing loss might still profit from a stapedectomy, if only to bring their hearing up to a level where a hearing aid could be of help.

The operation improves hearing in more than 90% of cases, although about 1% of patients experience loss of hearing from damage to the COCHLEA. Because of this risk, a stapedectomy is normally done on one ear at a time, although otosclerosis usually affects both ears. It is almost never used on a patient with hearing in only one ear.

Other less common complications from the surgery include change in taste from damage to the chorda tympani nerve, perforated eardrum, vertigo and damage to the ossicular chain. Temporary Bell's palsy (facial nerve paralysis) can occur immediately after the operation. Occasionally, vertigo persists and may require surgery. (See also FENESTRATION; STAPES MOBILIZATION.)

stapes   Commonly called the stirrup, this is the smallest bone in the body and is one of the three tiny bones that make up the OSSICLES in the middle ear. The head of the stapes joins the middle ossicle (anvil). Its base fits into the oval window located in the wall of the inner ear and, as it vibrates, plunges in and out of the oval window.

The condition of OTOSCLEROSIS immobilizes the stapes in the entrance to the inner ear by an overgrowth of spongy bone, interfering with the ability of the stapes to move freely and transmit sound to the inner ear, thereby causing deafness. The condition can be helped by a hearing aid but is cured only by surgery (STAPEDECTOMY). Although the operation improves hearing in about 90% of patients, about 1% of patients actually experience a deterioration of hearing. This is why—although otosclerosis normally affects both ears—a stapedectomy is usually only done on one ear at a time.

stapes mobilization   This operation for OTOSCLEROSIS was accidentally discovered during FENESTRATION (an operation creating a new oval window) when the stapes had been accidentally moved too much, loosening the otosclerosis and mobilizing the STAPES. After the operation, the patient had much better hearing than is normal after a simple fenestration.

But although this new type of operation seemed exciting at first, it was discovered that the otosclerosis continued to be active and would again fix the stapes to the OVAL WINDOW, losing all benefits of the mobilization. And for many patients, the otosclerosis had progressed too far and scarred or fixed their stapes too much to be helped with mobilization.

Mobilization today is used primarily for people who were born with problems of the stapes or oval window. In other patients, a STAPEDECTOMY is preferred to treat otosclerosis.

stenosis   A narrowing of the external ear canal as a result of various disease processes, including chronic OTITIS MEDIA (ear infection), inflammation, alergic reaction, injury or PERICHONDRITIS (an infection primarily of the cartilage covering the pinna).

stirrup   See STAPES.

substance abuse   The incidence of drug and alcohol abuse among deaf people is similar to the incidence among hearing people. However, deaf abusers historically have faced discrimination in treatment programs and services, with few professionals trained in chemical dependency and deafness, according to the National Information Center on Deafness.

There have been few studies of substance abuse in the deaf community, although it is generally believed that the problem is about the same as substance abuse in the hearing population: 1 in 10.

Deaf substance abusers generally have few ties with churches, organizations and clubs of the deaf community and live on the fringes of both the deaf and hearing societies. Substance abusers who are deaf high school students follow similar patterns.

Although treatment programs for substance abusers in the United States have proliferated since the 1930s, deaf people have found major barriers to existing treatment facilities. One of the biggest obstacles to treatment may be found in the deaf community itself, which has been reluctant in the past to admit that its members have a problem. Few referrals to substance abuse agencies come from the deaf community.

Further, deaf substance abusers find it difficult to admit to themselves that there is a problem, and self-referrals to treatment are lower in this population than in the general population.

A deaf person seeking treatment for a substance abuse problem, however, faces other hurdles: Most programs have been designed for hearing clients, and counselors lack an understanding of deafness, the deaf community and manual methods of communication. Agencies often can't afford to hire interpreters, and deafness experts aren't trained in substance abuse rehabilitation.

In 1973 the first treatment center for deaf alcoholics was established in St. Paul, Minneapolis, followed a year later by another in San Francisco.

In 1975, the first national conference on substance abuse in the deaf community was held in Cleveland, Ohio. During this time, inpatient treatment for deaf alcoholics, counseling programs and outreach projects were begun. In 1979 the quarterly *AID Bulletin* began to provide updated information to a national membership.

By 1985, alcohol treatment programs had begun in California, Illinois, New York, Ohio, Maryland, Minnesota and Massachusetts. These programs combine an outreach advocacy program run by specialists in substance abuse and deafness.

From the early 1970s on, programs for deaf alcoholics have featured outreach projects directed by substance abuse experts who understand the communication problems of deaf clients. When such treatment is therefore modified, deaf and hearing alcoholics recover at the same rate.

Sweden   There are an estimated 208,000 deaf and hard-of-hearing people in Sweden. There are approximately 200 hard-of-hearing babies born each year and of these, about 50 are profoundly deaf. About 87 per 100,000 Swedes are deaf, according to 1930 statistics, one of the higher prevalence rates among developed countries (which range from 300 per 100,000 to 35 per 100,000).

The first school for deaf children in Sweden was opened in Stockholm in 1809, influenced by other European schools and relying on the oral approaches. But unlike many other schools in Europe, Sweden retained an interest in manual education and taught either method to children depending on individual preferences.

Today, deaf Swedes can attend either large state schools for deaf children or local community schools, where many children are mainstreamed.

More than 90% of Swedish children go on to a "gymnasium" (higher education) after completing the required nine years of school; although there are no special classes for hard-of-hearing students in these gymnasiums, there is a special gymnasium for deaf students in Orebro, where they may take vocational courses or pre-university studies.

Swedish Sign Language   The language of more than 8,000 Swedish deaf citizens, Swedish Sign Language is unrelated to any other sign language in the world and is not derived from any other sign system.

Still, it shares many characteristics of other sign languages, including a complex structure; signs are made with the hands, while facial expression, body movement and posture are used to indicate clause and sentence type. In addition, lip movements are always used with FINGERSPELLING and may also be used with signs. Sweden's manual alphabet was invented in the early 1800s by Swedish educator Per Aron Borg, who later took this alphabet to Portugal where he established schools for deaf students.

Swiss Sign Language   Traditionally a country that favored the oral approach, sign language in SWITZERLAND today is slowly making a comeback in the deaf community.

In a country divided into three cultural sections (German, French and Italian), Swiss Sign Language varies widely from strictly sign language to mixtures of sign and spoken language.

Neither the German nor French areas of Switzerland have a manual alphabet. Because of this, the set of handshapes that make up the sign language is more restricted, and there is a tendency to mouth the equivalent word in the spoken language for those ideas that have no sign.

Research suggests that the various dialects of Swiss Sign Language have many similar characteristics in common with other sign languages, including the use of facial expressions, eye gaze and body posture.

In general, sign language is not widely used in the classroom, although both sign language and the pidgin forms of signing are used in the deaf community. There are still an insufficient number of sign language instructors and courses.

Switzerland   Life in Switzerland for deaf citizens is a complicated affair since the decentralized country recognizes four languages (German, French, Italian and Romansh) with a bewildering number of dialects, particularly in German and Romansh. Prevalence of deafness is rather high (94 out of 100,000) when compared to other countries, but almost equal to the rate in the United States (100 out of 100,000).

Although education varies among the 23 different cantons (states), in general hard-of-hearing students who use amplification attend regular schools, and deaf students are taught to speechread and speak. Schools are open to deaf students between ages 6 and 16.

The manual approach is not widespread in Switzerland, but deaf students sign outside of class. Although there are differences among local sign languages, most deaf people can make each other understood across dialects.

sympathetic vibration   A vibration in one object produced by vibrations of the same frequency in another object.

syntax   The study of the rules of sentence formation. (See also LINGUISTICS.)

T

Telecommunications for the Deaf, Inc. A consumer-oriented organization that sells caption decoders and a directory for deaf people. The group supports legislation and advocates the use of TELECOMMUNICATIONS DEVICES FOR THE DEAF, ASCII code, Emergency Access (911), telecaptioning and visual ALERTING DEVICES in the public, private and government sectors. Contact: Telecommunications for the Deaf, Inc., 8630 Fenton St., Ste. 604, Silver Spring MD 20910; telephone: (voice) 301–589–3786, (TDD) 301–589–3006. email: tdiexdir@ad.com

Telecommunications for the Disabled Act of 1982 See LEGAL RIGHTS.

Tele-Consumer Hotline Nonprofit, independent and impartial telephone consumer information service that provides free telephone assistance and publications on special telephone equipment, TDD directories, TDD/voice relay services, choosing a long distance company, selecting a phone, money saving tips and more. Contact: Tele-Consumer Hotline, 901 15th St. NW, Ste. 230, Washington DC 20005; telephone: 800–332–1124 (outside D.C.) or (voice and TDD) 202–223–4371.

temporomandibular joint syndrome (TMJ) Severe pain in the jaw, face and head, especially around the ears, that researchers believe is caused by the improper function of the jaw (temporomandibular) joints and their muscles and ligaments.

Other symptoms of TMJ include jaw and ear clicking or popping, "locking" jaws and pain in opening the mouth, and hearing loss.

Clenching and grinding the teeth, which cause the muscles to go into spasm, is the most common cause of TMJ. An incorrect bite, excessive tension, head injury or, rarely, osteoarthritis can also lead to TMJ.

Treatment involves the application of moist heat to relieve the muscle spasm and the use of muscle relaxant medication and pain relievers. In severe cases, joint surgery may be required.

tinnitus masker Masking is the technique of producing external "white noise" sounds that will mask the TINNITUS (ringing in the ears) and make it less distracting. Masking machines come in both in-the-ear and portable models that produce sounds ranging from random white noise to waterfalls to surf. Hearing aids can also function as maskers by amplifying external sounds. It takes time to find the correct method of treatment and to properly fit and adjust hearing or tinnitus instruments; the first fitting is seldom the final one. At best, masking only provides relief, not a cure.

Otherwise, many people find it helpful to use an electric fan to mask tinnitus, to tune a regular FM radio to an empty frequency to listen to the static. Others who suffer from tinnitus use an audio CD of nature sounds (ocean, jungle, whales, or rain) in autorepeat mode before going to bed.

In one recent masking study, 16% of patients reported relief using a hearing aid alone, 21% reported relief from a tinnitus masker alone and 63% reported relief from a combination hearing aid and tinnitus masker. In the latter case, it was important to adjust the hearing aid properly before attempting masking.

It is important for tinnitus patients to visit a tinnitus clinic to test ears for a specific tinnitus sound so that the right "white noise" can be matched up to it.

Simple Maskers   Simple tinnitus maskers generally provide a high frequency band of noise designed to mask the frequency of the tinnitus.

Hearing Aids   Although 90% of people with tinnitus also have a hearing problem, only a small percentage have ever used a hearing aid. If the pitch of the tinnitus is low, hearing aids usually help by raising the level of background noise and thereby masking the tinnitus. However, in cases of high-pitched tinnitus, even the highest-frequency hearing aids don't work very well as a masker since environmental noise is not high enough to mask the sound (environmental noise does not usually rise above 4,000 Hz).

Tinnitus Instrument   This is a combination hearing aid and simple masker, used in cases of high-frequency tinnitus and high-frequency hearing loss. It is useful because a simple masker does not work in cases of high-frequency hearing loss since the person cannot hear the frequencies required to mask the tinnitus. There are behind-the-ear and in-the-ear models, and they have independent volume controls.

TMJ   See TEMPOROMANDIBULAR JOINT SYNDROME.

total communication   This philosophy implies an acceptance, exposure and opportunity to use all possible methods of communication to help the deaf child learn to communicate. It is often confused with the SIMULTANE-OUS COMMUNICATION (Sim-Com) method, which combines both speech and sign at the same time.

Total communication provides exposure and opportunity to learn all modes of communication and allows the child to use whichever mode is easiest and with which he is best understood.

Rather than focus on one specific training method, parents and teachers who use a total communication approach try to decide which mode is best for a child in any one situation. Options can include SPEECHREADING, speech, SIGN LANGUAGE, auditory training and amplification, writing, audio-visual methods, FINGERSPELLING and graphics.

Total communication was first described by a California teacher and parent of a deaf child, who combined signing and fingerspelling with speech and speechreading. In 1968, the idea was picked up and introduced by the supervisor of a program for deaf students in Santa Ana and then adopted at the Maryland School for the Deaf in the same year.

Within 10 years, two-thirds of schools for deaf students in the United States had begun to use a total communication approach to education. At the same time, the approach was gaining acceptance around the world, and by the 1980s it was widely used to describe a philosophical attitude toward education for deaf students.

Historically, the proponents of particular systems have often disagreed with each other. Total communication has provided a compromise, adding to the increasing consensus that whatever system works best for the individual should be used to allow the hard-of-hearing or deaf person access to clear and understandable communication.

Still, schools that embrace total communication usually feature simultaneous communication, which combines the manual and oral approaches at the same time. This combination remains controversial since some oral approach proponents claim Sim-Com doesn't produce good speech and manual approach supporters complain about the manual English systems used with Sim-Com. (See also MANUALLY CODED ENGLISH.)

transliteration   Technically, there are two separate terms for sign language interpretation. Transliteration refers to the interpretation process between a hearing person and a person using a manual code of a spoken language (such as SIGNED ENGLISH). Sign language interpretation refers only to the process of interpreting between speech and a true deaf sign language (such as AMERICAN SIGN LANGUAGE). (See also SIGN LANGUAGE INTERPRETERS.)

TRIPOD   This organization provides a national toll-free hotline for parents and individuals wanting information about raising and educating deaf children. TRIPOD operates a parent/infant/toddler program, a Montessori preschool and an elementary mainstream program for hard-of-hearing students. Contact: TRIPOD, 1727 West Burbank Blvd., Burbank, CA 91506; telephone: (nationwide) 800–352–1124.

tuning forks   An instrument developed in the 19th century and used today by a specialist to determine the presence of a hearing loss. Because it emits a remarkably pure tone as it vibrates, the tuning fork has been a basic tool for people trying to learn how the mind interprets sound. The standard frequencies of tuning forks include 128, 512, 1024 and 2048 Hertz. Four tuning fork tests used most often today are the WEBER, RINNE and SCHWABACH.

While the tuning fork has been replaced by electronic sound makers in some tests, forks are still used to support results of more formal audiological testing. Still, the usefulness of tuning forks is limited for a number of reasons: There is no way to accurately measure the intensity of tone; sound is distorted if the fork is struck too hard; there are problems in isolating response of the ear; and they are hard to use with young children.

tympanoplasty   Surgery performed to repair the EARDRUM and/or OSSICLES (tiny bones in the middle ear). It is usually performed to treat conductive hearing loss, provided that the COCHLEA and AUDITORY NERVE can benefit from the improved conductive function.

Normally, sound waves move from the eardrum to the inner ear by the three bones called the ossicles (hammer, stirrup and anvil). Chronic otitis media can erode or fuse these bones, causing some degree of conductive hearing loss. Tympanoplasty is the only way to restore some of the lost hearing.

One form of tympanoplasty (also called MYRINGOPLASTY) involves the repair of a perforated eardrum in order to prevent recurring infections and improve hearing. The hole is closed with a graft (usually taken from the patient's own body)—which is usually a piece of connective tissue from the surface of the temporalis muscle adjacent to the ear or the outer, thin covering of the cartilage from the tragus.

OSSICULOPLASTY is the surgical repair of a defect in the transmission of sound by the middle ear ossicles, usually as a result of chronic ear infection (otitis media), cholesteatoma or temporal bone fracture. Under general anesthesia, an incision is made next to the eardrum. Using a microscope, the surgeon repairs the ossicles by reshaping the bones or replacing them with either a plastic, cartilage or donor ossicle. The bones are reset, and the eardrum is repaired.

Although the operation often improves hearing, there is no guarantee of success, which depends on the complexity of the problem. If the malleus or stapes is missing, for example, the solution is less predictable.

U

unisensory-auditory method   See AUDITORY-ORAL METHOD.

United Kingdom   The prevalence rate for profound prelingual deafness in the United Kingdom is estimated to be between .8 and 1.5 per 1,000 live births. About 62,000 people over age 16 have very severe hearing problems, and about 2.3 million have some degree of hearing difficulties. Approximately 30,000 people use BRITISH SIGN LANGUAGE as their main method of communication.

Early diagnosis (before age one) is emphasized in the United Kingdom; screening and subsequent diagnostic tests are free, as are HEARING AIDS, EARMOLDS, maintenance and batteries. Although only certain types of hearing aids are given to adults, children may be provided with any type of aid available. Once a child has been diagnosed, the family is placed in a home-based parent guidance program.

Education   The Royal Commission of 1889 recommended that every child who is deaf should be educated with the oral approach; consequently, schools throughout the United Kingdom adopted this method. It was not until 1968 that, concerned about the results of the oral approach, the government decided that, while oralism was still desirable, research into the manual approach should be conducted.

In 1982, the British Association of Teachers of the Deaf issued a proclamation promoting the oral approach but recognized that some children might benefit from additional help in other types of communication.

There are both residential and day schools available in the United Kingdom, and since 1979 the trend has been leading away from residential schools and toward placing children in regular schools with special help.

Many special schools for deaf children arrange for their students to attend technical colleges or other types of further education, and some schools offer advanced education specifically for people who are hard-of-hearing. The National Study Group on Further and Higher Education for the Hearing impaired in the United Kingdom publishes directories of available further education courses.

A few deaf students also go on to university or polytechnic schools, and specific facilities for deaf students are available at Sussex University and at the Colleges of St. Hilda and St. Bede of the University of Durham.

Continuing education for adult deaf people is also available through the Centre for the Deaf at the City Literary Institute in London.

Communication Services   Telephone communications are available for deaf people in the United Kingdom through a portable keyboard telephone

276

known as Vistel, replacing earlier teletypewriters. Vistel has an acoustic coupler to which any normal telephone handset may be attached. The message is typed on a conventional typewriter keyboard, displayed on a traveling display on the top of the equipment and sent over the phone lines to the receiver, who can read the same message on his or her own display.

In addition, deaf people in the United Kingdom can have access to Prestel, an interactive terminal with a large database of commercial and public service information. It provides thousands of pages of information with a TV, a Prestel decoder and a telephone.

Also available to deaf TV viewers is "teletext," a method of coding information in digital form in the unused lines of a TV picture. Teletext also offers the option to broadcast optional subtitles on ordinary TV programs at the press of a button.

In addition, special programs for deaf people are made available through the British Broadcasting system, called *See Hear,* a show including news and light entertainment in simultaneous speech, sign language and open subtitles. Other special BBC shows for deaf consumers include subtitles of daily news headlines, a news roundup and a series of educational programs in British Sign Language. In addition, some companies are producing special programs for deaf people in certain regional areas.

U.S. Deaf Skiers Association This group works with deaf members of U.S. ski teams involved in international competition and promotes recreational skiing for hard-of-hearing people. Contact: U.S. Deaf Skiers Association, Box USA, Gallaudet University, 800 Florida Ave. NE, Washington, DC; telephone (TDD): 202–651–5255.

utricle A small sac in the VESTIBULE of the inner ear.

V

vertigo A feeling of dizziness together with a sensation of movement and—most important—a feeling of rotating in space. It is this sense of rotation (either of the individual or the surroundings) that is an essential ingredient of true vertigo and distinguishes it from simple dizziness.

Vertigo is caused by a disturbance of the SEMICIRCULAR CANALS in the inner ear or the nerve tracts leading from them. It can occur in anyone when sailing, or an amusement ride, while watching a movie, or simply by looking down from a height. It also may be set off by motion sickness, brain disease, drugs (such as streptomycin) or damage to the AUDITORY NERVE.

However, there are more severe forms of vertigo caused by disease: labyrinthitis causes sudden vertigo accompanied by severe vomiting and unsteadiness in conjunction with an ear infection. Ménière's disease is also characterized by vertigo, sometimes severe enough to cause collapse. Sudden attacks of vertigo are usually assumed to be associated with labyrinthitis and are treated with bed rest and antihistamine drugs.

vestibular disorders A condition characterized by dizziness or balance problems that can be as mild as the momentary imbalance after a whirling carnival ride—or disruptive and debilitating. Dizziness or vertigo is among the 25 most common reasons Americans visit the doctor, and U.S. physicians report a total of more than 5 million dizziness or vertigo visits a year.

In many cases, the underlying cause of a vestibular disorder can't be determined. Otherwise, head trauma often causes vestibular disorders among people under age 50. Ear infections such as otitis media and inflammation of the inner ear (labyrinthitis) may also cause damage to the vestibular and hearing structures of the inner ear. Viruses may cause some vestibular disorders. High doses or long-term use of certain antibiotics can also cause permanent damage to the inner ear. Other drugs, such as aspirin, caffeine, alcohol, nicotine, sedatives, and tranquilizers (as well as many illegal drugs) can cause temporary dizziness but not permanent damage to the vestibular system. If the flow of blood to the inner ear or the brain is reduced or blocked (as in the case of a stroke), damage to the vestibular system can result. Rarely, a slow-growing tumor on the nerve that leads from the inner ear to the brain (an acoustic neuroma) may interfere with the normal function of the vestibular system.

The most frequently-reported symptoms of vestibular disorders are dizziness, unsteadiness or imbalance when walking, vertigo, and nausea. These symptoms may be quite mild or extremely severe, resulting in total

278

disability. Because the vestibular system interacts with many other parts of the nervous system, symptoms may also be experienced as problems with vision, muscles, and thinking, and memory.

In addition, people with vestibular disorders may suffer headache and muscular aches in the neck and back, increased tendency to suffer from motion sickness and increased sensitivity to noise and bright lights. Patients with vestibular disorders often report fatigue and loss of stamina and an inability to concentrate. Difficulty with reading and speech may occur during times of fatigue. When these symptoms are constant and disabling, they may be accompanied by irritability, loss of self-esteem, and/or depression.

Tests developed since 1984 enable physicians to diagnose some vestibular disorders that previously could not be documented. Modern diagnostic techniques for vestibular disorders rely on a combination of tests and a careful history of the problem. First, a doctor must complete physical examination to rule out other causes of dizziness caused by heart or central nervous system disorders. Then the patient will be referred to a specialist (an OTOLARYNGOLOGIST or neuro-otologist) for vestibular testing. Because the vestibular system is close to the hearing apparatus, vestibular testing includes hearing tests. Eye movements often hold clues to vestibular dysfunction, so to record eye movements, doctors use a technique called ELECTRONYSTAGMOGRAPHY. Balance is an essential component of vestibular functioning. During balance testing, patients may be asked to stand on special platforms that record the movement of the body. This kind of testing is called moving platform posturography.

Treatment for vestibular disorders varies according to the diagnosis. In mild cases, the symptoms may disappear their own as the vestibular apparatus heals or the nervous system learns to compensate for the disorder. If symptoms persist, some patients can be cured completely, but for others, symptoms can only be controlled and not eliminated entirely. Treatments may consist of drugs, diets, physical therapy or, in severe cases, surgery.

Although most vestibular disorders are treatable, some people with the disorders find they are temporarily or permanently unable to work or carry on normal activities. Social Security disability as well as many employee disability plans cover chronic, severe disability caused by vestibular disorders, but such payments can be received only if doctors attest to the disabling effects of the disorder.

Anyone troubled by symptoms of dizziness or imbalance should see a doctor; if vestibular disorders are suspected, the family doctor or the VESTIBULAR DISORDERS ASSOCIATION can recommend experts who specialize in diseases of the inner ear and who can perform the necessary tests.

Vestibular Disorders Association   A nonprofit organization established in 1983 to provide information and support to people suffering from inner-ear balance disorders (VESTIBULAR DISORDERS), including labyrinthitis, and MÉNIÈRE'S DISEASE. The Vestibular Disorders Association helps patients find knowledgeable doctors, distributes information about these disorders and provides videotapes, booklets, a quarterly newsletter and other materials about the problem.

vestibular nerve section   A surgical procedure that replaces LABYRINTHECTOMY (surgical excision of the entire inner ear) for incapacitating VERTIGO in patients with usable hearing in the diseased ear. The selective vestibular nerve section with preservation of hearing evolved from the earlier practice of severing the entire eighth cranial nerve.

vestibular system   This system—with its primary receptors located in the inner ear (the cristae of the three semicircular canals and the maculae of the utricle and saccule)—is responsible for our sense of orientation in space, for maintaining an upright balance and posture and for the ability to keep moving objects in focus.

There are five separate vestibular detectors, whose connections in the central nervous system allow the brain to integrate information from a variety of receptors in the eyes, the skin, muscles and joints. The vestibular receptor organs deal with the forces associated with head accelerations and changes in head position. As a result, nerves send messages to the brain centers that use these signals to develop a sense of orientation and to activate muscles that control automatic movements of the eyes, movement and posture.

Many of the vestibular pathways in the central nervous system are organized into reflex pathways, called the vestibular reflex systems, that stabilize and coordinate movements of the eyes, head and body.

Vestibular Development   Although the basic receptors and brain structures of the vestibular system are determined genetically, the development of vestibular function is a process that depends on use and interaction with the environment throughout life. These reflexes must be constantly adjusted in order to adapt to physical changes in the body's growing muscles and bones and to compensate for diseases or changes in the environment.

Research into the workings of the vestibular system is difficult because the fluid-filled receptor organs that detect motion and head position are encased in bone and therefore hard to study.

Vestibular Disorder Symptoms   The vestibular system is complex and highly interactive, capable of continual adaptations to changes in the body and the environment. Because it has many different parts, there are many separate symptoms when things go wrong, ranging from mild discomfort to total incapacitation.

These symptoms may seem unrelated to the ears but result from the complex interactions of different sensory modes that contribute to vestibular function and balance. The symptoms of balance disorders also vary depending on cause, location (one or both ears), age of the patient and so forth. To make things more complicated, the type of symptom— DIZZINESS versus imbalance, for example—may depend on the type of movement the patient is making at the time.

Primary symptoms of a vestibular system gone awry include: VERTIGO, sensation of falling, imbalance, lightheadedness, disorientation, giddiness and visual blurring. Secondary symptoms include nausea and vomiting, faintness, drowsiness, fatigue and depression.

Vestibular Diseases

Because vestibular signals interact with all of the major sensory systems and involve major brain centers, a large number of diseases can impair balance, especially among the elderly.

More than 90 million Americans have experienced dizziness or balance problems, and each year there are an estimated 97,000 new cases of MÉNIÈRE'S DISEASE, a disorder that affects the inner ear and causes episodes of vertigo, fluctuating hearing loss and TINNITUS.

There are many kinds of balance disorders, and motion sickness, with certain stimuli, can occur even in healthy people. Special environments (diving, high-speed flying and space travel) are situations for which humans are not genetically programmed, and therefore these reflexes must be overcome or reconditioned if humans are to be able to function in them.

viseme   A group of speech movements or shapes of the lips that are generally indistinguishable from one another. For example, one consonant category of visemes are the *p, b* and *m* sounds. These three consonants make up one viseme and are said to be homophonous.

However, researchers have not categorized vowels into visemes since no two vowels are produced with exactly the same movements. This does not mean, of course, that it is not possible to confuse the vowels when SPEECHREADING, as many do look similar.

visible speech   A system of sound writing (or phonetic transcription) that describes oral sounds through written symbols. Developed by Alexander Melville Bell, it was the first attempt to systematize speech training. Although the system did seem to work for Bell and his sons, it was too intricate for other scientists and was not enthusiastically endorsed.

Bell's system included 29 symbols, with 52 consonants, 26 vowels and 12 diphthongs (a complex sound made by gliding from the position for one vowel to another; for example in "boil" or "house") that, Bell claimed, could be used to represent all of the distinctive sounds of speech (and therefore, all languages) by expressing the movements of the articulators for individual speech sounds.

The elder Bell considered his system to be a way to improve elocution and did not originally design the method to be used for teaching deaf students, although educator GARDINER GREENE HUBBARD saw the possibilities for use with deaf students and arranged lectures for Bell to discuss his system. But it was ALEXANDER GRAHAM BELL who first really developed the system as a way to teach deaf students.

Because his first experience in teaching deaf students with visible speech seemed promising, the younger Bell accepted an invitation to teach the method in Boston. In 1871, Bell introduced the system in the United States at the Horace Mann School in Boston and at the Clarke School for the Deaf in Northampton, Massachusetts, where it was taught for 10 years before it was discarded.

voice-to-sign interpreting   Interpretation from a spoken language to a signed language. (See also SIGN LANGUAGE INTERPRETERS.)

Volta Bureau   The headquarters of the ALEXANDER GRAHAM BELL ASSOCIATION FOR THE DEAF, this bureau houses the association's extensive library containing literature on deafness.

The bureau was created and endowed by ALEXANDER GRAHAM BELL from money he received from the Republic of France, which had awarded him its Volta Prize for his inventions. Bell envisioned the bureau as the best way to increase and publicize information about deafness and presented the bureau to the association in 1909.

Much of the archival collection belonging to the association is still housed at the Volta Bureau.

W

Washoe   See NONHUMAN SIGNING.

wavelength   One of three measurements that describe a SOUND WAVE (the other two are amplitude and frequency). The wavelength is the longitudinal distance between the crests of two successive waves; the longer the wavelength of a sound, the lower its frequency.

Weitbrecht, Robert H. (1920–1983)   The inventor of the teletypewriter (TTY) for deaf people, which is the forerunner of the present-day telecommunications device for the deaf (TDD).

Weitbrecht was a deaf physicist who adapted a teletype model so it could be used to communicate over a telephone line with another teletype machine. Weitbrecht's modification was also called a TTY.

Because Weitbrecht's teletype was a surplus machine contributed by AT&T and there were only a limited number of these extra machines, only 25 TTYs were in use by deaf people by 1968. In that year, however, AT&T decided to donate surplus TTYs to deaf people and within several years had distributed several thousand.

white noise   A blend of audible frequencies over a wide range that can be used to convert disturbing silence into controlled quiet or to mask distracting noises. Often compared to the sound of escaping steam, white noise basically serves the same purpose as background music in restaurants. White noise has been used by dentists to mask the noise of the drill, which helps ease tension and pain. (See TINNITUS MASKER.)

Whitestone, Heather   Miss America for 1995, Heather Whitestone is totally deaf in her right ear and profoundly deaf in the other. Born in Dothlan, Alabama, February 24, 1973, she contracted a bacterial infection, *Haemophilus Influenzae* at the age of 18 months. She became deaf after taking antibiotics for the infection. But it was unclear whether the infection or the antibiotics were the cause of the problem.

Because her mother did not approve of sign language, she enrolled Heather in an oral program that emphasized teaching deaf students to speak. Heather's speech improved dramatically, but it also took her six grueling years to learn how to pronounce her last name correctly. As part of her therapy, she took ballet classes at the age of five, and eventually considered a professional career in ballet. She did not learn sign language until high school; no one else in her family signed.

When Heather was 15, her parents divorced. To pay for Heather's college education, her mother enrolled her in beauty pageants, which culminated in the Miss America pageant in 1995.

Wing's symbols   One of the first printed systems to help deaf children learn to speak, read and write syntactically correct sentences. Devised in 1883 by a deaf teacher named George Wing, it used numbers and letters to represent the different parts of speech in written language.

Specifically, Wing placed number and letter symbols over words, phrases or clauses. The symbols were grouped into the "essentials," "modifying forms," "correctives" and "special symbols." There were eight "essential" symbols: subject, transitive verb, intransitive verb, passive verb, object, adjective complement, noun and pronoun complement.

World Federation of the Deaf   This organization, formed by conference members during the 1951 World Congress of the Deaf, provides international visibility for deaf people and serves as an information exchange for deaf experts from around the world. Its main function is to hold international conferences, to help attain full citizenship for deaf people in all countries. To that end, it has represented their interests before various international groups.

One of the interesting developments contributed by this group is the creation of the first international sign language. Born out of the problem of communication presented by members from 57 different nations with many different sign languages and dialects, the federation first adopted French and English as its official languages. Since 1959, members have been trying to develop a true international sign language that can be understandable by all.

Its efforts resulted in GESTUNO, a sign language made up of 1,470 signs appropriated from existing sign languages that were the most easily-produced and the most natural referents.

The federation, which hopes to have gestuno accepted in other settings in addition to the annual congresses of the federation, now uses three sign languages at its plenary sessions: French and English sign language and gestuno.

World Games for the Deaf   The deaf athlete's Olympics. The World Summer and Winter Games for the Deaf have been held every four years since they began in Paris in 1924. The games are administered by the COMITÉ INTERNATIONAL DES SPORTS DES SOURDS (CISS), a group recognized by the International Olympic Committee.

In 1924, Belgium, Czechoslovakia, France, Great Britain, the Netherlands and Poland met at Pershing Stadium in Paris for the first World Games, where deaf athletes competed in track, swimming, soccer, shooting and cycling. Since then, the World Games have grown in size and number of events.

Today, the summer games are held one year after the Olympic Games followed by the winter games two years later. Host countries are chosen by a majority vote at the Comité six years in advance.

To be eligible, athletes who wish to complete in the games must have an average hearing level for speech greater than 55 decibels in the better ear, documented by audiogram submitted in advance. In addition, an AUDIOLOGIST makes spot checks of competitors and retests all event winners. Hearing aids cannot be worn during competition.

Summer game competitions include badminton, basketball, cycling, shooting, soccer, swimming, table tennis, team handball, tennis, track, volleyball, water polo and wrestling. Both male and female athletes may compete, although women are barred from wrestling, cycling, soccer and water polo. Gold, silver and bronze medals are given to the first three winners, and diplomas are awarded to the next six finishers.

Winter games consist of alpine and nordic ski events and speed skating.

Competitions are conducted under the same rules as the Olympic Games, although some modifications are used to make auditory cues visible. The games are opened with a parade of athletes and raising of the CISS flag. Although the Olympic torch is not used, the International Olympic Committee allows the Olympic flag to be flown.

In 1966, the International Olympic Committee awarded its Olympic Cup in recognition of CISS' service to the cause of sports and the Olympic spirit.

World Recreation Association of the Deaf, Inc./USA   This group promotes participation by hard-of-hearing people in a wide variety of recreational activities through its national and local chapters. Contact: World Recreation Association of the Deaf, Inc./USA, 1550 San Leandro Blvd., #196, San Leandro CA 94577; telephone: (TDD) 510–351–0397.

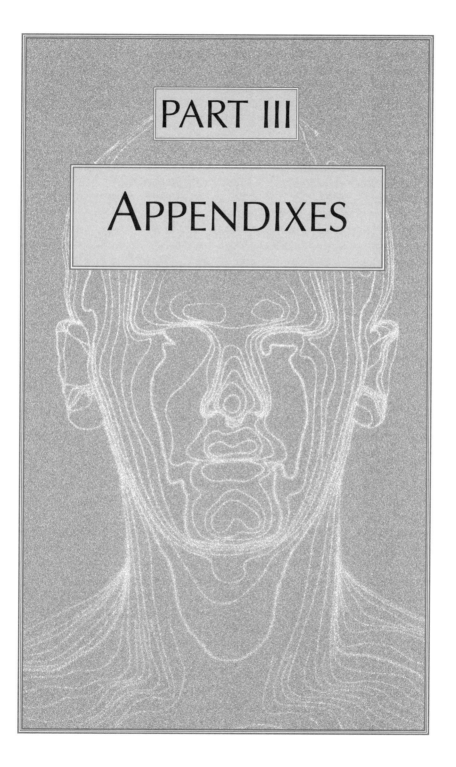

PART III

APPENDIXES

APPENDIX 1
GENERAL ORGANIZATIONS
AND RESOURCES

Academy of Dispensing Auditologists
3008 Millwood Avenue
Columbia SC 29205
803–252–5646
800–445–8629
http://www.audiologist.org

Acoustic Neuroma Association
P.O. Box 12402
Atlanta GA 30355
404–237–8023
http://www.anausa.org

Alexander Graham Bell Association
  for the Deaf
3417 Volta Place NW
Washington DC 20007–2737
202–337–5220 (voice/TDD)
http://www.agbell.org

American Academy of Audiology
8201 Greensboro Drive, Suite 300
McLean VA 22102
703–790–8466 (voice)
703–610–9022 (TDD)
800–AAA–2336
http://www.audiology.org

American Academy
  of Otolaryngology—Head and Neck
  Surgery
One Prince Street
Alexandria VA 22314
703'836–4444 (voice)
http://www.entnet.org

American Association of the Deaf-Blind
814 Thayer Avenue, Third Floor
Silver Spring MD 20910
301–588–6545
http://www.tr.wou.edu/dblink.aadb.htm

American Athletic Association of the
  Deaf, Inc.
1052 Darling Street
Ogden UT 84403
801–393–8710 (voice)
801–393–7916 (TTY)

American Deafness and Rehabilitation
  Association
P.O. Box 6956
San Mateo CA 94403
501–663–7074 (voice/TDD)
http://www.adara.org

American Hearing Research Foundation
55 E. Washington St., Suite 2022
Chicago IL 60602–2103
312–726–9670 (voice)

American Laryngological, Rhinological
  and Otological Society
555 N. 30th Street
Omaha NE 68131
402–498–6666

American Otological Society
2720 Tartan Way
Springfield IL 62707
217–483–6966
http://itsa.ucsf.edu/'ajo/AOS/AOS.html

American Society for Deaf Children
1820 Tribute Road, Suite A
Sacramento CA 95815
800–942–ASDC
http://www.deafchildren.org

American Speech-Language-Hearing
  Association
10801 Rockville Pike
Rockville MD 20852
301–897–5700 (voice/TDD)
800–897–8682 (helpline)
http://www.asha.org

American Tinnitus Association
1618 SW 1st Avenue
Portland OR 97201
503–248–9985 (voice)
http://www.ata.org

Association of Late-Deafened Adults
10310 Main Street
Box 274
Fairfax VA 22030
404–298–1596 (TDD)

Beginnings for Parents of Children
who are Deaf or Hard-of-Hearing
3900 Barrett Drive, Suite 100
Raleigh NC 27609
919–571–4843 (voice)
919–571–4843 (TDD)
800–541–4327
http://www.beginningssvcs.com/

Better Hearing Institute
5021 Backlick Road #B
Annandale VA 22003
800–EAR–WELL (voice)
703–642–0580 (voice)
http://www.betterhearing.org

Boys Town Research Registry for
  Hereditary Hearing Loss
555 North 30th Street
Omaha NE 68131
800–320–1171 (voice/TTY)
http://www.boystown.org/deafgene.org

Capital Communications for the Deaf
P.O. Box 149
McLean VA 22101
703–749–1876

The Caption Center
125 Western Avenue
Boston MA 02134
617–492–9225 (voice/TDD)
http://www.wgbh.org/caption

Captioned Media Program
1447 E. Main Street
Spartanburg SC 29307
http://www.cfr.org
800–237–6213 (voice)
800–237–6819 (TDD)

Children of Deaf Adults
P.O. Box 30715
Santa Barbara CA 93130
http://www.gallaudet.edu/rgpricke/coda

Cochler Implan Club International
5335 Wisconsin Avenue NW, Suite 440
Washington DC 20015–2034
202–895–2781 (voice)
202–895–2782 (TDD)
http://www.cici.org

Conference of Educational
  Administrators of the Schools
  and Programs for the Deaf
P.O. Box 1778
St. Augustine FL 32085
904–810–5200 (voice/TDD)

Convention of American Instructors
  of the Deaf
P.O. Box 377
Bedford TX 76095
512–441–2225
http://www.caid.org

Council on Education of the Deaf
Department of Education
Gallaudet University
800 Florida Avenue, NE
Washington DC 20002
202–651–5530 (voice/TDD)
http://www.educ.kent.edu/deafed/
  hane.htm

D.E.A.F., Inc.
215 Brighton Avenue
Allston MA 02134
617–254–4041 (voice/TDD)

Deaf Artists of America
301 North Goodman Street, Suite 205
Rochester NY 14607
716–325–2400 (voice/TDD)

Deafness Research Foundation
15 W. 39th Street, 6th Floor
New York NY 10018
212–768–1181 (voice, TDD)
800–535–DEAF
http://www.drf.org

DEAFPRIDE, Inc.
800 Florida Avenue, NE
Washington DC 20003–3660
202–675–6700 (voice/TDD)

Deaf Women United
215 Brighton Avenue
Allston MA 02134
617–254–4041 (voice/TDD)

The Ear Foundation
1817 Patterson Street
Nashville TN 37203
800–545–HEAR (voice/TDD)
http://www.earfoundation.org

Gallaudet Research Institute
800 Florida Avenue, NE
Washington DC 20002
202–651–5400
800–451–8834
http://gn.gallaudet.edu

Genetic Services Center
Gallaudet Research Institute
Gallaudet University

800 Florida Avenue, NE
Washington DC 20002
202–651–5258 (voice/TDD)
800–672–6720, ext. 5258
(voice/TDD)
http://gn.gallaudet.edu

Hard of Hearing Advocates
245 Prospect Street
Framingham MA 01701
508–875–8662 (voice)
http://hohadvocates.org

Hear Now
9745 E. Hampden Avenue, Suite 300
Denver CO 80231
800–648–HEAR (voice/TDD)
http://www.leisurelan.com/hearnow

Hearing Education and Awareness for
  Rockers (H.E.A.R.)
50 Oak Street, Suite 101
San Francisco CA 94102
415–431–3277 (voice)
http:/www.hearnet.com

Hearing Industries Association
515 King Street, Suite 420
Alexandria VA 22314
703–684–6048 (fax)

Helen Keller National Center for
  Deaf-Blind Youths and Adults
111 Middle Neck Road
Port Washington NY 11050
516–944–8900 (voice/TDD)
http://www.helenkeller.org

Holly Ear Institute
22101 Moross Road, MOB Suite 102
Detroit MI 48236–2172
313–343–7583 (voice)
313–343–8789 (TDD)
http://www.stjohn.org/hei

House Ear Institute
2100 W. Third Street #1D
Los Angeles CA 90057–1922
213–483–4431 (voice)
213–484–2642 (TDD)
http://www.hei.org

Hyperacusis Network
444 Edgewood Drive
Green Bay WI 54302
920–486–4667 (voice)
http://www.visi.com/minuet/
  hearing/hyperacusis

International Deaf/Tek
P.O. Box 2431
Framingham MA 01701–0404
508–620–1777 (voice)
508–620–1777 (TDD)
http://www.deaftek.org

International Foundation for
  Children's Hearing, Education
  and Research
871 McLean Avenue
Yonkers NY 10704

International Hearing Society
16880 Middlebelt Road, Suite 4
Livonia MI 48152
313–478–2610 (voice)
800–521–5247 (helpline)
http://www.hearingihs.org

Junior National Association of the
  Deaf Youth Programs
445 N. Pennsylvania Street, Suite 804
Indianapolis IN 46204
301–587–1788 (voice/TDD)
http://nad.org/jmad.htm

League for the Hard-of-Hearing
71 West 23rd Street
New York NY 10010
917–305–7700 (voice)
917–305–7999 (TDD)
http://www.lhh.org

National Association of the Deaf
  (NAD)
814 Thayer Avenue
Silver Spring MD 20910
301–587–1788 (voice/TDD)
http://nad.org

National Black Association for
  Speech-Language and Hearing
3605 Collier Road
Beltsville MD 20705
202–274–6162

National Board for Certification in
  Hearing Instrument Sciences
16880 Middlebelt Road, Suite 4
Livonia MI 48154
(734) 522–2900
http://www.hearingnbc.org

National Captioning Institute, Inc.
1900 Gallows Road, Suite 3000
Vienna VA 22182
703–917–7600
http://www.nciap.org

National Center for Law and the Deaf
Gallaudet University
800 Florida Avenue NE
Washington DC 20002
202–651–5373 (voice/TDD)
http://gngallaudet.edu

National Cued Speech Association
23970 Hermitage Road
Shaker Heights OH 44122
800–459–3529 (bookstore/information services)
http://www.cuedspeech.org

National Family Association for Deaf-Blind
111 Middle Neck Road
Sands Point NY 11050

National Fraternal Society of the Deaf
1118 S. 6th Street
Springfield IL 62703
312–392–9282 (voice)
312–392–1409 (TDD)
800–876–NFSD (voice/TDD)
http://www.nfsd.com

National Hearing Association
1010 Jorie Boulevard, Suite 308
Oak Brook IL 60521
312–323–7200

National Hearing Conservation Association
9101 East Kenyon Avenue, Suite 3000
Denver CO 80237
303–224–9022
http://www.hearingconservation.org

National Information Center for Children and Youth with Disabilities
P.O. Box 1492
Washington DC 20013
800–695–0285 (voice/TDD)
http://www.nincy.org

National Information Center on Deafness
Gallaudet College
800 Florida Avenue NE
Washington DC 20002
202–651–5051 (voice)
202–651–5052 (TDD)
http://www.gallaudet.edu/~nicd

National Information Clearinghouse on Children who are Deaf-Blind
345 North Monmouth Avenue
Monmouth OR 97361

800–854–7013 (TDD)
http://www.tr.wou.edu/dblink

National Institute on Deafness and Other Communication Disorders
31 Center Drive, MSC 2320
Bethesda MD 20892
301–496–7243 (voice)
301–402–0252 (TDD)
http://www.nih.gov/nidcd

National Organization for the Advancement of the Deaf, Inc. (NOAD)
18719 Set Point Lane
Humble TX 77346
281–812–2174
281–812–2174 (TDD)

National Rehabilitation Information Center
101 Wayne Avenue, #800
Silver Spring MD 20910
301–588–9284 (voice/TDD)
800–34–NARIC
http://www.ninds.nih.gov/patients/Feds/nric.htm

National Technical Institute for the Deaf
52 Lomb Memorial Drive
Rochester NY 14623–5604
716–475–6906 (voice)
716–475–6906 (TDD)
http://www.rit.edu/ntid

The National Theater of the Deaf
P.O. Box 659
Chester CT 06412
203–526–4971 (voice)
203–526–4974 (TDD)
http://www.thehartford.com/breakaway/deaf.html

Noise Pollution Clearinghouse
P.O. Box 1137
Montpelier VT 05601
802–229–1659
888–200–8332
http://nonoise.org/index.htm

Project ALAS
c/o D.E.A.F., Inc.
215 Brighton Avenue
Allston MA 02134
617–254–4041 (voice/TDD)

Quota International, Inc.
1420 21st Street NW
Washington DC 20036–5901
202–331–9694 (voice/TDD)

Rainbow Alliance of the Deaf
P.O. Box 14182
Washington DC 20044
202–779–6459 (TDD)
http://www.rad.org

Registry of Interpreters for the Deaf, Inc.
8630 Fenton Street, Suite 324
Silver Spring MD 20910
301–608–0050
http://www.rid.org

Self Help for Hard-of-Hearing People, Inc.
76910 Woodmont Avenue, Suite 1200
Bethesda MD 20814
301–657–2248 (voice)
301–657–2249 (TDD)
http://www.shhh.org

Sign Instructors Guidance Network (SIGN)
814 Thayer Avenue, #252
Silver Spring MD 20910
301–587–1788
Society of Hearing-Impaired Physicians
1999 Mowry Avenue, Suite L
Fremont CA 94538
510–797–2939

Society of Otorhinolaryngology and Head-Neck Nurses, Inc.
116 Canal Street, Suite A
New Smyrna Beach FL 32168

904–428–1695
http://www.sohnnurse.com

Telecommunications for the Deaf, Inc.
8630 Fenton Street, Suite 604
Silver Spring MD 20910
301–598–3786 (voice)
301–598–3006 (TDD)
http://www.tdi_online.org

Tele-Consumer Hotline
1910 K Street NW, Suite 610
Washington DC 20006
202–223–4371 (voice/TDD)
800–332–1124 (voice/TDD) (outside D.C.)
http://idi.net/hotline

TRIPOD
1727 W. Burbank Boulevard
Burbank CA 91506
800–352–8888
800–346–8888 (California only)
818–972–2080 (voice/TDD)
http://www.tripod.org

Vestibular Disorders Association
P.O. Box 4467
Portland OR 97208–4467
503–229–7705
800–837–8428
http://www.vesibular.org

APPENDIX 2
HEALTH CARE DELIVERY
AND SPECIAL SERVICES

National

Association of Medical Professionals
with Hearing Impairment
Frank Hochman, M.D.
2287 Mowry Avenue, Suite F
Fremont CA 94538

One of the primary aims of this association is to encourage and assist deaf students to enter medicine as a profession.

Promoting Awareness in Health Care, Medical & Deaf (P.A.H., M.D.)
Medical College of Virginia Chapter of AMSA
1008 West Avenue, #2
Richmond VA 23220
http://views.vcu.edu/amsa/pahmd.html

This on-line discussion group is a network of people dedicated to bridging the gap between the medical community and the deaf community. Physicians, nurses, social workers and others interested in health care among deaf persons participate.

SHHH Hospital Program
SHHH (Self Help for Hard of Hearing People, Inc.)
7910 Woodmont Avenue, Suite 1200
Bethesda MD 20814
http://www.shhh.org/

This is a complete guide to enable hospitals to provice services for people with hearing loss in health care settings and to comply with the Americans with Disabilities Act (ADA). The program includes a 56-page guidebook (*People with Hearing Loss and Health Care Facilities*), a staff training video (*I Only Hear You When I See Your Face*), one "Patient with Hearing Loss" brochure, 10 "Tips for Communication" cards, two "Tips for Staff" posters, and stickers of the International Symbol

of Access for Hearing Loss (50 1"x1" stickers; 5 5 1/2'x7' stickers). The complete Hospital Program is $70 for members and $80 for nonmembers. Components may be purchased separately from SHHH at the address above.

Regional

CALIFORNIA

Health Care Partnership and Acess Program for the Deaf
Greater Los Angeles Council on Deafness, Inc. (GLAD)
2222 Laverna Avenue

Los Angeles CA 90041
213–478–8000 TDD/Voice
http://www.gladine.org

GLAD provides outreach programs to deaf people, including education on AIDS, family planning, sexually transmitted diseases and substance abuse. LIFE SIGNS, a 24-hour medical sign language interpreter referral service, assists in any situations where an individual requires immediate medical care in an emergency room, emergency admittance to a hospital, urgent care center or any emergency matters with law-enforcement personnel.

Special Task Interpreters for the Deaf, Inc. (STID, Inc.)
P.O. Box 482
Atwood CA 92811
800–STIDVIP (784–3847) Voice/TTY
714–996–3774 Voice/TTY

STID provides trained interpreter/medical aides for medical office visits, 24-hour emergency room and urgent care centers, surgery, recovery, childbirth classes, labor, delivery and all diagnostic testing procedures. STID provides information, advocacy and assistance in medical situations as well as referrals for further support. STID provides continuity of care—the same interpreter is provided for all scheduled medical office visits and hospital procedures.

FLORIDA

Crystal Oaks of Pinellas
Health Care and Rehabilitation Center
for the Deaf and Hard-of-Hearing
6767 86th Avenue North
Pinellas Park FL 33782
813–548–5566 Voice/TTY

ILLINOIS

Silent Care
2711 W. Howard Street
Chicago IL 60645
773–275–2378 Voice/TTY

A specialized nursing home program responding to the needs of elderly deaf persons at certain long-term care facilities throughout Illinois, providing comprehensive long-term care services to members of the deaf community in a homelike environment. Two sites are currently under development: Lincoln Park Terrace, 2732 N. Hampden Court, Chicago, IL and Plaza Terrace, 3249 W. 147th Street, Midlothian, IL.

KANSAS

Hear for You
Olathe Medical Center
20333 West 151st Street
Olathe KS 66061
913–791–4311

Hear for You provides 24-hour interpreter services to deaf and hard-of-hearing patients and their families.

KENTUCKY

Heritage Hospice
337 West Broadway
P.O. Box 1213
Danville KY 40422
606–236–3367 Voice/TTY
800–718–7708 Voice/TTY

Heritage Hospice, a four-county rural hospice, is accessible to deaf patients and their families. HOSPICE provides

health care in the home under the direction of the patient's doctor.
http://www.mednexus.com/adverts/heritage/

MARYLAND

Deaf Services Program
Albert Witzke Medical Center
3411 Bank Street
Baltimore MD 21224
410–522–9534 Voice
410–522–9528 TTY

The Deaf Services Program makes all services of the Baltimore Medical System accessible to deaf patients through full-time sign language interpreters, health care coordination and health education in sign language, including childbirth education and prenatal care. The Deaf Services Program assists with arranging medical referrals and special tests, advocating for an interpreter at the facility of referral, and also provides information and referral to resources for nonmedical services.

MASSACHUSETTS

Deaf Family Clinic (DFC)
Department of Pediatrics
New England Medical Center
Boston MA
E-mail: defdoc@aol.co

The Deaf Family Clinic acts partly as an advocacy agency for deaf and hard-of-hearing children.

MINNESOTA

Health & Wellness Program Serving
Deaf and Hard of Hearing People
St. Paul-Ramsey Medical Center
640 Jackson Street
St. Paul MN 55101–2595
612–221–2719 Voice
612–221–3258 TTY

The Health and Wellness Program provides numerous services to deaf and hard-of-hearing people, including interpreting; sexual health and family planning; prenatal and parent education; sexual assault advocacy; and child abuse education, treatment, and prevention. Mental health and community education services for deaf, hard-of-hearing and deaf-blind people are provided under the direction of Ramsey's Psychiatric Department.

NEW YORK

Jacob Perlow Hospice-Deaf Services
  Project
Beth Israel Medical Center
New York NY
212–420–4129 TTY
212–420–4543 Voice
212–420–4131 Fax
Website: http://www.whitmore.org/
  hospicedeaf.html

The Jacob Perlow Hospice-Deaf Services Project provides specialized care to patients with end-stage disease and can assist deaf patients with deaf or hearing families and hearing patients with deaf family members. This culturally sensitive and linguistically appropriate hospice programs provides communication access to physicians, nurses, social workers, special therapists and chaplains through qualified and specially trained interpreters. Trained volunteers from the deaf, hard-of-hearing and adjoining American Sign Language community provide additional support.

APPENDIX 3
WHERE TO LEARN
COMMUNICATION SKILLS

Auditory Training Classes

Auditory training classes and instruction in listening skills help hard-of-hearing people learn to use their remaining hearing. For more information, call:

American Speech-Language-Hearing Association Helpline
800–638–8255 (voice/TDD)

Cued Speech

National Cued Speech Association
Cued Speech Center, Inc.
304 E. Jones Street 27601–1068
Raleigh NC 27622
919–828–1218
http://web7.mit.edu/cuedspeech/ncsainfo.html

Cue Speech Discovery
23970 Hermitage Road
Cleveland OH 44122
216–292–6213
http://www.isl.net/~cuedspmn

West Coast Cued Speech Programs
348 Cernon Street
Vacaville CA 95688
707–448–4060

Sign Language

The best way to learn sign is with a teacher in a class. Contact the following:

- local school system, community college or university extension program
- state or county department of public instruction, education or special education

- county vocational rehabilitation services (many states have a coordinator of services for the deaf)
- United Way
- recreation and community centers (YWCA, YMCA)
- adult education/continuing education centers
- religious organizations
- libraries
- deafness-related organizations or groups (see Appendixes A and C)
- state school for the deaf
- state office/commission or state association for the deaf (see Appendixes A and B)

In addition, each April the *American Annals of the Deaf* includes a comprehensive list of services, schools and classes for deaf students. These would be good contacts for information on the availability of sign language.

If there are no classes available, text and tape materials are available. Check your local library.

Speechreading

For more information, contact:

American Speech-Language-Hearing Association Helpline
800–638–8255 (voice/TDD)
http://www.asha.org/index.htm

Alexander Graham Bell Association for the Deaf
202–337–5220 (voice/TDD)
http://www.agbell.org

GLOSSARY

acoustic   Pertaining to sound or the sense of hearing.

acoustic feedback   See FEEDBACK.

acoustic nerve   See AUDITORY NERVE.

adenoids   The two lymph nodes above the tonsils at the back of the nose that are partly responsible for protecting the body's upper respiratory tract against infection.

ampulla   The expanded end of the semicircular duct contained in each semicircular canal of the inner ear.

anacusia   Term meaning total deafness (also "anakusis" or "anacusis).

antitragus   A bump on the pinna (outer ear) opposite the "tragus" found in front of the ear canal. The antitragus protects cartilage in the pinna near the opening of the ear canal.

anvil   The middle of the three bones (ossicles) in the middle ear that transmits sound vibration.

air-bone gap   The difference between air- and bone-conduction thresholds.

air conduction   Transmission of sound to the inner ear via the ear canal and middle ear.

auditory discrimination   The ability to tell one speech sound from another.

auditory nerve   The part of the eighth cranial nerve that carries information from the inner ear to the brain. It consists of two separate divisions, the vestibular nerve and the cochlear nerve.

auditory perception   The mental awareness of sound.

auditory training   The process of teaching a person with hearing loss to take full advantage of any sound cues that can still be heard. Auditory training can help those with hearing loss become aware of cues they might not otherwise notice. The type of auditory training depends on when the person lost hearing and the type of hearing loss.

aural   Pertaining to the sense of hearing or to the ear itself.

auricle   The outer part of the external ear, also called the pinna.

basilar membrane   A flexible membrane that is attached to the bony shelf and divides the coil of the cochlea lengthwise into two compartments; as sound disturbs the perilymph fluid on one side of the membrane, it is transferred through the basilar membrane to the organ of Corti on the other side, and on to the hair cells.

binaural   Pertaining to both ears.

bone conduction   The transmission of sound to the inner ear from vibrations reaching the bones of the skull.

bone conduction vibrator   A device used in bone conduction audiometry; it is placed on the mastoid bone behind the external ear to present pure tones during the test.

bone hearing level   A measurement that indicates how well pure tones are heard through the bones behind the ear.

CC   Acronym used to denote closed captioning on TV programs and videocassettes.

central hearing loss   A type of hearing loss caused by damage or impairment in the nerves or nuclei of the central nervous system, either in the pathways to the brian or in the brain itself.

cerumen Earwax secreted into the external ear canal.

cochlea The snail-shaped structure located behind the oval window the inner ear. It contains fluid and thousands of microscopic hair cells tuned to various frequencies, in addition to the organ of Corti, the receptor for hearing.

compliance The ability of the eardrum to accept and transmit sound vibrations from the external ear canal to the middle ear. Disorders of the eardrum or the middle ear decrease this ability.

conductive hearing loss A hearing deficit caused by a problem in the middle or outer ear. People with this type of medically treatable hearing loss usually have normal inner ears but specific problems in the outer or middle ear that prevent sound from getting into the inner ear in the normal way.

decibel Measure of the intensity (loudness) of sound. Zero decibels (dB) is the softest intensity of sound or speech that can be heard by a normal person; 100 dB is the most intense sound an audiometer can produce.

discomfort level The level at which pure tones (or speech) become too loud for the listener to hear comfortably.

discrimination In acoustics, this refers to the ability to understand speech once it is loud enough to hear.

distortion break The level at which sounds become unnatural as hearing aids are turned up.

eardrum A paper-thin covering stretching across the ear canal that separates the middle and the outer ears and that vibrates with sound; also called the "tympanic membrane." Blood vessels supplying the eardrum are extremely tiny, but inflammation can engorge them so that the entire membrane becomes reddish and opaque.

earlobe The fleshy, hanging lower portion of the outer ear (also called the lobule); it's the only part of the external ear that doesn't contain cartilage.

eighth cranial nerve See AUDITORY NERVE.

endolymph A viscous fluid contained in a small canal called the scala media.

epitympanum A smaller but continuous extension of the middle ear cavity that contains the bulk of the incus (anvil) and malleus (hammer). It is also known as the attic.

eustachian tube The air duct that connects the area behind the nose to the middle ear. It acts as a drainage passage from the middle ear, and maintains hearing by opening to regulate air pressure.

external auditory canal Also known as the ear canal (or "meatus"), this inch-long curved tube extends from the floor of the external ear inward to the eardrum. The outer third of the ear canal is cartilage, lined with thick skin, fine hairs, and modified oil glands. These glands produce earwax, which protects the inner portions of the ear from dirt and insects.

feedback A loud squeal from the amplifier of a hearing aid caused by a sound escaping around an ill-fitting earpiece which is then picked up and amplified. A hearing aid can deliver much louder sound without squeal if the earpiece fits well.

fenestra ovalis An opening in the inner wall of the middle ear into which the footplate of the stapes is embedded (also called the "oval window.")

flat hearing loss A hearing loss that is about the same at all important frequencies.

footplate In the ear, it is the base of the stirrup (stapes) that rests on the oval window.

frequency   The number of sound waves that pass a fixed point in a certain period of time and a measure of the number of cycles or vibrations during that time. Frequency is usually expressed as "hertz" (Hz).

frequency range   The measure of power that exists in certain pitch ranges and how far the amplification ability of a hearing aid extends into the high and low pitches.

hair cells   Sensory receptors in the inner ear that transform sound vibrations into the messages traveling to the brain.

hard of hearing   A term used to describe mild to moderate hearing loss. This term is preferred by the deaf community over "hearing impaired."

helicotrema   An opening in the basilar membrane at the top of the cochlear canal through which the scala tympani meets the scala vestibuli. Low-frequency vibrations of the oval window create waves in the perilymph of the scala vestibuli through the helicotrema.

helix   The curved border of the outer ear.

hertz (Hz)   A unit of vibration frequency adopted internationally to replace the term "cycles per second." One hertz is equal to one cycle per second; one kilohertz (kHz) is 1,000 hertz, and one megahertz is 1,000,000 Hz.

hypacusis   Another word for hard of hearing.

hyperacusis   An unusually acute sense of hearing.

hypoacusis   A synonym for hearing loss.

Hz   The abbreviation for "hertz."

incus   The middle bone of the three ossicles of the middle ear (also called the anvil).

inner ear   The interior section of the ear where sound vibrations and information about balance are translated into nerve impulses.

internal acoustic meatus   A passage in the temporal bone for the facial and auditory nerves.

loudness   The intensity factor of sound.

macula   A small sensory patch that is part of the body's delicate balance system, located inside both the saccule and utricle (small sacs in the vestibule). Each macula is covered with sensory hair cells and is connected to fibers from the vestibular branch of the hearing nerve.

malleus   One of the three bones of the middle ear, also known as the hammer.

mastoid bone   A prominent part of the temporal bone located behind the ear, honeycombed with air cells. It is connected to a cavity in the upper part of the bone called the mastoid antrum, which is in turn connected to the middle ear.

membranous labyrinth   A delicate closed system of ducts and sacs filled with a watery fluid called endolymph that is part of the body's balance system. The membranous labyrinth is suspended in the bony labyrinth of the otic capsule.

middle ear   The small cavity between the eardrum and the inner ear that houses the three tiny bones of the middle ear (the ossicles). The middle ear transmits the vibration of a sound to the fluid in the inner ear by the chain of these three tiny bones. Although the eardrum cuts off the middle ear from the outside, it's not completely airtight. A ventilation channel called the eustachian tube runs forward and down into the back of the nose.

mild to moderate hearing loss   Hearing loss generally considered to be in the 30 dB to 55 dB range.

modiolus   The central column of the cochlea in which the spiral ganglion of the hearing nerve is located.

monaural   Pertaining to one ear.

nerve deafness   A misleading term used to describe a sensorineural hearing loss.

ossicles   The three small bones of the middle ear (the malleus or hammer, the incus or anvil, and the stapes or stirrup). These bones help carry sound and speech from the eardrum to the inner ear.

otic capsule   The bony case enclosing the inner ear. Part of the otic capsule forms the inner wall of the middle ear.

otorrhea   The medical term for a discharge from the ear. This is usually fluid resulting from an ear infection, although it can include blood or cerebrospinal fluid following a skull fracture. A doctor should evaluate any otorrhea.

otoscope   An instrument used for examining the ear, to inspect the outer ear canal and the eardrum, and to detect certain diseases of the middle ear.

otospongiosis   Another name for otosclerosis.

outer ear   The portion of the ear that contains the external ear (or pinna).

oval window   A tiny opening in the body wall of the cochlea that is an entrance to the inner ear.

perilymph   The fluid (almost identical to spinal fluid) that is contained in the canals of the cochlea.

pinna   The part of the outer ear that we can see, also called the auricle.

presbycusis   A type of progressive sensorineural hearing loss associated with aging; it is one of the most common chronic problems among older people.

profound hearing loss   A hearing loss generally considered to be more than 90 decibels (dB).

pure tone   A sound at only one frequency (pitch) with no harmonics.

recruitment   An abnormal, rapid increase in loudness as the strength of the acoustic signal is increased.

Reissner's membrane   The thinnest membrane in the cochlea with the thickness of just two cells, this separates the perilymph and endolymph fluids.

resonance   The vibration of an object or air when certain pitches are made louder (such as when a person blows over the top of a bottle).

round window   An elastic membrane opening between the middle ear and inner ear.

scala media   A tubelike structure on top of the basilar membrane that follows the turns of the cochlea. Inside the entire length of the scala media is the sensitive mechanism of hearing called the organ of Corti.

scala tympani   A spiral fluid channel containing perilymph, located in the cochlea below the basilar membrane.

scala vestibuli   A spiral fluid channel containing perilymph located in the cochlea above the basilar membrane.

semicircular canals   Another name for the labyrinth, the organ inside the inner ear that is connected to the cochlea but does not contribute to the sense of hearing.   Instead, these three fluid-filled loops help maintain balance by sending information about the position of the head along the auditory nerve to the brain.

sensorineural hearing loss   A type of hearing loss that is caused by damage to the hair cells of the inner ear or the nerves that supply it.   It is unlike conductive hearing loss, which is caused by diseases or obstructions in the outer or middle ear.

sociocusis   Hearing loss caused by environmental noise.

stapedectomy   An operation to treat hearing loss caused by otosclerosis in which all or most of the stapes is replaced by a plastic prosthesis.

stapedial muscle   One of two intra-aural muscles in the middle ear, the stapedial muscle is attached to the top of the stapes and runs behind it.

stapedius   A small muscle in the inner wall of the middle ear that inserts into the neck of the stapes and is responsible for retracting the stapes.

stirrup   The common term for the stapes, one of the three ossicles in the middle ear.

tectorial membrane   A fine jellylike membrane on top of the hair cells of the organ of Corti.

tensor tympani   One of the two muscles in the middle ear attached to the upper portion of the handle of the malleus, crossed diagonally across the tympanum into the tensor canal.

tone control   A special device on a hearing aid that changes the pitch of amplified sound.

trigeminal nerve   The fifth cranial nerve ("facial nerve"), which supplies sensation to the face, scalp, nose, teeth, lining of the mouth, eyelid, sinuses, and front part of the tongue. About 60% of people have a sensorineural hearing loss related to an incompletely covered facial nerve canal in the middle ear. Rarely, the nerve interrupts the ossicular chain and causes a conductive hearing loss.

tympanic cavity   An air-filled space containing the ossicular chain located in the temporal bone. It's linked to the nasopharynx via the eustachian tube.

tympanic membrane, secondary   A membranous flap at the base of the cochlea that closes the scala tympani at the round window.

tympanic plexus   A group of nerves formed by branches of the facial and glossopharyngeal nerves and located on the mound between the round and oval windows. The tympanic plexus supplies sensation to the middle ear.

tympanum   The main part of the middle ear cavity that lies between the tympanic membrane and the lateral bony wall of the internal ear.

umbo   The point at which the malleus is attached to the eardrum; it is a prominent landmark for evaluating eardrum health.

vestibule   A portion of the labyrinth of the inner ear located between the cochlea and the semicircular canals.

Y cord   A special cord found on a body-type hearing aid that carries amplified sound to two receivers.

BIBLIOGRAPHY

Abercrombie, D. *Elements of General Phonetics.* Chicago: Aldine, 1967.

Aiello, B. *The Hearing-Impaired Child in the Regular Class.* Washington, D.C.: The AFT Teachers' Network for Education of the Handicapped, 1981.

Akens, David. *Loss of Hearing and You.* Huntsville, Ala.: Strode, 1970.

Albertini, J., B. Meath-Lang, and Caccamise, F. "Sign Language Use: Development of English and Communication Skills." *Audiology* 9 (1984): 111–126.

Allen, J. C., and M. L. Allen. "Discovering and Accepting Hearing Impairment." *Volta Review* 81, no. 5 (1979): 279–285.

Allen, T. E., and T. I. Osborn. "Academic Integration of Hearing-Impaired Students: Demographic, Handicapping and Achievement Factors." *American Annals of the Deaf* 129, no. 2 (1984): 100–113.

———, C. S. White, and M. A. Karchmer. "Issues in the Development of a Special Edition for Hearing-Impaired Students of the Seventh Edition of the Stanford Achievement Test." *American Annals of the Deaf* 128, no. 1 (1983): 34–39.

Altshuler, K. A. "Psychiatric Considerations in the Adult Deaf." *American Annals of the Deaf* 107, no. 5 (1962): 560–561.

———. "The Social and Psychological Development of the Deaf Child: Problems, Their Treatment and Prevention." *American Annals of the Deaf* 119, no. 4 (1974): 365–376.

———, W. E. Deming, and J. Vollenweider. "Impulsivity and Profound Early Deafness." *American Annals of the Deaf* 121, no. 3 (1976): 331–345.

———, and J. Rainer, eds. *Mental Health and the Deaf: Approach and Prospects.* Washington, D.C.: U.S. Department of Health, Education and Welfare, Social and Rehabilitation Services, 1968.

American Society for Deaf Children. *Position Statements on Education, Educational Options, Parental Involvement in Education, Communication, Total Communication.* Silver Spring, Md.: American Society for Deaf Children, 1983.

Angus, Jean Rich. *Watch My Words: An Open Letter to Parents of Young Deaf Children.* Cincinnati, Ohio: Forward Movement Publications, 1974.

Anthony, D., W. Dekkers, and C. Erikson. *Seeing Essential English: Code-breaker.* Boulder, Colo.: Pruett, 1978.

Archbold, S., et al. "Educational Placement of Deaf Children Following Cochlear Implantation." *British Journal of Audiology* 32@/5 (October 1998): 295–300.

Axon, P. R., et al. "Cochlear Ossification After Meningitis." *American Journal of Otolaryngology* 19, no. 6 (November 1998): 724–9.

Baker, C., and R. Battison. *Sign Language and the Deaf Community.* Silver Spring, Md.: National Association of the Deaf, 1980.

———, and D. Cokely. *American Sign Language: A Teacher's Resource Text on Grammar and Culture.* Silver Spring, Md.: T. J. Publishers, 1980.

Barnett, S. "Clinical and Cultural Issues in Caring for Deaf People." *Family Medicine* 31/1 (January 1999): 17–22. Review.

Battison, Robbin. *Lexical Borrowing in American Sign Language.* Silver Spring, Md.: Linstok Press, 1978.

Beard, Jonathan D. "Magnetic Implants Aid Hearing." *Popular Science* 245 (November 1994): 38.

Beck, B. "Self-Assessment of Selected Interpersonal Abilities in Hard of Hearing and Deaf Adolescents," *International Journal of Rehabilitation Research* 11, no. 4 (1988): 343–9.

Becker, G. *Growing Old in Silence.* Berkeley: University of California Press, 1980.

Bekesy, G. *Experiments in Hearing.* New York: McGraw-Hill, 1960.

Bellugi, Ursula, and D. Newkirk. "Formal Devices for Creating New Signs in American Sign Language." *Sign Language Studies* 30 (1981): 1–35.

Bender, R. *The Conquest of Deafness.* Cleveland, Ohio: Case Western Reserve, 1970.

Benzaia, Diana. "Hold on to Your Hearing." *Saturday Evening Post* 261 (January/February 1989): 40.

————. "Help Your Hearing." *The Saturday Evening Post* 261 (March 1989): 16.

Berendt, R. D., E. Corliss and M. Ojalvo. *Quieting: A Practical Guide to Noise Control.* U.S. Dept. of Commerce, National Bureau of Standards, Washington, D.C., 1976.

Berg, F. S. *Educational Audiology: Hearing and Speech Management.* New York: Grune & Stratton, 1976.

Bergman, M. *Aging and the Perception of Speech.* Baltimore, Md.: University Park Press, 1980.

Beynon, G. J., et al. "'Doctor, Do I Need A Hearing Aid?'" *Practitioner* 242/1587 (June 1998): 421.

Birch, J. *Hearing-Impaired Pupils in the Mainstream of Education.* Reston, Va.: Council for Exceptional Children, 1974.

Blackwell, P. *Teaching Hearing Impaired Children in Regular Classrooms.* Washington, D.C.: Center for Applied Linguistics, 1983.

Block, M., and M. Okrand. "Real-time Closed Captioned Television as an Educational Tool." *American Annals of the Deaf* 128, no. 5 (1983): 636–641.

Bodner-Johnson, B. A. "The Family Environment and Achievement of Deaf Students." *Exceptional Children* 52 (1986): 443–449.

Boettcher, F. A., and R. J. Salvi. "Salicylate Ototoxicity: Review and Synthesis." *American Journal of Otolaryngology* 12 (1991): 33–47.

Bonnickson, K. "A Functional Language Program That Works." *Volta Review* 87, no. 2 (1985): 67–76.

Bornstein, Harry. "A Description of Some Current Systems Designed to Represent English." *American Annals of the Deaf* 118 (1973): 454–464.

————. "Towards a Theory of Use for Signed English: From Birth Through Adulthood." *American Annals of the Deaf* 127, no. 1 (1982): 26–31.

————, and Karen Saulnier. *The Signed English School Book.* Washington, D.C.: Kendall Green Publications, Gallaudet University Press, 1987.

————, K. Saulnier, and Lillian Hamilton, eds. *The Comprehensive Signed English Dictionary.* Washington, D.C.: Gallaudet University Press, 1983.

Bottrill, I. "Diagnosing and Treating Ménière's Disease." *Practitioner* 242, no. 1587 (June 1998): 482–4.

Boughman, J. A., and K. A. Shaver. "Genetic Aspects of Deafness: Understanding the Counseling Process." *American Annals of the Deaf* 127, no. 4 (1982): 393–400.

Braddy, N. *Anne Sullivan Macy: The Story Behind Helen Keller.* New York: Doubleday, 1933.

Brasel, K., and S. P. Quigley. "Influence of Certain Language and Communication Environments in Early Childhood on the Development of Language in Deaf Individuals." *Journal of Speech and Hearing Research* 20 (1977): 95–107.

———. *Mainstreaming the Prelingually Deaf Child.* Washington, D.C.: Gallaudet University Press, 1978

Brietzke, C. E. "Listen Up!" *The Saturday Evening Post* 265 (September/October 1993): 36.

Brown, Mary Daniels. "The Ears: Your Personal Sound System." *Current Health II* 19 (November 1992): 6–11.

Bruce, Robert. *Alexander Graham Bell and the Conquest of Solitude.* Boston: Little, Brown, 1973.

Buchman, C. A., et al. "Cochlear Implants in the Geriatric Population: Benefits Outweigh Risks." *Ear Nose & Throat Journal* 78, no. 7 (July 1999): 489–94.

Caccamise, F., ed. "Sign Language and Simultaneous Communication: Linguistic, Psychological and Instructional Ramifications." *American Annals of the Deaf,* November 1978.

———, et al., eds. *Introduction to Interpreting for Interpreters/Transliterators, Hearing-Impaired Consumers, Hearing Consumers.* Silver Spring, Md.: Registry of Interpreters for the Deaf, 1980.

———, and D. Hicks, eds. *American Sign Language in a Bilingual Bicultural Context.* Silver Spring, Md.: National Association of the Deaf, 1980.

———, and W. Newell. "A Review of Current Terminology in Deaf Education and Signing." *Journal of the Academy of Rehabilitative Audiology* 17 (1984).

Caldwell, D. "Closed Captioned Television and the Hearing Impaired." *Volta Review* 83, no. 5 (1981): 285–289.

Calvert, D. *A Parent's Guide to Speech and Deafness.* Washington, D.C.: Alexander Graham Bell Association for the Deaf, 1984.

———, and S. R. Silverman. *Speech and Deafness.* Washington, D.C.: Alexander Graham Bell Association for the Deaf, 1983.

Casano, R. A., et al. "Inherited Susceptibility to Aminoglycoside Ototoxicity: Genetic Heterogeneity and Clinical Implications." *American Journal of Otolaryngology* 20, no. 3 (May–June 1999): 151–6.

Catford, J. *Fundamental Problems in Phonetics.* Bloomington: University of Indiana Press, 1966.

Chess, S., and P. Fernandez. "Impulsivity in Rubella Deaf Children: a Longitudinal Study." *American Annals of the Deaf* 125, no. 40 (1980): 505–9.

Chomsky, N. *Language and Mind.* New York: Harcourt Brace Jovanovich, 1968.

Chough, S. K. "Speech Is Not Equivalent to Personality Development." *Social Work* 22, no. 4 (1977): 310–312.

Christiansen, J. B., and D. P. Polakoff. "Characteristics of Social Workers and Social Work Programs at Residential and Day Schools for the Deaf." *American Annals for the Deaf,* June 125, no. 4, (1980): 482–7.

Clarke, B. R., and D. Ling. "The Effects of Using Cued Speech." *Volta Review* 78 (1976): 23–34.

Cohen, O. P. "Deaf Children from Ethnic, Linguistic and Racial Minority Backgrounds: An Overview." *American Annals of the Deaf* 135, no. 2 (1992): 67–93.

———. "At-Risk Deaf Adolescents." *Volta Review* 93, no. 5 (1991): 57–72.

Cokely, D. "When Is a Pidgin Not a Pidgin? An Alternate Analysis of the ASL-English Contact Situation." *Sign Language Studies* 38 (1983): 1–24.

———, and R. Gawlik. "A Position Paper on the Relationship Between Manual English and Sign." *Deaf American,* May 7–11, 1973.

Cole, E., and H. Gregory, eds. *Auditory Learning.* Washington, D.C.: Alexander Graham Bell Association for the Deaf, 1986.

Combs, Alec. *Hearing Loss Help.* Santa Maria, Calif.: Alpenglow Press, 1986.

Compton, Cynthia, and Fred Brandt. *Assistive Listening Devices.* Washington, D.C.: National Information Center on Deafness.

Connor, L., ed. *Speech for the Deaf Child: Knowledge and Use.* Washington, D.C.: Alexander Graham Bell Association for the Deaf, 1971.

Conrad, R. *The Deaf School Child.* London: Harper & Row, 1979.

Consumer Reports Editors. "Hearing aids." *Consumer Reports 1994 Buying Guide* 58 (December 15, 1993): 230–32.

———. "How to Buy a Hearing Aid." *Consumer Reports* 57 (November 1992): 716–21.

Consumer's Digest Editors. "New Generation Hearing Aids." *Consumer's Digest* 32 (September/October 1993): 76.

Corbett, E. E., Jr., and C. J. Jensema. *Teachers of the Deaf: Descriptive Profiles.* Washington, D.C.: Gallaudet University Press, 1981.

Craig, H. B. "Parent-Infant Education in Schools for Deaf Children." *American Annals of the Deaf* 128, no. 21 (1983): 82–98.

Craig, W. "Effects of Pre-School Training on the Development of Reading and Lipreading Skills of Deaf Children." *American Annals of the Deaf* 109, no. 3 (1964): 280–296.

Crammatte, A. B. *Deaf Persons in Professional Employment.* Springfield, Ill.: Thomas, 1968.

———. *Meeting the Challenge: Hearing Impaired Professionals in the Workplace.* Washington, D.C.: Gallaudet University Press, 1987.

———. *Questions and Answers About Employment of Deaf People.* Washington, D.C.: National Information Center on Deafness, 1988.

Crandall, K. E., and N. A. Orlando. "The Use and Learning of Spoken Language Systems." *American Annals of the Deaf* 125, no. 3 (1980): 335–448.

———. "A Comparison of Signs Used By Mothers and Deaf Children During Early Childhood." In *Proceedings of the Convention of American Instructors of the Deaf, 1975.*

Dale, D. M. *Individualized Integration: Studies of Deaf and Partially-Hearing Children and Students in Ordinary Schools and Colleges.* Springfield, Ill.: Thomas, 1984.

Daniloff, R., G. Schuckers, and L. Feth. *The Physiology of Speech and Hearing: An Introduction.* Englewood Cliffs, N.J.: Prentice-Hall, 1980.

Davidson, A., and J. Nuru. "Creating a Culturally Diverse Community: Academic Administrators as Agents for Change." *Gallaudet Today* 21, no. 2 (1990–1991, Winter): 18–23.

Daya, H., et al. "The Role of a Graded Profile Analysis in Determining Candidacy and Outcome for Cochlear Implantation in Children." *International Journal of Pediatric Otorhinolaryngology* 49, no. 2 (August 5, 1999): 135–42.

Day, P. S. "Deaf Children's Expression of Communication Intentions." *Journal of Communication Disorders* 19, no. 5 (1986): 376–386.

Delgado-Gaitan, C. *Literacy for Empowerment: The Role of Parents in Children's Education.* New York: Falmer Press, 1990.

Dichgans, M., et al. "Bacterial Meningitis in Adults: Demonstration of Inner Ear Involvement Using High-Resolution MRI." *Neurology* 52, no. 5 (March 23, 1999): 1003–9.

DiPietro, L. *A Look at Fingerspelling.* Washington, D.C.: The National Academy, Gallaudet University, 1976.

Discover Editors. "Sound: In Your Ear (Philips XP Peritympanic Device)." *Discover* 14 (October 1993): 71.

DuBow, S. "Courts Interpret Mainstreaming: How Residential Schools Can Adapt." *American Annals of the Deaf* 129, no. 2 (1984): 92–94.

Dunan, J. G. "Recent Legislation Affecting Hearing-Impaired Persons." *American Annals of the Deaf* 129, no. 2 (1984): 83–91.

Eisenberg, R. "The Development of Hearing in Man: An Assessment of Current Status." *ASHA* 12 (1970): 119–123.

Erting, C., and R. Meiesegeier, eds. *Social Aspects of Deafness.* Washington, D.C.: Gallaudet University Press, 1982.

Evans, L. *Total Communication: Structure and Strategy.* Washington, D.C.: Gallaudet University Press, 1982.

FDA Consumer Editors. "FDA Approves Marketing of Cochlear Implant for Children." *FDA Consumer* 24 (October 1990): 2–3.

Farrugia, D., and G. F. Austin. "A Study of Social-Emotional Adjustment Patterns of Hearing-Impaired Students in Different Educational Settings." *American Annals of the Deaf* 125, no. 5 (1980): 535–541.

Fasold, R. *The Sociolinguistics of Society.* Oxford, England: Blackwell, 1984.

Flexer, C. "Audiological Rehabilitation in the Schools," *ASHA* 32, no. 4 (April 1990): 44–5.

Fonseca, S. "Identification of Permanent Hearing Loss in Children: Are the Targets for Outcome Measures Attainable?" *British Journal of Audiology* 33, no. 3 (June 1999): 35–43.

Franck, Irene, and Brownstone, David. *The Parents' Desk Reference.* New York: Prentice Hall, 1991.

Freeman, Roger D., Clifton F. Carbin, and Robert J. Boese. *Can't Your Child Hear?* Baltimore: University Park Press, 1981.

Friedman, R. A., et al. "Maternally Inherited Nonsyndromic Hearing Loss." *American Journal of Medical Genetics* 84, no. 4 (June 4, 1999): 369–72.

Frishberg, N. "Arbitrariness and Iconicity: Historical Change in American Sign Language." *Language* 51, no. 3 (1975): 696–719.

———. *Interpreting: An Introduction.* Silver Spring, Md.: RID Publications, 1985.

Froehlinger, V. *Today's Hearing Impaired Child: Into the Mainstream of Education.* Washington, D.C.: Alexander Graham Bell Association for the Deaf, 1981.

Funk, B. "Being Ignored Can Be Bliss—How to Use a Sign Language Interpreter." *Deaf American,* 34, no. 6 (1982).

Furth, Hans G. *Thinking Without Language: Psychological Implications of Deafness.* New York: Free Press, 1966.

Galenson, E., and R. Miller, E. Kaplan, A. Rothstein et al. "Assessment of Development in the Deaf Child." *Journal of the American Academy of Child Psychiatry* 18, no. 1 (1979): 128–42.

Gannon, J. *Deaf Heritage: A Narrative History of Deaf Americans.* Silver Spring, Md.: National Association of the Deaf, 1981.

Garcia, W. J., ed. *Medical Sign Language.* Springfield, Ill.: Thomas, 1983.

Geeslin, Ned. "After Live Aid and Farm Aid, Hearing Aid May be Next for Unwary Victims of Rock." *People Weekly* 31 (January 23, 1989): 95–6.

Gelfland, S. *Hearing: An Introduction to Psychological and Physiological Acoustics.* New York: Dekker, 1981.

Gerkin, K. P. "The High-Risk Register for Deafness." ASHA 26, no. 3 (1984): 17–23.

Gibbs, K. W. "Individual Differences in Cognitive Skills Related to Reading Ability in the Deaf." *American Annals of the Deaf* 134, no. 3 (July 1989): 214–8.

Gilbert, L., ed. "Deafness and Aging in the USA." *Gallaudet Today* 12, no. 2 (Winter 1982).

Glick, F. P., and D. Pellman. *Breaking Silence.* Scottsdale, Ariz.: Herald Press, 1982.

Goldstein, M. H., Jr. and A. Proctor. "Tactile Aids for Profoundly Deaf Children." *Journal of the Acoustical Society of America* 77, no. 11 (1985): 258–265.

Graff, Stewart and Polly Anne. *Helen Keller: Toward the Light.* New York: Dell, 1971.

Greenberg, M. T. "Family Stress and Child Competence: The Effects of Early Intervention for Families with Deaf Infants." *American Annals of the Deaf* 128, no. 4 (1980): 407–417.

———, and R. Calderon. "Early Intervention for Deaf Children: Outcomes and Issues." *Topics in Early Childhood Special Education* 4 (1984): 1–9.

Gregory, S. *The Deaf Child and His Family.* New York: Wiley, 1976.

Groce, N. *Everyone Here Spoke Sign Language.* Cambridge, Mass.: Harvard University Press, 1985.

Grosjean, F. *Life With Two Languages: An Introduction to Bilingualism.* Cambridge, Mass.: Harvard University Press, 1982.

Gustason, G., E. Pfetzing, and E. Zawolkow. *Signing Exact English.* Silver Spring, Md.: National Association of the Deaf, 1980.

Hagborg, W. J. "A Sociometric Investigation of Sex and Race Peer Preferences Among Deaf Adolescents," *American Annals of the Deaf* 134, no. 4 (October 1989): 265–7.

Hairston, E., and L. Smith. *Black and Deaf in America: Are We That Different?* Silver Spring, Md.: T. J. Publishers, 1983.

Halmagyi, et al. "Gentamicin Toxicity." *Otolaryngology-Head and Neck Surgery* 111 (1994): 571–4.

Hardie, N. A., et al. "Sensorineural Hearing Loss During Development: Morphological and Physiological Response of the Cochlea and Auditory Brainstem." *Hearing Research* 128/1–2 (February 1999): 147–65.

Hardy, R., and J. Cull, eds. *Educational and Psycho-Social Aspects of Deafness.* Springfield, Ill.: Thomas, 1974.

Harner, S. G. et al. "Transtympanic Gentamicin for Meniere's Syndrome." *Laryngoscope* 108, no. 10 (October 1998): 1446–9.

Haring, Norris, ed. *Exceptional Children and Youth.* Columbus, Ohio: Merrill, 1981.

Harris, G. *Broken Ears, Wounded Hearts.* Washington, D.C.: Gallaudet University Press, 1983.

Harris, S., M. Casselbrant, A. Ivarsson, and O. Tjernström. "Hearing Threshold Measurement in Menieres Disease" *Audiology* 1984 23(1): 46–52.

Haybach, P. J. "Tuning Into Ototoxicity." *Nursing* 23(6) (1993): 34–40.

Heffner, R. *General Phonetics.* Madison: University of Wisconsin Press, 1960.

Henggeler, S. W., and P. F. Cooper. "Deaf Child-Hearing Mother Interaction." *Journal of Pediatric Psychology* 8 (1983): 83–95.

Hester, T. O., et al. "Stapes Footplate Fistula and Recurrent Meningitis." *Otolaryngology/Head Neck Surgery* 121, no. 3 (September 1999): 289–92.

Higgins, P. *Outsiders in a Hearing World: A Sociology of Deafness.* Beverly Hills, Calif.: Sage Publications, 1980.

Hochberg, I., H. Levitt, and M. J. Osberger, eds. *Speech of the Hearing Impaired: Research, Training and Personnel Preparation.* Baltimore, Md.: University Park Press, 1983.

Holborow, C. "Deafness as a World Problem." *Advances in Oto-Rhino-Laryngology* 29 (1983): 174–182.

Hughes, Gordon B., M. D., and Lawrence Koegel, M.D. "Ototoxicity." In *Textbook of Clinical Otology.* New York: Thieme-Stratton, 1985.

Hull, R., and K. Dilka, eds. *The Hearing Impaired Child In School.* Orlando, Fla.: Grune & Stratton, 1984.

Jacobs, L. *A Deaf Adult Speaks Out.* Washington, D.C.: Gallaudet University Press, 1980.

———. "The Community of the Adult Deaf." *American Annals of the Deaf* 119, no. 11 (1974): 41–46.

Jamison, S. L., ed. *Signs for Commuting Terminology.* Silver Spring, Md.: National Association of the Deaf, 1983.

Jeffers, J., and M. Barley. *Speechreading (Lipreading).* Springfield, Ill.: Thomas, 1971.

Jensema, C., and J. Mullins. "Onset, Cause, and Additional Handicaps in Hearing-Impaired Children." *American Annals of the Deaf* 119, no. 6 (1974): 701–705.

Johnson, I., et al. "Who Benefits from Cochlear Implantation?" *Practitioner* 242, no. 1587 (June 1998): 434, 437–8, 444.

Kampfe, C. M. "Parental Reaction to a Child's Hearing Impairment," *American Annals of the Deaf* 134, no. 4 (Oct. 1989): 255–9.

Kannapell, B., Lillian Hamilton, and H. Bornstein. *Signs for Instructional Purposes.* Washington, D.C.: Gallaudet University Press, 1969.

Kaplan, H. *Anatomy and Physiology of Speech.* New York: McGraw-Hill, 1971.

Karchmer, M. A., et al. "The Functional Assessment of Deaf and Hard of Hearing Students." *American Annals of the Deaf* 144, no. 2 (April 1999): 68–77.

Katsuki, J., et al. "Application of Theory of Signal Detection to Dichotic Listening." *Journal of Speech and Hearing Research* 27 (1984): 444–448.

Kettrick, Catherine. *American Sign Language: A Beginning Course.* Silver Spring, Md.: National Association of the Deaf, 1984.

King, S. "Comparing Two Causal Models of Career Maturity for Hearing-Impaired Adolescents," *American Annals of the Deaf* 135, no. 1 (Spring 1990): 43–9.

Klane, J. "Are Your Workers Protected to Deaf?" *Occupational Health and Safety* 67, no. 10 (October 1998): 90–4, 96.

Klein, Larry. "Progress in Hi-Fi Hearing Aid Design." *Radio-Electronics* 61 (February 1990): 24–5.

Klima, E., and U. Bellugi. *The Signs of Language.* Cambridge, Mass.: Harvard University Press, 1979.

Kluwin, T. N. "The Grammaticality of Manual Representations of English in Classroom Settings." *American Annals of the Deaf* 126 (4) (June 1981): 417–421.

———. "A Rationale for Modifying Classroom Signing Systems." *Sign Language Studies* 23 (1979): 99–136.

Koegel, L. "Ototoxicity: A Contemporary Review of Aminoglycosides, Loop Diuretics, Acetylsalicylic Acid, Quinine, Erythromycin, and Cisplatinum." *American Journal of Otology* 6, no. 2 (1985): 190–8.

Kothman, V. "Classroom Auditory Trainers." *Hearing Aid Journal* Dec. 1981, 8–9, 41–43.

Krebs, D. E., K. M. Gill-Body, P. O. Riley, and Parker, S. W. "Double-Blinded, Placebo-Controlled Trial of Rehabilitation for Bilateral Vestibular Hypofunction: Preliminary Report." *Otolaryngology-Head and Neck Surgery* 109 (1993): 735–41.

Kretschmer, R., and L. Kretschmer. *Language Development and Intervention with the Hearing Impaired.* Baltimore Md.: University Park Press, 1978.

Ladefoged, P. *A Course in Phonetics.* New York: Harcourt Brace Jovanovich, 1975.

Lash, J. *Helen and Teacher: The Story of Helen Keller and Anne Sullivan Macy.* New York: American Foundation for the Blind, 1980.

Lass, N. *Speech and Language: Advances in Basic Research and Practice.* Vol. 8. New York: Academic Press, 1982.

———, *Speech, Language and Hearing.* Philadelphia: Saunders, 1982.

Levine, E. *The Ecology of Early Deafness: Guide to Fashioning Environments and Psychological Assessments.* New York: Columbia University Press, 1981.

———, and E. Wagner. "Personality of Deaf Persons." *Perceptual and Motor Skills* 39 (1974): 1167–1236.

Levitt, H. "Hearing Impairment and Sensory Aids." *Journal of Rehabilitation Research and Development* 23, no. 1 (1986): xiii–xviii.

Locke, J. *Phonological Acquisition and Change.* New York: Academic Press, 1984.

Libbey, S. S., and W. Pronovost. "Communication Practices of Mainstreamed Hearing-Impaired Adolescents." *Volta Review* 82, no. 4 (1980): 197–213.

Liben, L. S., ed. *Deaf Children: Developmental Perspectives.* New York: Academic Press, 1978.

Ling, D. *Early Intervention for Hearing-Impaired Children: Oral Options.* San Diego, Calif.: College-Hill Press, 1984.

———. *Early Intervention for Hearing-Impaired Children: Total Communication Options.* San Diego, Calif.: College-Hill Press, 1984.

———. *Speech and the Hearing Impaired Child.* Washington, D.C.: Alexander Graham Bell Association for the Deaf, 1976.

Liston, S. L. "Beethoven's Deafness." *Laryngoscope* 99, no. 12 (Dec. 1989): 1301–4.

Lubinski, R. B. "A Review of Recent Research on Verbal Communication Among the Elderly." *International Journal of Aging and Human Development* 9 (1978–79): 237–245.

Luey, H. S., and M. Per-Lee. *What Should I Do Now: Problems and Adaptations of the Deafened Adult.* Washington, D.C.: Gallaudet University Press, 1983.

Luterman, D., et al. "Identifying Hearing Loss: Parents' Needs." *American Journal of Audiology* 8/1 (June 1999): 13–8.

Luterman, D. M., ed. *Deafness in Perspective.* San Diego, Calif.: College-Hill Press, 1986.

———. *Counseling Parents of Hearing Impaired Children.* Boston: Little, Brown, 1979.

———. *Deafness in the Family.* Boston: Little, Brown, 1987.

Markowicz, H. "American Sign Language: Fact and Fancy." Washington, D.C.: The National Academy, Gallaudet University, 1977.

Marshall, L. "Auditory Processing in Aging Listeners." *Journal of Speech and Hearing Disorders* 46, no. 3 (August 1981).

Martin, F. N. *Introduction to Audiology.* Englewood Cliffs, N.J.: Prentice-Hall, 1981.

McArthur, Shirley H. *Raising Your Hearing-Impaired Child: A Guideline for Parents.* Washington, D.C.: Alexander Graham Bell Association for the Deaf, 1982.

McFarland, W., and B. P. Cox. *Aging and Hearing Loss.* Washington, D.C.: National Information Center on Deafness/American Speech-Language-Hearing Association, 1987.

Meadow, K. P. *Deafness and Child Development*. Berkeley, Calif.: University of California Press, 1980.

———. Greenberg, M. T., and C. Erting. "Attachment Behavior of Deaf Children with Deaf Parents." *Journal of the American Academy of Child Psychiatry* 22 (1983): 23–28.

———, M. T. Greenberg, C. Erting, and H. Carmichael. "Interactions of Deaf Mothers and Deaf Pre-school Children: Comparisons with Three Other Groups of Deaf and Hearing Dyads." *American Annals of the Deaf* 126, no. 4 (1981): 454–468.

Mendelsohn, J. Z., and B. Fairchild. *Years of Challenge, A Guide for Parents of Hearing-Impaired Adolescents*. Silver Spring, Md.: National Association of the Deaf, 1982.

Miller, S. T., et al. "Better Use of Hearing Aid in Hearing-Impaired Adults." *Journal of the American Geriatric Society* 46, no. 9 (September 1998): 168–9.

Mills, J. H., and J. A. Going. "Review of Environmental Factors Affecting Hearing." *Environmental Health Perspectives* 44 (1982): 119–127.

Moeller, M. P. "Parents' use of Signing Exact English: a descriptive analysis," *Journal of Speech and Hearing Disorders* 55, no. 2 (May 1990): 327–37.

Moore, D. R., et al. "Conductive Hearing Loss Produces a Reversible Binaural Hearing Impairment." *Journal of Neuroscience* 19, no. 19 (October 1, 1999): 8704–11.

Moore, B. *An Introduction to the Psychology of Hearing*. 2d ed. New York: Academic Press, 1982.

Moores, D. *Educating the Deaf: Psychology, Principles, and Practices*. 3d ed. Boston: Houghton Mifflin, 1987.

Morlet, T., et al. "Auditory Screening in High-Risk Pre-Term and Full-Term Neonates Using Transient Evoked Otoacoustic Emissions and Brainstem Auditory Evoked Potentials." *International Journal of Pediatric Otorhinolaryngology* 45, no. 1 (September 15, 1998): 31–40.

Murphy, Kate. "Hearing Aids Get Smart—and Better-Looking." *Business Week*, May 8, 1995, p. 116.

Mutton, P. "Early Identification of Deaf Babies." *Lancet* 352/9145 (December 19–26, 1998): 1951–2.

Naiman, D., and J. Schein. *For Parents of Deaf Children*. Silver Spring, Md.: National Association of the Deaf, 1978.

Nash, J., and A. Nash. *Deafness in Society*. Lexington, Mass.: Heath, 1981.

National Center for Law and the Deaf. *Legal Rights of Hearing-Impaired People*. Washington, D.C.: Gallaudet University Press, 1986.

National Information Center on Deafness. *Communicating with Deaf People*. Washington, D.C.: Gallaudet University Press, 1987.

Neisser, A. *The Other Side of Silence: Sign Language and the Deaf Community in America*. New York: Knopf, 1983.

NIH. "Early Identification of Hearing Impairment in Infants and Young Children." *NIH Consensus Statement Online* 11, no. 1 (March 1993): 1–24.

———. "Cochlear Implants in Adults and Children." *NIH Consensus Statement Online* 13, no. 2 (May 15–17, 1995): 1–30.

Nikolopoulos T. P., et al. "Age at Implantation: Its Importance in Pediatric Cochlear Implantation." *Laryngoscope* 109, no. 4 (April 1999): 595–9.

Nix, G. W. "The Right To Be Heard." *Volta Review* 83, no. 4 (1981): 199–205.

———. *Mainstream Education for Hearing Impaired Children and Youth*. New York: Grune & Stratton, 1976.

Norris, C. H. "Drugs Affecting the Inner Ear: A Review of Their Clinical Efficacy, Mechanisms of Action, Toxicity and Place in Therapy." *Drugs* 36 (1988): 754–72.

Northcott, W. H. *The Hearing Impaired Child in a Regular Classroom.* Washington, D.C.: Alexander Graham Bell Association, 1973.

Odkvist, L. M., C. Moller and K. A. Thomas. "Otoneurologic Disturbances Caused by Solvent Pollution." *Otolaryngology-Head and Neck Surgery* 106, no. 6 (1992): 687–92.

O'Donoghue, G. M., et al. "Speech Perception in Children After Cochlear Implantation." *American Journal of Otolaryngology* 19, no. 6 (November 1998): 762–7.

———. "Cochlear Implants in Young Children: The Relationship Between Speech Perception and Speech Intelligibility." *Ear Hear* 20, no. 5 (October 1999): 419–25.

Ogden, P., and S. Lipsett. *The Silent Garden: Understanding the Hearing Impaired Child.* New York: St. Martin's Press, 1982.

Orlans, H. *Adjustment to Adult Hearing Loss.* San Diego, Calif.: College-Hill Press, 1985.

Osberger, M. J. "Audiological Rehabilitation with Cochlear Implants and Tactile Aids." *ASHA* 32, no. 4 (April 1990): 38–43.

Ozdamor, O., N. Kraus, and L. Stein. "Auditory Brainstem Responses in Infants Recovering from Bacterial Meningitis." *Archives of Otolaryngology* 109 (January 1983): 13–18.

Panara, R.F. "Cultural Arts Among the Deaf." *The Deaf American* 32, no. 9 (1980): 9–11.

———, and J. Panara. *Great Deaf Americans.* Silver Spring, Md.: T.J. Publishers, 1983.

Parasnis, I. "Visual Perceptual Skills and Deafness." *Journal of the Academy of Rehabilitative Audiology* 16 (1983): 148–160.

Perrin, E., et al. "Evaluation of Cochlear Implanted Children's Voices." *International Journal of Pediatric Otorhinolaryngology* 47, no. 2 (February 15, 1999): 181–6.

Pimental, A. T. "A Barrier-Free Environment for Deaf People." *The Deaf American* 32, no. 5 (1980): 7–9.

Poizner, H. "Visual and Phonetic Coding of Movement: Evidence from American Sign Language." *Science* 212 (1981): 691–693.

Port, Otis. "They're Bearing the Gift of Sound." *Business Week,* February 6, 1995, p. 152–3.

Porter, A. "Sign-language Interpretation in Psychotherapy with Deaf Patients." *American Journal of Psychotherapy* 53, no. 2 (Spring 1999): 163–76.

Prasher, D., et al. "The Role of Otoacoustic Emissions in Screening and Evaluation of Noise Damage." *International Journal of Occupational Medicine and Environmental Health* 12/2 (1999): 183–92.

Quigley, S. P., and R. E. Kretshmer. *The Education of Deaf Children: Issues, Theory and Practice.* Baltimore, Md.: University Park Press, 1982.

Rainer, J. D., K. Z. Altshuler, and F. J. Kallmann, eds. *Family and Mental Health Problems in a Deaf Population.* Springfield, Ill.: Thomas, 1969.

Ramsdell, D. A. "The Psychology of the Hard of Hearing and Deafened Adult." In *Hearing and Deafness,* 499–510. New York: Rinehart & Winston, 1978.

Reardon, W. "Prevalence, Age of Onset, and Natural History of Thyroid Disease in Pendred Syndrome." *Journal of Medical Genetics* 36, no. 8 (August 1999): 595–8.

Reardon, W. "Sex-linked deafness," *Journal of Medical Genetics* 27, no. 6 (June 1990): 376–9.

Rezen, Susan, and Carl Hausman. *Coping with Hearing Loss.* New Jersey: Barricade Books, 1993.

Rupp, R. "The Roles of the Audiologist." *Journal of the Academy of Rehabilitation Audiology* 10, no. 1 (1977): 10–17.

Rutman, D. "The Impact and Experience of Adventitious Deafness," *American Annals of the Deaf* 134, no. 5 (Dec. 1989): 305–11.

Rybak, L. P. "Hearing: The Effects of Chemicals." *Otolaryngology–Head and Neck Surgery* 106, no. 6 (1992): 677–86.

Sataloff, Joseph, M.D., and Paul L. Michael, Ph.D. *Hearing Conservation.* Springfield, Ill.: Thomas, 1973.

Sattler, J. *Assessment of Children's Intelligence and Special Abilities.* 2d ed. Boston: Allyn and Bacon, 1982.

Schaeffer, Benson, Arlene Musil, and George Kollinzas. *Total Communication: A Signed Speech Program for Nonverbal Children.* Springfield, Ill.: Research Press, 1980.

Schildroth, A. N., and M. A. Karchmer, eds. *Deaf Children in America.* San Diego, Calif.: College-Hill Press, 1986.

Schleuning, A., R. M. Johnson, and J. A. Vernon. "Masking and Tinnitus." *Ear and Hearing* 6, no. 2 (March–April 1980): 71–72.

Schowe, B. *Identity Crisis in Deafness.* Tempe, Ariz.: Scholars Press, 1979.

Scott, P. M., and M. V. Griffiths. "A Clinical Review of Ototoxicity." *Clinical Otolaryngology* 19 (1994):3–8.

Scouten, E. L. *Turning Points in the Education of Deaf People.* Danville, Ill.: Interstate, 1984.

Schroedel, J. G., and W. Schiff. "Attitudes Towards Deafness Among Several Deaf and Hearing Populations." *Rehabilitative Psychology* 19 (1972): 59–70.

Solow, S. *Sign Language Interpreting: A Basic Resource Book.* Silver Spring, Md.: National Association of the Deaf, 1981.

Soviero, Marcelle M. "Signal Processing for Ears (Digital Hearing Aid System Developed by Janet Rutledge)." *Popular Science* 239 (July 1991): 30.

Spradley, Thomas S., and James P. Spradley. *Deaf Like Me.* Washington, D.C.: Gallaudet University Press, 1978.

Stone, H. "Hearing Loss and Mental Health." *Shhh* 3, no. 6 (November/December 1982).

Sullivan, P., and M. Vernon. "Psychological Assessment of Hearing-Impaired Children." *School Psychology Review* 8, no. 3 (1979): 271–290.

Switzer, M. E., and B. R. Williams. "Life Problems of Deaf People: Prevention and Treatment." *Archives of Environmental Health* 15 (1967): 249–256.

Tomblin, J. B., et al. "A Comparison of Language Achievement in Children with Cochlear Implants and Children Using Hearing Aids." *Journal of Speech-Language Hearing Research* 42, no. 2 (April 1999): 497–509.

Turkington, Carol A. "Cochlear Implants: Delivering Sound to the Deaf." *The World Book Health and Medical Annual.* Chicago: World Book, Inc., 1996.

———. *The Hearing Loss Sourcebook.* New York: Penguin, 1997.

Turner, C. W., et al. "Speech Audibility for Listeners with High-Frequency Hearing Loss." *American Journal of Audiology* 8, no. 1 (June 1999): 47–56.

Valente, Michael. "Programmable Aids Improve Hearing." *USA Today* 122 (October 1993): 12–13.

Van Cleve, J. V., ed. *Gallaudet Encyclopedia of Deaf People and Deafness.* New York: McGraw-Hill, 1987.

Van Naarden, K., et al. "Relative and Attributable Risks for Moderate to Profound Bilateral Sensorineural Hearing Impairment Associated with Lower Birth Weight in Children 3 to 10 Years Old." *Pediatrics* 104/4 Pt 1 (October 1999): 905–10.

Warner, David. "An Unexpected Phone Bill: Business Phones Must Be Able To Be Used By Persons With Hearing Aids." *Nation's Business* 81 (May 1993): 72.

Wax, Teena, and Loraine DiPietro. *Managing Hearing Loss Later in Life.* Washington, D.C.: National Information Center on Deafness/American Speech-Language-Hearing Association, 1987.

Wilbur, R. *American Sign Language and Sign Systems.* Baltimore, Md.: University Park Press, 1979.

Wilcox, S. A., et al. "Connexin26 Deafness in Several Interconnected Families." *Journal of Medical Genetics* 36, no. 5 (May 1999): 383–5.

Williams, Rebecca. "Enjoy, Protect the Best Ears of Your Life." *FDA Consumer* 26 (May 1992): 25–7.

Williamson, W. D., M. M. Desmond, N. LaFevers, L. H. Taber, F. I. Catlin, and T. G. Weaver. "Symptomatic Congenital Cytomegalovirus: Disorders of Language, Learning and Hearing." *American Journal of Diseases of Children* 136 (1982): 902–905.

Wong, D., et al. "PET Imaging of Cochlear-Implant and Normal-Hearing Subjects Listening To Speech and Nonspeech." *Hearing Research.* 132, no. 1–2 (June 1999): 34–42.

Woodward, J. "Historical Bases of American Sign Language." In *Understanding Language Through Sign Language Research,* edited by R. Siple. New York: Academic Press, 1978.

Wright, T. "Bacterial Meningitis and Deafness." *Clinical Otolaryngology* 24, no. 5 (September 1999): 385–7.

Yeo, K. L., et al. "Outcomes of Extremely Premature Infants Related to Their Peak Serum Bilirubin Concentrations and Exposure to Phototherapy." *Pediatrics* 102, no. 6 (December 1998): 1426–31.

Yoken, C., ed. *Interpreter Training: The State of the Art.* Washington, D.C.: The National Academy of Gallaudet College, 1980.

Yoshinaga-Itano, C., et al. "The Development of Deaf and Hard of Hearing Children Identified Early Through the High-Risk Registry." *American Annals of the Deaf* 143, no. 5 (December 1998): 416–24.

———. "Identification of Hearing Loss After Age 18 Months Is Not Early Enough." *American Annals of the Deaf* 143, no. 5 (December 1998): 380–7.

Youniss, J. *Parents and Peers in Social Development.* Chicago: University of Chicago Press, 1980.

Suggested Readings For Children and Parents

FOR CHILDREN:

Arthur, Catherine. *My Sister's Silent World.* Chicago: Children's Press, 1979.

Blatchford, Claire. *Yes, I Wear A Hearing Aid.* New York: Lexington School for the Deaf, 1976.

Glazzard, Margaret H. *Meet Camille & Danielle: They Are Special Persons.* Lawrence, Kaus.: H&H Enterprises, 1978.

Hlibok, Bruce. *Silent Dancer.* New York: Messner, 1981.

LaMore, Gregory S. *Now I Understand.* Washington, D.C.: Gallaudet University Press.

Peterson, Jeanne W. *I Have A Sister, My Sister Is Deaf.* New York: Harper & Row, 1977.

Rosenberg, Maxine. *My Friend Leslie: The Story of a Handicapped Child.* New York: Lothrop, Lee & Shepard, 1983.

Scott, Virginia. *Belonging.* Washington, D.C.: Gallaudet University Press, 1986.

Walker, Lou Ann. *Amy, the Story of a Deaf Child*. New York: Lodestar Books/Dutton, 1985.

Wolf, Bernard. *Anna's Silent World*. New York: Lippincott, 1977.

FOR PARENTS:

Angus, Jean R. *Watch My Words: An Open Letter to Parents of Young Deaf Children*. Cincinnati, Ohio: Forward Movement Publications, 1974.

Benderly, Beryl L. *Dancing Without Music: Deafness in America*. New York: Anchor Press/Doubleday, 1980.

Featherstone, Helen. *A Difference In The Family, Living With a Disabled Child*. New York: Penguin Books, 1981.

Ferris, Caren. *A Hug Just Isn't Enough*. Washington, D.C.: Gallaudet University Press, 1980.

Forecki, Marcia C. *Speak to Me*. Washington, D.C.: Gallaudet University Press, 1985.

Frederickson, Jeannette. *Life After Deaf*. Silver Spring, Md.: National Association of the Deaf, 1985.

Glick, Ferne P., and D. Pellman. *Breaking Silence: A Family Grows With Deafness*. Scotsdale, Pa.: Herald Press, 1982.

Harris, George. *Broken Ears, Wounded Hearts*. Washington, D.C.: Gallaudet University Press, 1983.

Ling, Daniel, ed. *Early Intervention for Hearing-Impaired Children: Oral Options*. San Diego, Calif.: College Hill Press, 1984.

Luterman, David. *Deafness in the Family*. Boston, Mass.: Little, Brown, 1987.

Meadow, Kathryn P. *Deafness and Child Development*. Berkeley, Calif.: University of California Press, 1980.

Mendelsohn, Jacqueline Z., and Bonnie Fairchild. *Years of Challenge, A Guide For Parents of Hearing Impaired Adolescents*. Silver Spring, Md: National Association of the Deaf, 1982.

Ogden, Paul, and Suzanne Lipsett. *The Silent Garden: Understanding the Hearing Impaired Child*. New York: St. Martin's Press, 1982.

Schwartz, Sue, ed. *Choices in Deafness: A Parents' Guide*. Kensington, Md.: Woodbine House, 1987.

Spradley, Thomas S., and James P. Spradley. *Deaf Like Me*. Washington, D.C.: Gallaudet University Press, 1985.

Tweedie, David, and Edgar Shroyer, eds. *The Multihandicapped Hearing Impaired: Identification and Instruction*. Washington, D.C.: Gallaudet University Press, 1982.

INDEX

Page numbers in **boldface** indicate extensive treatment of a topic.